The Intimate State

The Intimate State

How Emotional Life Became Political in Welfare-State Britain

Teri Chettiar

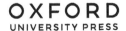

OXFORD
UNIVERSITY PRESS

Oxford University Press is a department of the University of Oxford. It furthers
the University's objective of excellence in research, scholarship, and education
by publishing worldwide. Oxford is a registered trade mark of Oxford University
Press in the UK and certain other countries.

Published in the United States of America by Oxford University Press
198 Madison Avenue, New York, NY 10016, United States of America.

© Oxford University Press 2023

All rights reserved. No part of this publication may be reproduced, stored in
a retrieval system, or transmitted, in any form or by any means, without the
prior permission in writing of Oxford University Press, or as expressly permitted
by law, by license, or under terms agreed with the appropriate reproduction
rights organization. Inquiries concerning reproduction outside the scope of the
above should be sent to the Rights Department, Oxford University Press, at the
address above.

You must not circulate this work in any other form
and you must impose this same condition on any acquirer.

Library of Congress Cataloging-in-Publication Data
Names: Chettiar, Teri, author.
Title: The intimate state : how emotional life became political in
welfare-state Britain / Teri Chettiar.
Description: New York, NY : Oxford University Press, [2023] |
Includes bibliographical references and index.
Identifiers: LCCN 2022029891 (print) | LCCN 2022029892 (ebook) |
ISBN 9780190931209 (hardback) | ISBN 9780190931230 |
ISBN 9780190931223 (epub)
Subjects: LCSH: Interpersonal relations—Great Britain. | Interpersonal
relations—Political aspects—Great Britain. | Welfare state—Great Britain.
Classification: LCC HM1111 .C546 2023 (print) | LCC HM1111 (ebook) |
DDC 302—dc23/eng/20220812
LC record available at https://lccn.loc.gov/2022029891
LC ebook record available at https://lccn.loc.gov/2022029892

DOI: 10.1093/oso/9780190931209.001.0001

1 3 5 7 9 8 6 4 2

Printed by Integrated Books International, United States of America

Contents

Acknowledgments   vii

Introduction. Making Relational People: The Politics of Emotional Life in Post-1945 Britain   1

PART I: THE WELFARE STATE'S INTIMATE PLACES AND PEOPLE

1. Democracy as Therapy: Psychiatry and the Social Environment in Interwar and Wartime Britain   25

2. The Welfare State Begins at Home: "Deprived" Children and Britain's Future after the War   52

3. Problem Mothers: Maternal Neglect, Mental Illness, and the Fragility of Female Maturity   80

4. "More than a Contract": Marriage Welfare Services and the Politics of Intimacy   112

PART II: SEXUAL REVOLUTION AND INTIMACY REIMAGINED

5. Pursuing Connection: Queer Romance and Friendship during Britain's Sexual Revolution   143

6. Inherently Unstable: Adolescent Sexuality at the Boundary of Private Life   170

7. "Home Is for Many a Very Violent Place": Healing from Family Violence in 1970s Britain   197

Epilogue: Intimacy in the Age of the Individual   233
Notes   241
Select Bibliography   279
Index   303

Acknowledgments

In researching and writing this book, I have (very happily) accrued many personal and professional debts. Many years have passed since I first began to conceive this book as a PhD student and, during that time, I have been incredibly fortunate to have many generous and inspiring colleagues and friends help shape it.

This book's origins owe much to the encouraging and supportive faculty in the History Department at Northwestern University who so generously gave their time and scrupulous attention to help make me a historian: Alex Owen, Ken Alder, Deborah Cohen, Francesca Bordogna, and (the late) Bill Heyck. I also benefited enormously from the interdisciplinary scholarly communities attached to the Science in Human Culture Program and The Sexualities Project at Northwestern, which offered tremendous opportunities for intellectual engagement and research funding.

While researching the dissertation that forms the core of this book, I spent two very memorable and productive years in London, primarily at the Wellcome Trust Centre for the History of Medicine, which was then fortuitously housed a few floors above the Wellcome Library and Archives. Words cannot express my gratitude to Rhodri Hayward, who became an unofficial advisor during those years and to Roger Cooter, Lindsay Fitzharris, Bill MacLehose, and the incredibly dynamic community of graduate students, postdocs, and faculty at the Wellcome in 2009–2010.

During a three-year postdoctoral fellowship at the Humboldt University in Berlin, I was fortunate to be part of two highly engaged communities of historians of science. In addition to the lively intellectual culture and generous mentorship of Anke te Heesen's *Lehrstuhl*, I am also deeply grateful for the exciting intellectual community in Department II at the Max Planck Institute for the History of Science under Lorraine Daston's direction. Conversations with John Carson, Cathy Gere, Rebecca Lemov, Shigehisa Kuriyama, Felicity Callard, Jenny Bangham, Elena Aronova, Michael Stanley-Baker, Rohan Deb Roy, and many more insightful interlocutors helped to enlarge and enrich my understanding of the relationship between science, politics, and culture that became a significant focus of this book. During those years, I also benefited from participating in Laura Lee Downs's collaborative research group on the history of welfare and social care at the European University Institute in Florence. Laura's boundless intellectual interests helped inspire me to further pursue questions surrounding the politics of family, social protection, and state-supported care.

As a postdoctoral fellow at the University of Chicago, I was very fortunate to workshop chapters at both the Fishbein Centre and the Society of Fellows. I am especially grateful to Tara Zahra, who read and commented on two chapters, and to Bob Richards, Nima Bassiri, Aaron Benanav, and Isabel Gabel for their support and invaluable advice. During those years, Kirsten Leng, Guy Ortolano, Emily Callaci, Steve

Rosenberg, Marsaura Shukla, Caroline Rusterholz, and Yuliya Hilevych also offered brilliant feedback at critical points in the book's re-conceptualization.

I could not ask for more supportive colleagues at the University of Illinois and owe special debts of gratitude to Antoinette Burton, Dana Rabin, Clare Crowston, Leslie Reagan, Ken Cuno, Rana Hogarth, Tamara Chaplin, Kristin Hoganson, and Carol Symes. Each has gone above and beyond to help orient me as a new faculty member and, in the process, become a better thinker and writer. I owe particular thanks to Antoinette Burton for organizing a highly productive book manuscript workshop with Deborah Weinstein and Jordanna Bailkin over Zoom early on in the pandemic. I could not have asked for three more exceptionally perceptive readers. Our three-hour conversation was both profoundly stimulating and enormously helpful in creating the final version of this book.

I wish to thank University of Illinois, Urbana-Champaign (UIUC)'s Office of Research Advising (especially Maria Gillombardo and Cynthia Oliver) and UIUC's Campus Research Board for funding a crucial final trip to archives in the UK in 2019. My sincere thanks also go to the UIUC History Department office staff, especially Tom Bedwell, who have made the final stages of writing manageable alongside a busy teaching schedule. I am also deeply appreciative of the many librarians and archivists who helped this book come into being, especially archivists at the Wellcome Library and Archives, the Hall-Carpenter Archives at LSE, and the Planned Environment Therapy Trust.

Over the course of many years of thinking and writing about intimacy and families, my life has undergone several major changes—I not only became a mother, I also lost a father. To my parents Ramen Chettiar and Anne McGrath, and my siblings Nadiya Chettiar, Natasha Chettiar, and Nathan Chettiar: I could not have asked for a better set of "first" relationships. I continue to be genuinely grateful for (and equally astonished by) our shared unwillingness to let the past define who we become. To my father, who sadly will not read this book, your imprint as a parent and truly caring physician is ubiquitous.

As my network of family expands, I am thankful to have formed genuinely enriching family relationships with Stuart Dunbar, Ted Bois, Nozue Yasui, Maureen Meter, Jack Henning-Sepkoski, and David Sepkoski. Maureen, especially, has been a pillar of support: I have much to thank you for, not least for helping with childcare at key moments when I needed to write. To David, thank you for everything that you have given to this book, both on its pages and off.

To Sid Chettiar-Sepkoski, I dedicate this book this you. I am grateful to be your mother and for getting to experience, and regularly be infected by, your unflagging love of life. Thank you for helping me to discover so much more about what this book is about than I once dreamed possible.

Introduction

Making Relational People: The Politics of Emotional Life in Post-1945 Britain

Children need their mothers' love. This belief is now so deeply entrenched that we hardly question it. During the Second World War (WWII), British child psychiatrist John Bowlby, in collaboration with economist and Labour politician Evan Durbin, made it his mission to promote this seemingly self-evident psychological truth and helped make it widely accepted. And even more than highlighting the advantages of a mother's love for her child's health and wellbeing, Bowlby and Durbin heralded its benefits for wider society. Both ardent proponents of social democracy, they presented mother love as the single most important prerequisite for nurturing responsible democratic citizens. In their eyes, the intimate bond between mother and child was not only important, it was paramount. It was the gateway to a world in which every individual would grow up to become a loving parent, an attentive spouse, a helpful neighbor, a cooperative colleague, and a dedicated community-minded citizen.

The importance of a loving mother-child relationship, including its proposed wider social and political consequences, was passionately endorsed in Bowlby's best-selling 1951 report *Maternal Care and Mental Health*, sponsored by the World Health Organization.[1] Publishers and reading publics alike saw the message as so timely and important that the following year, Bowlby's report was abridged and circulated to wider audiences with the more accessible title *Child Care and the Growth of Love*.[2] It quickly sold four hundred thousand copies in Britain alone and was translated into fourteen languages. Across the Western world, Bowlby's message helped shape generations of childcare. The impact of his argument that a mother's love was necessary for healthy psychological development was both immediate and far-reaching. Orphanages lost significant public support; foster care and adoption were instead prioritized. At the same time, Bowlby's findings supported the blaming of countless mothers for their children's perceived shortcomings and helped fuel a ubiquitous internalization of maternal shame. Despite the seemingly powerful hold of individualism in twentieth-century Britain, the priority that Bowlby assigned to intimate relationships resonated for many. Most obviously, his proclamation that human beings are fundamentally relational by nature, and that our lives are powerfully

The Intimate State. Teri Chettiar, Oxford University Press. © Oxford University Press 2023.
DOI: 10.1093/oso/9780190931209.003.0001

shaped by this fact, offered psychological legitimacy to the post-WWII ascendance of social democracy. This "psychopolitical" turn was one of the most important transformations of Western political life in the second half of the twentieth century.

Although Bowlby remains an iconic figure with respect to the 1950s cultural fixation on mother love, he was not alone in fervently promoting the intertwined and wide-ranging psychological and political benefits of loving, intimate relationships in the decades following WWII. This book argues that British audiences were primed to positively receive Bowlby's work because his findings confirmed what many already suspected. In the same post-WWII moment that Bowlby's publications were being avidly discussed by both lay and scientific audiences, marriage therapy pioneer Henry Dicks was similarly promoting the wider importance of marital intimacy in determining the democratic and egalitarian "psycho-social climate of the future."[3] And only a decade after Bowlby and Dicks stressed the far-reaching social benefits of intimate mother-child and marriage relationships, gay rights campaigner and psychosexual counselor Antony Grey insisted that queer people's access to stable and lasting intimate relationships was not only an important goal of queer liberation but the necessary foundation for a truly liberated, "sexually sane" society.[4] A few years later, at the height of Britain's late-1960s sexual revolution, Marxist radical psychiatrist David Cooper would similarly insist that true social revolution would only come about through attention to the "micro-social"—that is, close personal relationships. Intimate authentic human connection, in addition to income redistribution, were in his view the true foundations for the liberated and humane "good society," and he argued that it was the neglect of intimate life that had led to the Soviet Union's failed revolution.[5] At first glance, social democracy, queer liberation, and antipsychiatry may appear to be widely disparate concerns. All, however, came to identify interpersonal intimacy as the key to social liberation. A shared commitment to the inescapable political consequences of intimate relationships binds these preoccupations together.

This book tells the story of how intimacy came to take on unprecedented and far-reaching social and political value during the heady and transformative decades following WWII. Long before second-wave feminists adopted the rallying cry "the personal is political" in the late 1960s, intimate emotional life was ascribed profoundly consequential political meaning by many of Britain's most prominent mental health professionals, social scientists, politicians, and social reformers. This book tracks the birth of an ideal of intimate relationality, traces the evolution of that ideal's quintessential forms and its widespread allure, and examines the many efforts that were made in the decades after 1945 to transform a widely experienced desire for intimacy into a lived reality.

How did the intimacy that was presumed to be shared between mothers and children and husbands and wives become highly politicized in Britain after WWII? I argue that it was intimacy's associations with emotional health and individual wellbeing—increasingly valued in the post-WWII decades—that endowed it with urgent political consequence. Cutting-edge psychiatric findings routinely presented human social and psychological development as primarily shaped by close bonds, especially those formed in early life. Respected behavioral scientists—Harry Harlow in the United States and Konrad Lorenz in Europe—also confirmed this in animals ranging from Rhesus monkeys to geese.[6] In the wake of a devastating total war, mental health professionals and the public alike fretted over the developmental fates of the many children who had recently (even if only temporarily) lost the security of a two-parent family home.

A commitment to protecting children's emotional health featured prominently in political planning for Britain's future at the end of WWII. The deep uncertainties of the postwar period made children across all socio-economic classes, as citizens of the future, key figures in the British socio-political imaginary.[7] A series of post-WWII social reforms that contributed to the creation of the welfare state—including, most prominently, the passage of the Children's Act in 1948—was geared explicitly toward ensuring children's healthy emotional development within stable family environments.[8] The new redistributive British welfare state invested in child-centered health and social service enterprises ranging from child guidance to innovative in-patient psychiatric treatments for post-partum depression to the prevention of divorce through marriage counseling services. All this work was meant to ensure that British children would not experience lives deficient in emotional connection. It was on this basis that government sponsorship of these mental health programs was rationalized.

Why were children's emotional lives considered an essential part of a revolutionized state mandate dedicated to eliminating structural poverty and unemployment? And why did this take hold in a place that was predominantly associated with a dogged resistance to emotional expression and a "stiff upper lip" response to hardship? At the time, British children were seen as blameless victims of a war-riven, economically unstable world. Even more worrying—fueled by the growing influence of child development experts—children were believed to be potential victims of their own unruly undeveloped emotions, and the entire nation (and possibly world) was seen as suffering acutely as a result. The latest war stood as only the most recent devastating example of what several respected mental health professionals proposed was an outcome of the dysfunctional development of entire societies. Aiming to protect children from experiencing a lack—or "deprivation"—of emotional relationships, Britain's post-WWII welfare government responded to the perceived threat that unmet emotional needs had the power to negatively determine individual and national destinies alike.

After WWII, a wide range of state-sponsored initiatives directed toward guaranteeing children's emotional health focused on improving access to loving family life. The space for engineering the desired relational subject after the war was the male-breadwinning, female-homemaking nuclear family. This model of the family was widely seen as intimacy's "natural" home since it was believed to offer maximum opportunities for a mother to lovingly bond with her child. British households became crucial sites of state intervention under the guiding assumption that they needed to be brought back to a state that they had presumably looked and, more importantly, *felt* like before the disastrous dislocations caused by war and economic depression.

This idealized model of healthy emotional life was actively pursued in multiple ways—in government policy responding to child homelessness, in psychiatric efforts to treat post-partum mental illness, and in state-supported marriage counseling programs. The goal of Britain's new welfare state was to make intimate bonds available to those who presumably lacked them—a large number that included orphans, neglectful mothers and their children, and unhappily married men and women. Innovative state-supported initiatives were intended to generate stable and lasting emotional intimacy and consciously sought to capitalize on the power of nurture as a positive alternative to eugenicists' attempts to direct nature through heredity.

Underwriting these post-WWII initiatives was the belief that the two-parent family was "natural," an assumption at odds with contemporary reality. In 1945, the divorce rate was ten times what it had been in 1900; the number of children born out of wedlock had more than doubled since 1939. The male-breadwinning, female-homemaking family was far from reality for most British people in the decades following WWII. Even as late as 1971, when the marriage rate was on the rise, the census showed that fewer than one-third of British families included two married parents.[9] Despite the relative rarity of the two-parent nuclear family, it was this household form that captured the British imagination as the place where intimacy naturally thrived. Advocates of the nuclear family believed that by removing the financial barriers that interfered with emotional closeness between husbands and wives and mothers and children—allowing for ample time and private space as core supportive elements to emotional intimacy—the welfare state could be directed to not only maintain full employment and universal healthcare, but to ensure that all Britons had access to an emotionally healthy and fulfilling family life.

Emotional intimacy continued to be invested with immense social significance well beyond the postwar apex in the 1950s of the British obsession with the nuclear family ideal. Despite growing challenges to the inconsistencies and limits to the universalizing aspirations of British social democracy in the late 1960s and 1970s—in addition to criticisms of the power imbalances inherent to male-breadwinning, female-homemaking families and a resurging dominance of biological understandings of mental illness—intimacy remained highly prized and widely sought after. If anything, its perceived value grew. In the 1960s and 1970s, the relational language and goals of marriage and family therapists had helped shape new personal expectations about the importance of intimate relationships and animated those movements for social and sexual reform that are centrally associated with Britain's sexual revolution and cultural backlash against the family. Petitions to expand citizens' sexual freedoms—including the decriminalization of homosexuality, the public provision of birth control, and the abolition of the legal age of sexual consent—were rationalized by reformers as promoting the necessary conditions for cultivating "healthy" emotional relationships. Activists' campaigns sought to bring the law into conformity with citizens' emotional needs, increasingly framed as "rights."

Just as the project of attaching the intimacy ideal to the white middle-class British family gained traction, it was challenged by efforts to make intimate relationality more inclusive and accessible to a wider range of people, including queer people, teenage mothers, and divorce seekers. Individuals whose lives bore little resemblance to the male-breadwinning, female-homemaking ideal sought inclusion within the intimacy paradigm. The second half of *The Intimate State* focuses on the many ways that the postwar intimacy ideal was embraced by groups of people for whom it had not originally been intended. This ideal, moreover, came to be appropriated for radically different ends. Rather than resulting from a revolutionary shift in social mores and rising cultural permissiveness, I argue that those 1960s social reforms associated with Britain's "sexual revolution" were underwritten by the post-WWII ideal of emotionally healthy citizenship.

While state-supported, expert-driven interventions into citizens' emotional development initially centered on children, they soon came to encompass adult emotional development as well. From the perspective of emotional development, childhood came to be seen as an increasingly expansive stage of life, and a psychosocial infantilization was variously applied to sexual minorities, single mothers, neglectful parents, and many others who did not easily fit within the male-breadwinning, female-homemaking family ideal. This could be seen in psychosocial therapies aimed at helping emotionally "stunted" women afflicted with post-partum mental illness and marriage counseling that focused on enabling spouses in dysfunctional relationships to arrive at emotional adulthood. Although Britain's child- and family-centered initiatives had initially been relatively modest in number after the war, the post-WWII agenda to stabilize interpersonal emotional life had a transformative impact on British understandings of "adulthood," which increasingly became an emotional category rather than a demographic designation.

This book explores how intimacy was politicized for a variety of transformative ends. In some instances, it served the goal of future-making in the present. This was the case for political preoccupations related to the welfare state's role in ensuring optimal conditions for healthy child development. For the 1970s sexual reformers who advocated wider access to birth control for teenagers and lowering the age of sexual consent, intimacy in adolescent relationships was seen as a guarantee for stable and lasting monogamous relationships in adulthood. For others, like the LGBTQ+ activists who appear in this book, intimate romance and friendships were seen as both individually *and* socially healing and pursued not only for personal ends but also as a way of solving Britain's homo- and transphobic marginalizing culture now in the immediate present. Making traumatized adults capable of creating and sustaining intimacy in the present was, for some radical reformers, the only genuine path to political change. These were attempts, to invoke Michel Foucault, "to define and develop a way of life" in the present.[10] Homosexuality, for example, was presented as a more highly evolved form of relationality that transcended the emotionally cordoned-off world of the nuclear family, rather than purely a sexual orientation. Intimate modes of supportive queer friendship, or relationality writ large, were seen as helping heal the damaging impact of stigma, as well as ending the damaging exclusions of the heteronormative social world.

Although the intimacy ideal was given legitimacy, urgency, and a sense of real-world everyday importance by the British welfare state, its popular appeal was not single-handedly created through government efforts. By the end of the 1950s, it had become clear that intimate relationships and their promise of emotional health and wellbeing were not only appealing to the state, or to the formal infrastructures of power and public life. Notably, the guarantees of intimacy—including full self-realization and emotional fulfillment—had become desirable for large numbers of British people, including those for whom the narrow post-WWII model of intimacy had not originally been intended. By the late 1960s and early 1970s, queer people, divorce seekers, and young people below the legal age of sexual consent campaigned for expanded access to the intimacy ideal—in the form of loving child-producing marriages in some cases and, in others, publicly recognized romantic relationships—to benefit from its many alluring promises.

The Welfare State

What is specifically British about this story? After all, similar developments unfolded in the United States after WWII, where marriage counseling and family therapies of various kinds came to prominence against a similar backdrop of an early Cold War cultural idealization of the male-breadwinning, female-homemaking nuclear family.[11] While many similar developments contributed to an emotionalization of family life after 1945 on both sides of the Atlantic, what was unique about the British case was the powerful presence of a universal state welfare system that helped make new family-oriented mental health initiatives possible and gave them a wider social reach. For example, in the United States, marriage counseling was largely provided in the decades after WWII to private fee-paying clients and to Protestant and Catholic Church parishioners. In Britain, most marriage reconciliation services were provided by the state. This meant that Britain's "marriage welfare" services were not only able to reach a much broader cross-section of the population but were also explicitly given political valence.

The British welfare state was initially intended to eliminate poverty and involuntary unemployment in the aftermath of WWII. It was meant to prevent citizens from falling into abject poverty during times of challenge.[12] For this reason, at first glance it may seem surprising that the protection of family stability would have fallen under its mandate. However, as some historians of the British welfare state have pointed out, what was new and revolutionary in this moment was not the nationalization of already-existing social insurance. Although nine-tenths of the immediately best-selling Beveridge Report—the influential founding document of Britain's welfare state drafted by economist and Liberal politician William Beveridge—were dedicated to eliminating "want" through social insurance proposals, the blueprint for the welfare state and its enactment in the final half of the 1940s was much more than this. What was new was the totalizing vision that was being aspired to: the goal of eliminating "Want, Disease, Ignorance, Squalor, and Idleness" signaled that British citizens should never experience these identified "evils." This was groundbreaking. It presented a complete alteration of traditional liberal notions of freedom, which had focused on individual autonomy: citizens' right to speak, write, buy, and sell as they saw fit. Freedom was revised to focus not only on experiences from which citizens, as full members of Britain's political community, should be exempt for reasons of physical safety and wellbeing. In addition, there was an *emotional* dimension to the travails that the state was imagined as needing to prevent. It is this new focus on preventing emotional harm that this book illuminates and explains.

By highlighting the new and transformative priority that was attached not only to eliminating financial insecurity, but also to eradicating *emotional* insecurity after 1945, *The Intimate State* presents a new view of the early decades of the British welfare state. Rhodri Hayward has argued that the avoidance of an emerging anxiety epidemic played a significant role in structuring welfare state reform.[13] *The Intimate State* similarly argues that the social policy of the post-WWII years was focused on ensuring that citizens were guaranteed the emotional security that was presumed to be provided most effectively by families—and by adult female family members especially.

One of this book's central interventions lies in its revelation of the surprising flexibility and durability of the political goal of ensuring citizens' emotional security. Emotional health only became a more prominent objective during the 1950s and 1960s, even as the welfare state had undergone periods of partial retrenchment (as early as 1951 when, for example, the Conservative government removed dental work and eyeglasses from the list of government-sponsored health provisions). By the end of the 1960s, the pursuit of emotional security had broadened to include individual emotional fulfilment and self-realization as endpoints of healthy psychological development in adults. Emotional health had thus become the basis for individual and social wellbeing for many early believers and new stakeholders alike.

This book does not assume the welfare state to be a unitary and cohesive entity. It is treated, rather, as a wide-ranging set of policy aspirations directed toward a common goal of social protection for the most vulnerable, and as insurance against inevitable instabilities for the entire population. *The Intimate State* engages with a rich and nuanced ongoing conversation among historians and sociologists of the British welfare state (and welfare states more broadly), many of whom argue that the welfare state itself is an abstraction rather than a concrete entity with easily identifiable characteristics.[14] For example, Derek Fraser—echoing Richard Titmuss—has characterized the "classic" British welfare state as nothing more than the social policy of a particular moment (rather than the exemplary model of *the* welfare state).[15] Nonetheless, although there is disagreement among scholars over its precise chronological origins and key identifying features, all agree that the postwar British welfare state was geared toward the provision of security at an apex of insecurity that had been building since the emergence of industrial capitalism. I argue that insecurity was treated as having crucial emotional aspects in both its nature and origins after 1945.

The individuals and groups who launched Britain's family welfare services and embarked on new research into children's and families' emotional lives were also often motivated by a political agenda. The two most prominent British child psychiatrists of the post-WWII era, Bowlby and Donald Winnicott, argued that the psychological foundations of democracy and authoritarianism were rooted in specific kinds of family structures and dynamics. For its founders, partnership with the welfare state in creating an expanded network of child guidance clinics and marriage and family therapy services was meant to not only address a host of worrying social problems like juvenile crime, divorce, and neglectful parenting, but to also support the mature psychological development that they believed made stable democracy possible. Experts' guiding rationale in viewing the family as an irreducible emotional "unit" and foundation for mental health may strike the contemporary reader as not only unfamiliar, but also maddeningly resistant to easy location within a "progressive" versus "conservative" political binary.

Expanding the Meaning of Health

The areas of welfare activity at the heart of this book were meant to protect citizens' "health" in its broadest possible sense. In the modern world, health has become essential to how we understand, organize, and participate in society and social relations.[16] It is in the name of "health" that states have intervened in populations to both promote and prevent certain activities, lifestyles, and behaviors—such as sanitation and compulsory vaccination programs to prevent the spread of infectious disease, birth control initiatives to positively impact infant and maternal health, and genetic screening and baby wellness schemes to ensure that all citizens are provided with the healthiest possible start in life. Supporting health has functioned both as a way of surveilling private behavior and decision-making and of helping individual citizens to have the best life possible in a world dominated by precarity and risk.

Many scholars and commentators consider citizens' equal access to health for both personal benefit and the public good as foundational to modern state-provided welfare. For this reason, Britain's National Health Service (NHS) has been looked upon since its 1948 origins as the "best of Britain." It is considered by most British people to be the crown jewel of the welfare state and has survived waves of reform and retrenchment even up to the present day. The NHS is more popular than any other British institution, surpassing the royal family and the BBC in the public mind. In the recently compiled "People's History of the NHS," nurse Dame Elizabeth Anionwu described it as "British to the core."[17] Other contributors emphasized its importance in similar terms. Playwright Alan Bennett stressed that "It's part of being English,"[18] while another interviewee proclaimed it, "A great reflection of the best of our society."[19] The equation of the NHS with the "best of Britain" reveals how central health has been to assumptions about the caretaking role of the state in citizens' lives, particularly when they are at their most vulnerable.

The Intimate State focuses specifically on the British investment in mental and emotional health to produce the best possible individual and collective national futures. As the book shows, after 1945, mental health professionals' psychosocial approach to the treatment of psychoneuroses popularized individual mental and emotional health as the bedrock for creating a democratic egalitarian society made up of responsible citizens. Citizens' trustworthiness in this moment of social reconstruction was gauged according to their "healthy" mature emotional development, as seen in their capacity to form and maintain stable intimate relationships. This expansive relational understanding of "health" was, in part, inherited from the preceding interwar decades when eugenic-inspired programs, directed toward improving the health of populations, also began to target a wide range of environmental circumstances for their impact on hereditary outcomes. As a result, allied work performed in the interest of health by Britain's social services are an important part of the story presented in this book. Though far from unimportant, I discuss areas of welfare state activity pertaining more centrally to education, housing, and law and order only when they were envisioned as playing important roles in supporting individual and social health.

As much as health has featured in positive assessments of the modern welfare state, it has also served as a basis for normalizing behavior and surveilling citizens' lives. Historians of sexuality have noted that health replaced morality in the modern secular world as the basis for intervening in private behaviors.[20] *The Intimate State* takes a similar approach in examining not only the perceived benefits of state-supported health initiatives aimed at improving citizens' emotional wellbeing, but also how the post-WWII public framing of "emotional health" often stood as a moral ideal for the conduct of citizens' private lives. When prescriptions were made in the name of emotional health, the understanding was that these benignly served the individual's own good.

Post-1945 concerns about emotional instability were connected to a broadening of the domain of psychiatry from treating "the mentally abnormal" into addressing problems of "normal everyday life" that accelerated in the decades following WWII.[21] As the 1968 annual report for the National Association for Mental Health (NAMH) stated:

> Mental health does not affect just a small minority of abnormal people. It covers a very wide field ... There is juvenile delinquency, drugtaking, alcoholism, marriage breakdown and suicide ... All of these ... are caused by or result in mental stress. None of us is immune from mental stress.[22]

Emotional disturbances were believed to lead to serious social problems and "health" thus became integral to a wide range of discussions relating to social change during these decades. It provided a seemingly irrefutable gauge for making moralizing assessments of private behavior and evaluating the state's obligation toward citizens.

Recent scholarship has shed light on how certain non-asylum-based twentieth century "psy" agendas—such as mental hygiene, psychiatric epidemiology, and the antipsychiatry movement—have aspired to function as political theory and, in some cases, have been influential in shaping national health, family, education, and labor policies.[23] Similarly, *The Intimate State* examines how British family welfare services were developed in connection to explicit discussions about Britain's future. Not only mental health professionals, but also politicians and activists, saw their value in terms of both contributing to citizens' right to emotional health and helping create future responsible democratic citizens.

Revealing the political interests that have supported the contemporary authority of the "psy" sciences serves a critical agenda that explicitly challenges the modern liberal conception of freedom. I owe a great intellectual debt to Michel Foucault, Nikolas Rose, Jan Goldstein, and others for opening space for examining both the political underpinnings and uses of the human sciences.[24] However, *The Intimate State* approaches the politics of modern "psy" thought and practice somewhat differently. Rather than treating the permeation of "psy" concepts and practices throughout British society as an outcome of false consciousness, it seeks to understand *why* these ideas and practices were persuasive enough to be *chosen* by many people. To this end, it focuses on the post-1945 appeal of the human sciences as a promising basis for resolving what Hannah Arendt described as the post-WWII "crisis of authority" at the same time as it tracks the growing cultural valuation of intimate emotional relationships.[25] Challenging the historical claim that individualism triumphed in the twentieth century, *The Intimate State* reveals the political and personal importance of close personal relationships in decades that are more typically associated with rising affluence, consumer culture, and individual self-expression.[26]

From Childhood to Adulthood: The Politics of Life Stages

One of the goals of *The Intimate State* is to explain why the male-breadwinning, female-homemaking nuclear family became so central to the post-1945 political order and social imaginary. Why was its promotion a major political priority? Susan Pedersen has shown that the British welfare state was modeled upon the dynamics of social dependency and care for the young and vulnerable provided within the male-breadwinning, female-homemaking family. Women and children were denied direct insurance provisions and given access to state-provided social and health services as the financial dependents of male taxpayers. *The Intimate State* builds on Pedersen's insights but focuses more specifically on the rationale behind the state's promotion of women and children as dependents, despite open criticism by several women's organizations. I argue that to fully grasp the privilege accorded to the nuclear family in the mid-twentieth century decades it is vital to consider widespread anxieties surrounding children's perceived emotional vulnerability.

A preoccupation with children's malleability was certainly not new to the postwar period; however, it acquired greater political urgency following the popularization of theories of psychological development that prioritized "nurture" and environment over hereditary "nature." In recent decades historians have revealed that the modern transformation of the wage-earning child-worker into the emotionally priceless child-student (or nascent citizen) was underwritten by a middle-class idealization of the child as an emblem of the future.[27] This idealization was not, however, always understood in psychological terms. For instance, concern for the health of mother and child at the turn of the twentieth century grew out of a commitment to the healthy physical development of children into future workers and soldiers. It was primarily during the interwar decades of the twentieth century—the dawn of what Maria Montessori called the "century of the child"—that Freud's observations about the child's psychological significance as the "father of the man" and children's potential psychological development into future criminals, alcoholics, homosexuals, neurotics, unemployed welfare recipients, and political dissidents became a source of great anxiety.[28] This interwar psychologization of children also had important social dimensions. This can be seen in child development experts—including Susan Isaacs, Cyril Burt, Ian Suttie, and even John Bowlby—stressing that "maladjusted" children were shaped by the social environments that they inhabited. They focused especially on poverty-stricken environments like overcrowded orphanages and slums as major causes of juvenile delinquency.

While new theories of child development formulated during the 1920s and 1930s identified the middle-class nuclear family as the ideal context for children's healthy social development, they stopped short of identifying the child as embedded within a larger family "system" and instead treated children as autonomous self-contained individuals. This changed after WWII. Wartime studies detailing the effects of family separation on evacuated and orphaned children highlighted symptoms of aggression, bedwetting, and tantrums, which were interpreted as evidence for children's psychological need for continuous contact with their families—especially their mothers—as they matured emotionally. Whereas Ellen Key, an early advocate for child-centered education, had emphasized the broader political importance of childhood in 1909 when she declared that "man is not fixed; he can recreate himself," in 1946 Bowlby pursued a similar line of reasoning but with a single-minded focus on the family as the venue for healthy child development.[29] He concluded that the child's emotional attachment to their mother in infancy blossomed into the highest human qualities in adulthood—including "very strong altruistic sentiments"—when mother and child developed an uninterrupted loving relationship.[30]

By the early 1950s, child psychiatrists, pediatricians, and psychoanalysts, including Bowlby, Winnicott, and Anna Freud popularized the view that child development was relational at its core and that children were in danger of becoming socially and emotionally stunted if "deprived" of continuous mother love.[31] Concerns about the negative emotional effects of "maternal deprivation" especially impacted women, who were seen as performing essential emotional work within their families. Parenting literature thus sought less to instruct on specific parenting techniques than to help mothers learn to follow their instincts to bond with their children and become more in touch with their innate relational impulses.

Being a mother of young children in a culture saturated with child development theories was guilt-inducing—presenting as it did new possibilities for maternal blame and internalized shame. At the same time, maternal care carried tremendous socio-political importance given the heightened expectations of its long-term psychological impact. These expectations did not disappear even when Bowlby's theory of "maternal deprivation" came under fire in the 1960s and 1970s, but instead surprisingly intensified. Even the radical feminist periodical *Spare Rib* and the women's refuge organization National Women's Aid Federation promoted the emotional importance of maternal care and women's special talents at child rearing, pointing out that the emotional labor of parenting had long been performed much more expertly by women than men.[32]

By the 1970s, as *The Intimate State* shows, beliefs about the emotional fragility and the relational needs of children had been naturalized and extended to certain groups of adults as well. Emotional development had come to be seen as perpetually under threat of premature stunting by damaging life events, especially those involving troubled family relationships. The definitive markers of emotional adulthood included successfully choosing and sustaining a lifelong heterosexual monogamous child-producing partnership and the capacity to provide one's children with a stable family. Those who had strayed from this idealized model of private life were pathologized as emotionally immature. The possibility of cure—rather than full social banishment (as was the projected outcome of moral prohibitions)—was offered through expert-assisted strategies for encouraging healthy developmental maturity. The major features of adulthood had thus come to be marked by specific interpersonal emotional qualities and capacities. "Emotional maturity" became a neutral-sounding term for right behavior and sound decision-making.

Emotional development was appealed to as the basis for marking out the appropriate timing of a range of life experiences, including sex, marriage, parenthood, employment, and home ownership. A key component of the social value of "emotional maturity" was its apparent directedness toward a particular kind of future (even if people making such decisions were only passively adhering to social conventions). Jack Halberstam notes that "heteronormative time/space constructs" that demarcate "reproductive time and family time" are future directed.[33] He points out that queer subjects, or those who live outside of the logic of capitalist accumulation, including "ravers, HIV-positive barebackers, rent boys, sex workers, homeless people, drug dealers, and the unemployed" are marked by their disregard for the future.[34] Living in the present has meant—and continues to signify to many—living irresponsibly in accordance with instinct, chaos, and a lack of concern for the future.

The Intimate State examines what it meant for the British welfare state to effectively map plans for Britain's future onto human developmental time. The child stood as a present-day foothold into the future in intimacy projects that sought to produce emotional security and fulfillment along a time axis that followed the long and often turbulent progression from infancy to emotionally mature adulthood. Where the past ended and the future began was continually revised in the post-1945 decades as adults were increasingly infantilized as not yet mature—rather than, say, having either a defective hereditary disposition or an irredeemably immoral character—until they had established stable heterosexual marriages and embarked on the project of rearing two healthy, emotionally secure children. Married men and women in stable child-producing relationships supported this political project by appropriately orienting their lives toward the future. And parents who aspired to raise their children in accordance with the advice of child development experts further contributed to the project of "engineering" similar future-oriented people. The future that was being imagined and worked toward was not near—particularly when compared to the impatient speed of modern life in the mid-twentieth century, as seen in the exponential advances in information technology, arms and space races, transportation, and other sectors since the 1950s. And it was continually deferred with each re-articulation of the ever-expanding markers of adulthood and the lingering immaturities that were newly identified as obstacles to healthy citizenship.

Gender, Class, and the Creation of Intimate Subjects

What was the specific locus for producing meaning about the good mother, the loving family, healthy childhood, and mature adulthood? These ideals were grounded in cutting-edge, post-WWII psychological and social science, and I argue that we need to look to specialized therapeutic sites like psychiatric hospitals, child guidance clinics, marriage therapy interview rooms, and children's hospital wards to answer that question. These were spaces where key cultural scripts became legible and invested with authority. *The Intimate State* thus focuses on the labor-intensive psychopolitical enterprises that sought to make intimacy into a tangible reality. The participants in these projects were diverse. They included politicians, policymakers, and psychiatrists whose work produced Britain's continuously developing welfare state. They also included grassroots actors such as child welfare advocates, sexual law reformers, and mothers of young children who wanted to see the emotional lives of British citizens not only protected but also improved—and even, for some, liberated.

The sites and actors that appear in this book are diverse. All, however, saw the solution to their problems—whether related to tackling emotional deprivation in children or sexual liberation for LGBTQ+ people—in the cultivation of "healthy" emotional relationships. They focused on improving the relational potential of the people they served. The therapeutic projects and political initiatives that I examine were fueled by the belief that human beings are fundamentally relational, and they each sought to hone this as a basis for social improvement. The relational subject who was meant to emerge out of these therapeutic initiatives was set against the "anti-social" or "affectionless" subject whose emotional development had been stunted through an absence of stable loving relationships in their early years. Some of these people had lost or been taken from their mothers, but more often they had mothers who faced financial struggle and were unable to provide around-the-clock care. Their mothers may have been unmarried, or they may have had spouses who were unable to take on the role of full-time breadwinner. As the book will show, the anti-social "affectionless" subject was a moving target—at times, they were Nazi soldiers, and, at others, the urban poor, juvenile delinquents, neglectful mothers, and violent husbands.[35] What they all had in common was an inability to form stable relationships.

Although the post-WWII project of making intimacy into a universally accessible reality was meant to apply to all British citizens irrespective of race, gender, or class, neither practice nor theory was consistent with this. Those state-funded services like marriage therapy and child guidance that targeted family stability were initially grounded in a vision of white middle-class Britishness that not so subtly communicated to citizens of all backgrounds the race- and class-specific meaning of "healthy" humanity. It supported expectations of the inherent health of monogamous coupling publicly recognized through marriage and active yet restrained child-production that kept families at a size small enough to accommodate the financial ideal of private home ownership. Emotional security was not free—it cost a significant amount of money to secure both the time and space to ensure that children were given ready access to a stable and presumably loving emotional environment.

The assumptions of white middle-classness were seldom explicit. For example, the lack of attention to socio-economic and cultural background as relevant details in case reports is startling. When mentioned, it was typically in passing. Case reports from the Marital Unit at the Tavistock Clinic, one of Britain's flagships for psychoanalysis, focused solely on clients' family relationship histories. One case report from the early 1950s, describing a middle-class Jewish woman who was married to a working-class Christian man and experiencing marriage problems, only mentioned the couple's religious and class background to give a quick sense of their differing family experiences and expectations.[36] In the mid-1970s, at the queer befriending organization Friend, a self-identified black lesbian writing in for advice was told that her sexual minority status was far more significant to her experience of social oppression than her racial background.[37] Neither of these examples stands out as unusual in the sources examined: religion, ethnicity, and class were consistently positioned in the background to allow the facts surrounding emotional life to be analyzed and improved. The intimacy ideal was meant to teach white middle-class people and others presumed to be aspiring to white middle-classness how to embrace and enact the right kind of "civilized" values in the post-1945 decades.

Within the male-breadwinning, female-homemaking nuclear family, women were understood to make essential emotional contributions. As the chief generators of emotional connection within their families, they were expected to provide their children with emotional care and maintain intimate relationships with their husbands.[38] The conscious practiced effort that this often involved was presented by some second-wave feminists as comparable to skilled work. However, comparisons between emotional forms of domestic labor and paid work were more often undermined as a result of two dominant concerns: first, the worry that emotional care would be cheapened if it was commodified or made transactional and second, the belief that the capacity for intimate relationships was a natural outcome of mature femininity and therefore an intrinsic feature of healthy female adulthood.[39]

This psychopolitical project not only implicated British mothers in ensuring that children grew up to be emotionally mature adults; it also politicized femininity more broadly for its presumably natural capacity for relational emotion. In endowing healthy mature femininity with effortless relationality and, in turn, making emotional life the basis for stable democracy, women's work at home attending to their children was given tremendous social significance. Moreover, the recipient of maternal care was implicitly gendered male. This was a male subject formed in relationship to an idealized adult woman: women's presumed innate aptitude for intimacy made fully mature men—"independent *and* society-minded"—possible.[40] Mature femininity—with its associations with a natural capacity for marital stability and effortless emotional bonding with children—had become a form of nature that was to be aspired to, making deviations from this highly specific (and for many impossible) life path increasingly costly.

The politics of emotional intimacy did not (and do not) stop there. Egalitarianism is presumed to be present in relationships founded in intimacy. This might be contrasted with the inequality that is at the heart of another interpersonal emotion, compassion. Lauren Berlant notes that compassion is an emotion rooted in a kind of privilege—suffering is presumed to be somewhere else, at some distance from the individual experiencing compassion.[41] Intimacy, on the other hand, involves equality, a flattening of social relations—between generations (parent and child) and between genders (man and woman)—as both a proxy for (and way of concealing) an absence of equality elsewhere. The presumption of equality in the capacity to experience intimacy and even the possibility that intimacy might do away with distinctions of race and class (in cross-class and inter-racial relationships) invested the promise of interpersonal connection with great socio-political consequence. Intimacy-building projects allowed Britons to imagine a future that was equal, free, and in harmony with longstanding liberal values (and surprisingly so, since traditional liberal values are more typically associated with reason rather than emotion).

In addition to situating gender at the heart of its inquiry, *The Intimate State* interrogates modern British heteronormative preoccupations with intimacy as a primary feature of socially acceptable sexuality. Non-intimate, non-future-directed sexuality has been, and continues to be, associated with deviance.[42] Historians of sexuality have shown heterosexuality to be far more than a matter of object choice. In the post-1945 era, heterosexuality has been connected to an emotional style—private, intimate, mutually enriching—that has also been imagined as providing stability to large democratic capitalist communities. As Gayle Rubin points out, sexuality that falls outside of the range of social acceptability—such as non-monogamous homosexuality, sadomasochism, fetishism, and transsexuality—has been imagined to be "devoid of all emotional nuance" and for this reason, "repulsive."[43]

Building on this insight, *The Intimate State* argues that by the mid-1960s, private life did not become increasingly separate from public life but was made more intensely visible to the outside world as a way of performing highly attuned emotional awareness. Respondents to social surveys in the late 1960s were more than twice as likely as they were in the early 1950s to rank emotional intimacy as the most important basis for a successful long-lasting relationship.[44] Evidence of a shifting set of priorities in marriage in which emotional over material factors were increasingly valued could be seen across the socio-economic classes. However, expectations of love and compatibility were usually linked to a specific kind of middle-class lifestyle. This was neatly summed up in a report from the Royal College of Psychiatrists in 1976 as involving "a complex commitment of two partners who are together capable of preparing for, and building, a family, so that 'going steady,' mutual respect and helpfulness, maintaining work, finding lodgings, buying a cot and a pram, handling the two sets of grandparents amicably may be better criteria of maturity than physical or intellectual attainment."[45] The report fittingly concluded that, "Sexual activity is now recognized to serve ends other than reproduction."[46]

The Personal Is Political: Intimate Relationships at the Intersection of Public and Private Life

Why did the British invest so much in the emotional life of its citizens at the precise moment they did, in the decades after WWII? This vision of the transformative consequences of emotional health was initially dreamed up at a moment when war, mass murder, and the pursuit of unbridled national power (often disturbingly conflated with racial power) were recent experiences that the future was being imagined against. Only a brief time before that, millions of Britons had directly experienced the catastrophic effects of economic depression, including unprecedented involuntary unemployment and a depth of poverty that was exposed as a recurring fact of life under industrial capitalism. A combination of these recent experiences and the advice of psychological experts made a focus on emotional relationships—given their untested open-ended promise for positive change—seem like a crucial component of any plan for moving toward a recovered new world.

Between 1945 and 1979—what might be described as Britain's psychopolitical era—intimate relationships were fundamental to remaking both public and private life in Britain. The story that this book presents and the core initiatives that it describes sought to move modern life in a more community-oriented, anti-individualist direction, attending to all citizens equally as fundamentally motivated by a will to develop interpersonal connection. The activities and initiatives that this book examines were motivated by a common belief that private life was at its core emotional and that close personal relationships provided the foundation for public life.

The prominent and pioneering child psychiatrists, marriage therapists, therapeutic community creators, and social and sexual reform activists who appear in this book believed that harmonious relationships would work against social fragmentation and re-invigorate public life by setting an empathic sense of social responsibility on a solid foundation—the healthy and fully developed personality. Their focus on intimate relationships did not constitute a disavowal of modernity, but rather are part of a history of appeals for a larger—more expansive—modernity.[47] These were projects that took human emotional potential seriously. Interpersonal life was seen as the basis for every social phenomenon, large and small, from democracy to international war to sexual stigma to marriage woes.

At the heart of *The Intimate State* is an exploration of how modern emotional subjectivities were formulated between WWII and the rise of neoliberalism, as Britain became a post-imperial, post-industrial, democratic society. Ian Hacking's work has insightfully revealed the creative and dynamic ways that psychiatric classifications have "made up people."[48] Emphasizing the extent to which people who are classified participate in transforming their classifications, Hacking has provided a useful alternative to Foucault's far less agentive model by arguing that the process of creating diagnostic labels involves the named as much as those who do the naming. From E.P. Thompson to Michel de Certeau to Joan Wallach Scott, scholars have for many decades been preoccupied with the potential for agency in everyday life.[49] Do social structures determine who we become and the kinds of decisions that are available to us? To what extent are we, in fact, active participants in becoming the kinds of people that we are? Can we actively and consciously resist social forces and claim some measure of freedom and authenticity as integral to who we are? *The Intimate State* argues that experts did not single-handedly produce new emotional subjectivities but rather offered a compelling language and set of concepts explaining the wide-ranging benefits of complex human relationships that many British men and women were drawn to and appropriated. These were people who wanted to become more emotionally satisfied and fully realized individuals and hoped that the theories and practices of social psychiatrists and relationship therapists would help them to achieve this goal. Furthermore, new kinds of post-1945 political subjects saw the potential for new levels of freedom and social justice through the kind of relationship work that socially oriented mental health professionals promoted.

Not everyone, however, benefited from intimate relationships becoming so explicitly and visibly identified as social imperatives. Many people's agency was damagingly compromised by harmful social messaging. The notion that interpersonal intimacy came easily to women and was essential for successful child-rearing was neither welcomed nor experienced as liberatory by all. By the early 1960s, large numbers of mothers of young children were guiltily confessing to struggling under the enormous weight of gendered social expectations that women were naturally nurturing and adept at intimacy. Many married heterosexual people (especially women) described to their marriage counselors feeling not only dissatisfaction, but also shame, at their marriages not living up to an ideal of intimate companionship that was free of conflict, diverging interests, and leisure time spent apart. Queer people who approached counseling and befriending services in the 1960s and 1970s seeking help finding partners for unattached sex were often met not with support but with diagnoses of socially induced pathologies stemming from stigma around queer sexuality.

Wartime and immediate postwar attention to mental and emotional health transformed the meaning and scope of politics in Britain. Examining the pursuit of intimacy through a variety of therapeutic initiatives and political movements for reform, *The Intimate State* argues that emotional life—seen as intersubjective at its core—became a primary terrain on which social politics were articulated and imagined in Britain for several decades after 1945. Intimate emotional relationships were imagined to be simultaneously the foundation for collective political stability and a right of all individual citizens. But more broadly, *The Intimate State* also contributes to tracing the history of a new and enduring emotionally directed political culture on both sides of the Atlantic after 1945—one that continues to recognize both intimate relationships and emotional wellbeing as fundamental to citizens' wholeness as humans. In both Britain and North America, this continues to inform, on the one hand, the politics surrounding equal access to marriage, parenthood, and family, and, on the other, increasing concerns about trauma and other forms of serious mental and emotional damage caused by institutional sexism, racism, homophobia, and transphobia. In relating this story of how emotional life became political in Britain after 1945, *The Intimate State* highlights the complex contingency of the many circumstances, encounters, values, and lived experiences that have helped produce the distinctly emotional political and cultural landscape that many (in Britain and beyond) inhabit today.

Structure of the Book

The Intimate State takes its chronological point of departure in 1920s Britain, when a growing number of physicians, psychologists, and social scientists active in the child guidance and mental hygiene movements began to explore the many ways that an individual's social environment determined both their degree of mental health and their capacity for responsible democratic citizenship. The first chapter focuses on the crucial set of developments in interwar and WWII British medicine and psychiatry that made it possible to forge a new, and much more proximate, relationship between the politics of democratic citizenship and the private world of intimate emotional relationships. It focuses especially on key areas of wartime psychiatric activity that established a broad range of social applications for British psychiatry in guiding post-WWII reconstruction. These included the world's first "therapeutic community" at Northfield military hospital; the development of new social psychological techniques for officer selection and enemy interrogation; and psychosocial research using German prisoners of wars (POWs) that investigated how the appeal of Nazi ideology was rooted in childhood family experiences. The latter study became the basis for a post-WWII program of "denazification" focused on eliminating authoritarian psychological influences from positions of German state power. While much scholarship has focused on the importance of eugenics in shaping twentieth-century politics focused on the family, the book's opening chapter sheds light on the roots of a profoundly influential departure in the environmental politics of the family during the mid-twentieth century decades that resisted biological or hereditarian determinism.

Chapter 2 moves the focal point from wartime innovations in group psychiatry aimed at adult male soldiers to a post-WWII preoccupation with the deep impact of environment on children's emotional development. This chapter explores how the wartime discovery of widespread emotional "deprivation" in children—and fears attached to its long-term psychological effects—transformed post-WWII British political culture by making it a basic duty of the modern state to ensure citizens' emotional health. Although there had been concerns about emotional deprivation before WWII in relationship to the underlying cause of the rising incidence of juvenile delinquency, this discussion exploded during and immediately after the war in the wake of the perceived failures of the evacuation of close to 735,000 urban children to the British countryside (a significant proportion of whom reportedly showed signs of emotional distress). This chapter reveals how concerns about Britain's future after 1945 became tied to the developmental futures of British children. Alongside its agenda of eliminating poverty and guaranteeing full employment, Britain's new welfare state was tasked with ensuring that all children be reared within "family-like" environments and given the best possible shot at emotional health. Concern for children's emotional development framed the government's approach to adoption, foster care, daycare provision, and children's in-patient treatment in hospitals. The protection and promotion of family intimacy came to be seen as one of the functions of the new welfare state. This not only helped reinvent the family as first and foremost a set of intimate relationships, it also introduced a new emotional component to the rights and responsibilities of modern democratic citizenship.

Chapter 3 examines the impact of this prominent new concern for children's healthy emotional development on mothers as the chief providers of emotional care. It investigates new rehabilitative programs designed to tackle the increasingly visible problems of child neglect and post-partum mental illness, focusing on the joint admission of mothers and their young children at the Cassel Hospital for Functional Nervous Disorders in London. Although staff at the Cassel sought to humanize "bad" mothers and establish greater empathy for their emotional distress, they were reluctant to challenge post-WWII expectations that childcare was the "natural" central preoccupation of female adulthood. Instead, treatment at the hospital—set within an innovative "therapeutic community"—focused on helping mostly young married female patients resolve their "emotional immaturity" through an intensive, around-the-clock therapeutic regime centered on patients' appropriately loving relationships with their children. This chapter argues that new post-WWII visibility surrounding the emotional burdens of motherhood ended up further reifying, rather than undermining, the presumption that women were, by nature, relational "experts" and better suited to childcare than men.

Chapter 4 continues to examine the rising value attributed to intimate family relationships in the post-1945 decades by focusing on the important role that marriage counseling and therapy services played in promoting its wide-ranging benefits for both individual emotional health and national wellbeing. Initially launched under the aegis of preventive mental health, Britain's post-WWII network of state-supported "marriage welfare" services was fueled by concerns about the effects of divorce on children's emotional development. This chapter explores the implications of state support for relationship therapy services and uncovers how the expansive social health objectives of marriage therapy pioneers actively contributed to the welfare-state project of creating a "classless" social democratic society. Citizens' access to loving relationships was cast as the great social equalizer as marriage therapists argued that human beings were primarily shaped through their desire for emotional, rather than socio-economic, wellbeing. This chapter also investigates the *unintended* political effects of marriage therapy, revealing how therapists' language and concepts helped create a new public discourse of relationship "breakdown" and provided persuasive (ostensibly scientific) arguments for liberalizing the divorce law. Tracking divorce reformers' mobilization of marriage therapists' psychosocial understanding of intimate relationships in framing and legitimizing their demands for change, I investigate the effects of the popular dissemination of this new psychiatric view in shaping public expectations and related political discourses surrounding emotional fulfillment and psychological freedom.

Although post-WWII psychological initiatives like marriage counseling and aversion therapies had contributed significantly to the social and legal marginalization of LGBTQ+ people, beginning in the early 1960s, activists supporting homosexual law reform looked to psychosexual counseling as a powerful tool for progressive social change. Chapter 5 examines the launching of counseling and befriending services by British queer activist organizations at the height of Britain's so-called "sexual revolution."[50] Seeking to remedy the many serious social and emotional problems that homosexual, bisexual, and trans populations faced, supporters of homosexual law reform and queer liberation activists alike saw in counseling a promising solution to the harmful psychological effects of social exclusion and internalized homo- and transphobia. However, as this chapter demonstrates, although the meaning and markers of psychological "health" were expanded and revised, many features of Britain's dominant constellation of sexual values were retained as goals, and even internalized by social reformers themselves. These included the valorization of stable intimacy and pathologization of promiscuity. This chapter reveals that British counseling aimed at queer people, in its pursuit of resolving the emotional suffering uniquely experienced by sexual minorities, focused on cultivating clients' psychological capacity to choose and sustain intimate relationships. Moreover, the chapter argues that this goal was connected to broader political objectives related to queer equality and socio-sexual liberation that have since been forgotten.

Chapter 6 investigates another set of activist campaigns prioritizing access to intimate relationships, but this time directed at the freedoms of young people: the sexual expression of teenagers and queer men under the age of twenty-one. It examines how the longstanding psychiatric pathologization of adolescence as a period of emotional instability became the basis for closing a series of explosive controversies surrounding teenage sexuality in the 1970s. Young people were considered in many quarters to be more physically and intellectually mature than they had been in previous generations, and this was reflected in the lowered age of majority from twenty-one to eighteen by 1970. Psychiatrists maintained, however, that adolescents' rate of emotional development had not kept pace. Although teenagers became directly involved in the campaign to lower the legal age of sexual consent, their petitions were rejected by 1981 on the grounds that sexual activity had the potential to pathologically disrupt adolescents' delicate emotional development. This chapter argues that this set of political confrontations further hardened conceptions of young people as emotionally immature, incapable of making responsible sexual choices, and vulnerable to emotional harm, thus requiring the protection of the criminal law. By the end of the 1970s, the democratic and emotionally enlightened "good society" had come to be equated with the guarantees of privacy and sexual freedom. I argue that this freedom, however, was rooted in associations between adulthood and emotional maturity, and legitimated through its exclusion of children as the proper recipients of the protection of the state. The explicit infantilization of adolescents and young queer men, who were effectively deemed children in an emotional sense, provided a compelling rationale for not offering consistent sex education in British schools and NHS-provided birth control to young women, as well as for maintaining age-based restrictions in the laws surrounding sexual consent.

Chapter 7—the book's final chapter—tracks the surprising durability of the intimacy ideal in the face of the "discovery" of family violence in white middle-class families in the 1970s. This chapter focuses on key areas of backlash against the middle-class nuclear family as a pathological site of physical *and* emotional violence, with emotional violence highlighted as particularly damaging because of its lasting psychological impact. Most importantly, it was understood that emotional violence led to the passing down of trauma from one generation to the next. This chapter explores influential exposés of the routineness of middle-class family violence produced by antipsychiatrists, second-wave feminists, and activists associated with the battered women's refuge movement. It reveals that the mother-child relationship took on even greater emotional significance as the basis for a fulfilling private life *despite* political movements that attempted to destabilize other traditional normative views of gender roles. Even within these critical movements themselves, both the satisfactions of private life and the humane "good society" were presented as rooted in interpersonal emotional bonds that began in infancy. This chapter demonstrates the enduring preoccupation with emotional relationships in this era of privacy and permissiveness, especially spotlighting the intensified importance of mothers' emotional labor and presumed natural capacity for emotional connection even though intimacy in families was increasingly exposed as having a dangerous, dark side.

Finally, the epilogue brings the narrative to a close with a brief exploration of how the changing neoliberal climate in the 1980s coincided with state efforts to eject emotional life from the sphere of politics. The nuclear family continued to hold enormous social currency, however the British government no longer presented itself as playing a decisive role in its private affairs. If anything, the opposite of this was now the explicit goal. In this new world of private freedoms, intimacy was presumed to have finally (and rightfully) been unmoored from the public world of politics. The epilogue demonstrates that despite the presumed incompatibility of neoliberal values and quintessentially private experiences associated with personal relationships, intimacy continued to retain its connection to the (often elusive) promise of a meaningful life.

PART I
THE WELFARE STATE'S INTIMATE PLACES AND PEOPLE

PART I

1
Democracy as Therapy
Psychiatry and the Social Environment in Interwar and Wartime Britain

> A co-operative, peaceful, and nonpersecutory society demands that personal and social relations within it be based on the principles of freedom and democracy ... if it can be demonstrated that liberty and democracy are necessary for its existence, they cease to be merely desirable in themselves but are seen to be social and psychological techniques having as their purpose the creation of a society with certain particular valued attributes.
> —John Bowlby, "Psychology and Democracy," 1946

> The widest view will look upon group therapy as an expression of a new attitude towards the study and improvement of human inter-relations in our time. It may see in it an instrument, perhaps the first adequate one, for a practicable approach to the key problem of our time: the strained relationship between the individual and the community ... Perhaps someone taking this broad view will see in it the answer in the spirit of a democratic community to the mass and group handling of totalitarian regimes.
> —S.H. Foulkes, "On Group Analysis," 1946

At the height of the Second World War (WWII), Britain's newly constituted MI19 initiated an extensive psychological study of German prisoners of war to provide strategic insight into the enemy that would help ensure victory and bring the war to a timely end. The MI19 was the division of the British Directorate of Military Intelligence responsible for compiling information from enemy prisoners of war who were known or suspected to be working for either Germany or Japan. The study, which took almost three years to complete, was meant to piece together a definitive "psychological assessment of the ideas, feelings, and impulses which animate the human beings composing the enemy's Armed Forces,"[1] and also identify "those traits of personality which were characteristic of men holding Nazi beliefs and convictions."[2] It more broadly promised to "throw some light on the connections which exist between character structure and political ideology."[3] Russian-born British psychiatrist Henry Dicks, who was fluent in German, was charged with the task along with his collaborator American sociologist Edward Shils, who served with both the British Army and US Office of Strategic Services during WWII. Both men oversaw countless hours of interviews with more than two thousand POWs being held captive in London.

Dicks and Shils were interested in assessing the extent to which authoritarianism was present in German families. The questions asked were deeply personal and probing. They focused primarily on POWs' childhoods and upbringing—questions that elicited strong emotional responses, even reducing some soldiers to tears. At the end of the study, they concluded that German fathers' excessive influence over their sons' upbringing alongside the denigration of "feminine" tenderness had cultivated "aggressive," "sadistic," and "inhuman" attitudes, as well as "destructive impulses," in the majority of German men.[4] They argued that Nazi fears of "enemy encirclement" and the scapegoating of Jewish people had emerged out of an "impotence feeling implicit first of all in their family life."[5] Dicks concluded that the type of personality forged within German families not only informed Nazi state philosophy but also contributed to its widespread appeal.

That the British War Office would charge a psychiatrist and a sociologist with the important task of unraveling the internal logic of "the enemy mind" was neither an exceptional nor unusual basis for counter-offensive attack during WWII. The Office of Strategic Services (the forerunner of the CIA) had similarly enlisted anthropologists Margaret Mead and Ruth Benedict to "crack" the "cultural code" supporting enemy action.[6] However, unlike the comparatively relativist stances of Benedict and Mead, Dicks and Shils's study of Nazi personality treated German culture not as a benign variant but as a pathological deviation.

Describing his work as "psychological warfare," Dicks viewed the ardent Nazi's personality as a social psychiatric problem in need of cure. Noting that some POWs arrived at cathartic realizations during their imprisonment—given their removal from Wehrmacht culture—Dicks concluded that "it should be the task of our psychological warfare to cause more and more men to pull out of the group sadism and review their situation in these individual reflections."[7] As the main adviser for the German Personnel Research Branch (GPRB) after the war, Dicks was given further opportunity to pursue his politico-therapeutic agenda during Germany's denazification. He introduced psychological tests to uncover authoritarian personality traits in the selection of civil servants. In his view, the removal of such personalities from positions of state power would help transform German cultural values.

Dicks's view of authoritarianism as a pathology that could be cured was not unusual among British mental health professionals at this time. During the war, several prominent British psychiatrists launched initiatives that blended politics and psychiatry believing that stable democracy was fundamentally connected to mental health. Wilfred Bion created the world's first democratic "therapeutic community" for war neuroses at a psychiatric hospital in Birmingham. Maxwell Jones created a similar democratic treatment experiment targeting "effort syndrome," a psychosomatic heart condition in soldiers. S.H. Foulkes pioneered group therapy as a form of treatment that worked on boosting soldiers' collective morale. John Bowlby oversaw psychological testing for effective democratic leadership in military officer selection. Tom Main introduced strategies for cultivating morale in Britain's battle schools. Main's psychological contributions de-emphasized aggression in warfare and instead worked to establish feelings of protectiveness toward family back home.

This chapter explores how democracy came to have powerful associations with mental health in Britain. Arguments supporting the benefits of egalitarian democratic community often proceeded from a psychopolitical standpoint, and some of the most vocal champions of democracy claimed to speak as scientists rather than politicians. I illuminate how in Britain during the war health and politics were often seen as constituting a unified agenda, centered on the dynamics of intimate interpersonal life. British psychiatrists and officials at the British War Office were not only concerned that war might introduce neuroses in soldiers and civilians—given the massive numbers of shell-shocked soldiers during WWI—but that motivations for war might themselves *result* from neuroses that were rooted in childhood family dysfunction. According to this view, war was neither an inevitable feature of group life nor the product of rational political decisions. It was a symptom of social disease.

Pioneers of the emerging sub-discipline of social psychiatry in the middle decades of the twentieth century saw themselves as mavericks working against a pervasive, and, in their view, far too narrow, view of health as simply the absence of illness. Although social psychiatry is now a lesser-known therapeutic subfield, in the mid-twentieth century its innovators were not marginal figures. They were leaders in their fields and often politically well connected. Historian Joanne Meyerowitz explains the current amnesia surrounding social psychiatry in the United States as resulting from the ascendance of biological explanations for a wide range of human behaviors since the 1960s. As she puts it, this has caused us to forget "the competing biopolitics of twentieth-century social constructionists."[8] In 1940s and 1950s Britain, social psychiatrists and their allies saw psychiatry's future focused on interpersonal life, rather than psychopharmacology or neuroscience.

How did this psychopolitical agenda arise in the first place? In this chapter, I argue that its origins lay in social therapies that found democratic social environments to have a positive impact on health—mental *and* physical—between the mid-1920s and the end of WWII. I therefore begin by examining interwar developments in both the comprehensive health center and the psychiatric hospital that provided new and compelling democratic models for understanding health and illness. I then focus on the wartime emergence of social psychiatry by examining two key areas of innovation during the war, both under the leadership of the British War Office: the world's first "therapeutic community" at Northfield military hospital and psychiatric studies of German POWs that helped produce new causal connections between German family life and Nazi ideology. Stressing the key impact of practical interventions in community life, I argue that social psychiatrists' psychopolitical ambitions were actualized through practical efforts aimed at making social interactions thoroughly democratic.

This chapter focuses on crucial developments in British psychiatry that made it possible to forge new, much more proximate, connections between public life and the ostensibly private world of intimate relationships. While much work has gone into revealing the prominent place of eugenics in shaping an intentionally modern, future-oriented, and biologically informed politics centered on the family during the first half of the twentieth century, this chapter sheds light on the roots of a profoundly important and influential departure during the mid-twentieth century decades. Even before eugenics came into disrepute—in the wake of public recognition of Nazi abuses—many British and American mental health professionals turned their attention away from heredity and toward the psychologically transformative effects of the social environment in producing a range of "antisocial" individuals, including neurotics, criminals, and followers of totalitarian rule.[9] Family relationships were particularly spotlighted and scrutinized for the ways that they contributed to the shaping of personality.

Each of the health initiatives examined in this chapter sought to understand the impact of social life on human psychological development. They provide necessary context for understanding widespread interest in the family after WWII. Why did the family capture the psychiatric imagination as the healthiest of all possible social forms? Why were other modes of social organization—such as the urban neighborhood, the workplace, the trade union, the military unit, the social club, or the socialist style of community modeled at the kibbutz—so comparatively unpopular (although each of these was also studied)?[10] The answer lies, in substantial part, in concerns about the fragility of liberal democratic values in an age of looming totalitarianism. What was the relationship between the individual and their social world? Were they inevitably in conflict or inextricably bound to one another? Were democratic citizens, as psychiatrist John Bowlby and economist Evan Durbin stressed, certain *kinds* of people who were reared in specific family environments? This chapter explores the moment when psychiatrists first began to actively experiment with the effects of social environments on human development and gesture in the direction of the family as not only the mediating point between individuals and society but as itself constitutive of both. Moreover, it sheds light on an important moment of possibility, helping us to understand how the family—now so often understood to be a carrier for conservative moral values—briefly, for a few decades, stood at the center of a future-oriented and consciously modern democratic social politics and for much longer as the quintessential ideal (however fraught) of meaningful interpersonal intimacy.

Psychiatry and the Social Environment in Interwar Britain

Although social psychiatry only became a branch of psychiatry after WWII, its intellectual heritage can be traced back to late-nineteenth- and early-twentieth-century developments in crowd, group, and social psychology. The earliest psychological explanations for troubling group phenomena (such as fads and riots), produced in the wake of the rise of mass democracies and affordable publishing, were concerned about the powerful influence of group life on less educated, unpropertied, and newly enfranchised members of society.

Early psychological speculation viewed group life as having dominated primitive stages of human evolution. There was no consensus, however, on whether this earlier human past had been predominantly cooperative or violent. Writing in 1889, in the wake of the French Revolution's centenary, crowd psychologist Gustave Le Bon linked group behavior to revolutionary violence.[11] In the opening decades of the twentieth century, British neurosurgeon and early social psychologist Wilfred Trotter instead saw an instinctive human desire for social belonging as the basis for peaceful social progress.[12] Despite these differences, Le Bon, Trotter, and Sigmund Freud, who published his landmark work on group psychology in 1921, all saw the group as continuing to exert a powerful psychological hold on individuals in modern civilized societies.[13] They believed that when people gathered in groups, rational skepticism fell away.

The psychological propensity for war was a major preoccupation of several leading British psychoanalysts after WWI, including Edward Glover, John Rickman, and John Bowlby. All commonly viewed war as the outcome of primitive aggression and an evolutionary holdover that interfered with the development of wholly civilized societies. Directed at audiences around the world, these psychological studies praised internationalism as the most promising path toward a globally peaceful future. The venues for addresses on the psychology of war reflected their pacifist internationalist orientation. Glover—who had early in his career worked as a physician in a Scottish prison hospital and had since devoted himself to understanding connections between war and crime—delivered a series of lectures on war prevention to the International Federation of League of Nations Societies in Geneva in 1931.[14] Rickman also presented social psychological research on Russian culture and politics at several international meetings in the 1930s—including the International Federation of the League of Nations Societies—and led a study of "tensions affecting international understanding" for UNESCO in 1948.[15]

Interwar transformations in asylum legislation and psychiatric practice had perhaps even greater influence in laying the foundations for the mid-century social "revolution" in psychiatry. In the second half of the nineteenth century, the British asylum population doubled and all treatment options—which were meagre in most asylums, but when they existed included baths, sedatives, and at times occupational therapies—had failed to stem the rise in insanity. In the wake of mental hospital overpopulation, some looked to improvements in patient housing at smaller hospitals and clinics as the way forward in genuinely treating less severe cases. By 1930, the passage of a new Mental Treatment Act formally acknowledged the mentally ill person's vulnerability to their social environment and aimed to make hospital treatment accessible to patients afflicted with a broad range of "mild" forms of mental illness. The 1930 Act empowered local authorities to provide both inpatient and outpatient hospital care to sufferers of all types of mental illness (and not only severe psychotic afflictions) and develop "after-care" rehabilitative services to prevent discharged patients' relapse.[16] The act abolished the language of the "lunatic" and the "asylum" and replaced these with "patient" and "mental hospital" to signal their aim to treat rather than confine.[17]

The Mental Treatment Act of 1930 resulted from concern about an ongoing rise in the incidence of mental illness, especially among lower-income groups. Worries about the psychiatric impact of the urban slum featured especially prominently in discussions in major medical journals in the early decades of the twentieth century. Whereas psychiatrists in the late nineteenth century were preoccupied with heredity and worried that the rise in insanity might indicate nationwide degeneration, some of Britain's most influential psychiatrists had radically changed their understanding of insanity in the early twentieth century. In 1908, Henry Maudsley—a major proponent of the late-nineteenth-century view that mental illness was inherited and incurable—donated £30,000 to create a small hospital specializing in the treatment of "mild" mental disorders. He saw the research and teaching hospital as playing a crucial role in separating out curable cases of mental illness from the harmful influence of the mass of incurable "degenerates" (which he estimated numbered as high as 90% of the asylum population).[18] This early move toward the development of a psychiatric hospital reflected the view that the large asylum was itself a pathogenic space.

In a similar spirit, in 1905 Helen Boyle, an Irish physician who would later become the first female president of the Royal Medico-Psychological Association, launched a small hospital for women suffering from "nervous" illness in Brighton. Boyle explained that the impetus for founding this small therapeutic hospital had come from her years working at Claybury Asylum in East London, where she had encountered large numbers of low-income women suffering from incurable insanity. Boyle hypothesized that most of these women's mental afflictions could have been prevented had they been removed from their slum conditions much earlier and vehemently defended the poor against accusations of hereditary degeneracy. In her view, mental illness was caused by the crowded, run-down neighborhoods that the poor inhabited, which needed to be escaped for treatment to be possible.

Boyle and Maudsley were not alone in their concern for the pathological mental effects of overcrowded and unhygienic environments. Discussions in medical journals surrounding the abolition of asylum certification overwhelmingly linked treatment to the small modern hospital. Certification was seen as an outdated obstacle to early treatment since it rested upon symptoms of mental illness being so florid and obvious that a judge could not fail to miss them. It was therefore limited to fully developed cases of insanity:

> We seem to prefer to allow men to drift into advanced and ofttimes incurable insanity before granting to them proper means for obtaining relief. There is no place for the poor man to go for treatment when he feels that his mind is becoming unhinged, even if he is willing and anxious to do so. Such a patient must wait until his

mind has become so far disordered that a certificate can be signed, which would convince a British jury of his insanity; then, and not till then, is he considered a proper subject for treatment.[19]

The rationale for the construction of updated mental hospitals in the 1930s conflated concerns about the rising incidence of mental illness with critiques of various British social environments. Between the late 1920s and late 1930s, *The Lancet* published a series of discussions of "suburban neurosis," focusing on the negative mental effects of social dislocation resulting from slum clearance and alienating impact of suburban life. In 1938, *The Lancet*'s assistant editor, Stephen Taylor, described the suburb as another kind of slum, a "slum which stunts the mind."[20] Discussions surrounding the construction of therapeutic mental hospitals focused not only on architectural planning details but also touched on the mental effects of urban versus rural locations. During the interwar decades, psychiatrists vastly preferred to see mental hospitals situated in rural settings far from the noise and excitement of towns. Urban critique often ran through descriptions of healthy hospital life.

The 1930 Mental Treatment Act made psychiatric hospitalization voluntary and played an important role in making the intention behind British mental hospitals genuinely therapeutic. Physicians successfully made the case that that the legal authorities who had guarded entry to the asylum did not possess necessary skills to discern the subtle symptoms of a "mild" mental disorder. They were presented as far less capable than afflicted individuals themselves of identifying most cases requiring treatment. With the institution of voluntary admission in 1930, the doors of mental hospitals were opened to people who believed that they suffered from embryonic forms of insanity. By actively seeking out hospitalization, the modern, psychiatrically literate, mental patient not only demonstrated an ability to exercise autonomous therapeutic judgment but also agreed that they required medical protection from the social worlds they inhabited.

The introduction of voluntary admission to mental hospitals was meant to achieve several interrelated treatment objectives. First, it officially recognized the reality of "nervous" illnesses as an incipient stage in the development of insanity. Second, it made treatment available to lower-income sufferers of neurotic disorders who could not afford treatment in a private hospital or clinic. Finally, it sought to transform the asylum into a place of treatment rather than a stigmatized place of confinement. Voluntary admission met a real need. This can be seen in the steady rise in the numbers of voluntary patients admitted over the course of the 1930s and 1940s. Whereas voluntary admission had not been considered possible in the latter half of the nineteenth century because administrators believed that no one would willingly seek out asylum treatment, in 1935 24% of mental hospital admissions were made on a voluntary basis. By 1945 this figure had risen to more than 50%.[21] The passage of the Mental Treatment Act in 1930 was described by physicians in the months and years that followed as "the greatest practical advance which so far has been made,"[22] and as "vital" in extending the psychiatric hospital's "tentacles into the outside world."[23] It ushered in new ways of understanding mental illness, even if therapy largely remained focused on physical, rather than psychological, methods until after WWII.

As further evidence of psychiatrists' growing focus on the social environment, in the late 1930s several mental hospitals across the country experimented with various social therapies. Staff at hospitals experimented with group psychotherapy, group forms of occupational therapy, and even created patient-led "therapeutic social clubs." Explicitly therapeutic environments established continuity between the patient's pre-admission and hospital lives. They were seen as affirming the afflicted individual's social identity beyond the hospital. At Runwell Hospital in the late 1930s—under the medical direction of former kibbutz resident Joshua Bierer—patients engaged in a range of occupations, from gardening to carpentry to participation in "parliamentary" committees assisting with hospital management. The height of mental hospitalization in Britain coincided with decades when the social environment was highlighted as having paramount importance in restoring mental health.

Psychiatric literature emphasizing patients' vulnerability to their social environment grew considerably during the interwar decades. The numbers of cases of "mild" mental illness were rising rapidly and this was interpreted as indicating that mentally afflicted people required greater protection from harmful social influences in the transformed postwar world. This particularly became a concern following the Feversham Committee's comprehensive study of Britain's mental health services showing that, "only 43% of Britons show[ed] no indication of nervous illness."[24] By 1939, support for the creation of more mental hospitals to house the growing patient population was as pervasive in the mainstream news media as it was in professional circles. At the heart of the social and cultural transformations that made voluntary admission desirable was an affirmation of a persistent Victorian ethic of self-help. This was, however, a version of self-help that saw the social environment as playing a central role in the delicate processes of mental adjustment.

The Peckham Experiment: Democratic Community as the Foundation for Health

During the same moment that voluntary hospitalization was being endorsed as necessary to both democratize and elevate mental health nationwide, the founders of the Pioneer Health Centre in South London, Innes Pearse and George Williamson, were promoting democratic social milieus as essential for health. Although they were both pathologists by training, in the 1920s and 1930s Pearse and Williamson had come to view health as about more than contagious infectious illness. To secure health, a thriving community life was key, and they explicitly positioned themselves against the eugenicist focus on breeding restrictions. In their view, reducing health to the narrow logic of inheritance was misguided.

After more than five years of fundraising and planning, on May 3, 1935, Pearse and Williamson saw the Pioneer Health Centre open its doors to the families of the working-class South London district of Peckham. The center had been painstakingly designed to deal with the pervasive yet "invisible" problem of "lack of health" that the prime minister had recently declared affected most British people.[25] The Pioneer Centre was meant to provide an alternative to the disease-focused orientation of Britain's hospitals. Its medical directors approached health as resulting from organisms' state of being harmoniously adjusted to their environment. Poor health was reasoned to result from Britain's overpopulated urban neighborhoods, which Pearse described as "antisocial and inhuman."[26] The Pioneer Health Centre was created to be a place where health—in its most expansive possible sense—would flourish.

Following its opening in 1935, the center's premises received high praise in a range of popular and professional publications. *The Observer* likened it to a "great ship of health ... moored peacefully in its field among the squat dark houses crowded around it," and "a place that breathes the clean health it hopes to induce in its members."[27] With its large windows and its open plan, every aspect of the center's design was meant to function as an antidote to the "socially disintegrated" conditions of 1930s urban industrial Britain, especially prominent in low-income neighborhoods.[28] Pearse argued that since "the first causes of sickness and social disorder had been found in the arid soil of social life," the center provided an ideal space for a "living society" to develop.[29]

The Pioneer Health Centre's medical directors allowed all member families—who joined as a "membership unit"—total freedom in their use of the building, which featured an Olympic-size swimming pool, a gymnasium, a dance hall, a cafeteria, several spacious lounge areas, and a range of "adaptable spaces" that could support a variety of events, including public lectures, theater performances, and boxing matches—between 2pm and 10:30pm every day. In exchange for a small weekly fee, each family was given regular health "overhauls" and full access to the center's many activities. The building's open plan and glass walls, which afforded complete visibility everywhere except the medical examination areas and changing rooms, were meant to both encourage sociability and allow medical staff to observe everything that went on.

The center's ethos was overtly anti-authoritarian. Williamson and Pearse saw all forms of authority, regulation, and instruction as running counter to the goal of healthy vitality:

> Civilization hitherto has looked for the orientation of society through an imposed "system" derived from some extrinsic authority ... The biologist conceives an order emanating from the organism living in poise with its environment. Our necessity, therefore, is to secure the free flow of forces in the environment so that the order inherent in the material we are studying may emerge. Our interest is in that balance of forces which sustains naturally and spontaneously the forms of life we are studying.[30]

As a result, some of the center's visitors were put off by its absence of rules and apparent chaos. When Williamson's sister Edith Williamson, a senior medical officer,

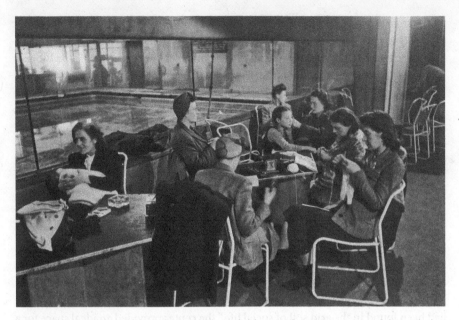

Figure 1.1. Parents could easily watch their children in the swimming pool through the glass walls of the Pioneer Health Centre cafeteria.
Source: Picture Post/Getty images. Photo credit: Kurt Hutton/Stringer.

first visited four months after the center's opening, she was shocked at its lack of direction. She expressed her "intense disappointment" to her brother:

> It is a fine building—a grand idea—but the place seems lost, rudderless, no soul, no direction ... I hated to see children of four asleep in their mothers' arms at 10pm while mother has a beer. True, it is better than being outside a pub; but it is bad. I dislike the crying babies trying to sleep in the cafeteria amidst the noise, and in prams too short for them; the older children flying round without aim or object.[31]

She pleaded with Williamson to hire additional staff to instruct the center's working-class members on how to use the building's facilities more responsibly. Williamson remained resolute in response, insisting that his sister had not correctly interpreted what she had seen. What appeared to be chaos, he explained, was an early stage of a new social organism's development: "it looks ugly—so do all embryos."[32] Any imposition of rules on the center's growing membership, he maintained, would extinguish the sense of personal responsibility that any healthy society both nurtured and needed:

> Our discoveries ... point to Responsibility as the biological characteristic of organism. Authority and responsibility are mutually antipathetic: and, indeed, as they grow strong and adult, they are antagonistic. I am sorry biology is like

that ... There is both discipline and system in Authority—oh yes! But there is NO order. I don't want machine-made men, or barracks-made men; I am looking for world-made men; natural men.[33]

Williamson and Pearse approached the center as the world's first biological "study in the *living* structure of society," which they believed would furnish crucial findings about the creation of healthy populations.[34] Much more than a local health center, the Peckham Experiment—as it came to be known—was conceived as a field station for observing "natural" unimpeded behavior in an open and flexible social environment, as opposed to an "artificial" environment like densely populated South London, which the center's directors believed inhibited authentic action. What Williamson's sister had seen as working-class disorder, the center's directors instead interpreted as true social life, which developed spontaneously out of interactions between the group's unique members.

Pearse and Williamson's ambitious research agenda had resulted from a trial-and-error process of discovery. Between 1926 and 1929, they had operated a small health center on Peckham's bustling Queen's Road. When they first began their work in 1926, the health center idea was still very new. It was not until 1936 that a new public health act would empower local councils to provide medical services for their lower-income residents.[35] By 1938, only a few health centers had opened in London—the most well-known was in the Labour district of Finsbury and built for the "common working man." All apart from Peckham focused exclusively on providing a comprehensive range of outpatient medical services, including physical therapy and massage, dental services, and gynecological exams.

The Pioneer Centre's unique focus on disease prevention initially drew its inspiration from Marie Stopes's birth control clinics that had recently begun making contraceptive devices available to working-class communities to curb family size and promote infant and maternal health. Additionally, Pearse and Williamson's years of experience in pathology research at the Royal Free Hospital in North London and interest in epidemiology informed their preoccupation with the contagiousness of ill-health. Pearse later noted that she and Williamson became more interested in the proportion of a population that showed resistance to an infection than in studying the transmission of infection itself. They speculated that, disease "susceptibility ... was not 'normal'; it was an acquired characteristic."[36]

Their initial objective in introducing a local health center was to provide regular compulsory check-ups for Peckham residents and treatment of all symptoms, however minor.[37] Varicose veins, intestinal disorders, and skin irregularities were frequently mentioned problems. Regular "overhauls" revealed that once problems had been treated, they often recurred and, additionally, new conditions cropped up. During the first year, results continually showed that not more than "10% of persons of all ages were without discoverable pathological conditions ... [and] some 60% ... had one or more disorders of which they were unaware, or oblivious."[38] They saw this as evidence for working-class urban Peckham's pathological influence, particularly resulting from its densely populated streets and cramped housing.[39] They therefore made the health center available to members as an informal meeting place every afternoon and evening of the week. They purchased sewing machines for women to use and provided a nursery to offer mothers breaks from childcare. Within a few months, the health center had become a social hub for Peckham residents while offering its medical directors "ample opportunity ... of making observations."[40]

As Pearse and Williamson became increasingly focused on cultivating health, the center's board of executives and consultants expanded. Their interest in the benefits of environmental reform toward positive evolutionary change was shared by many biologists and physicians in the 1920s and 30s, and the Peckham Experiment attracted the financial and intellectual support of several contemporary luminaries, including Chief Medical Officer of Health Sir Frederick Menzies, Royal Society president and Nobel Prize winner Frederick Gowland Hopkins, Secretary of the Royal Zoological Society Julian Huxley, and pioneering social psychologist Wilfred Trotter. Although it served only a small urban locality, the center's findings were seen as offering insight into methods for improving the human species. By 1929, their growing body of patrons made it possible to plan the construction of a larger center that would better accommodate their developing vision of a space that would, "influenc[e] the social life of our members" and "widen their environment."[41]

The purpose-built premises, ready for use in May 1935, were a stunning modernist achievement. Walter Gropius described the Peckham Experiment as "an oasis of glass in a desert of brick."[42] *The Times* stated that it was "destined architecturally to become a local landmark."[43] *The Edinburgh Evening News* remarked that nowhere had they seen "the new more graphically and beautifully expressed than at the Pioneer Health Centre at Peckham."[44] On the cutting-edge of modern functionalist design, the center's architect Sir Owen Williams—an engineer by training—had developed a reputation for having his buildings' form perfectly satisfy their function. Peckham's resemblance to Williams' multi-story factories was unmistakable, inspiring journalist John Comerford to muse that the new Pioneer Health Centre's functionalist exterior likely caused passersby to mistake the building "for some modern, enlightened factory."[45]

While the center's exterior had distinct visual appeal, Pearse and Williamson were most pleased with its internal layout, designed as it was to "invite new interests and social contacts at every turn of its ample, confluent open spaces."[46] At the building's center was a large community pool, which was ringed by a gymnasium, a cafeteria, a lecture theater, a children's play area, and several lounges. The simple open design of every room was meant to reflect the center's democratic ethos:

> No place was designed for any one purpose or reserved for any one group. The theatre and the gymnasium were used also for dancing, boxing, Christmas and wedding parties. Even the nursery school could in the evening become the meeting place of the whist club, a parents' school committee, or a classical music or

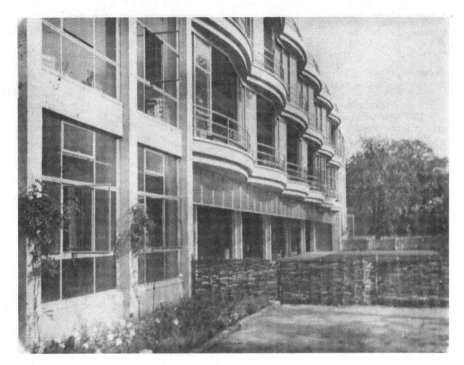

Figure 1.2. View of the Pioneer Health Centre's exterior.
Source: Southwark Council Archives; reproduced by permission.

debating group. The use of the floor-space at any one time was determined by the wishes of members and not by "the authorities."[47]

A contributor to *The Architectural Review* admired how perfectly Peckham's design manifested its social vision: "by means of open planning ... the function of each part is quite clearly subsidiary to the function of the whole ... Freedom in fact is the salient characteristic of the plan."[48]

Visibility and freedom of movement were seen as the most important precursors to a thriving social life. They made the center a "focus of infection" as the founders believed that "there is nothing so infectious as the sight of some one absorbed in some activity."[49] For example, Pearse and Williamson would note that as Mrs. Smith glanced in the direction of the swimming pool and saw Mrs. Chapman learning to swim, she became more inclined to also try out the pool herself. They thought that it was especially important for children that all activities were "carried on in full view of all the members" as this fostered the "habit of taking advantage of opportunity, of launching out whenever possible."[50] The building's open plan allowed all health center members, regardless of age, to move about freely "infecting the less vigorous with their health."[51]

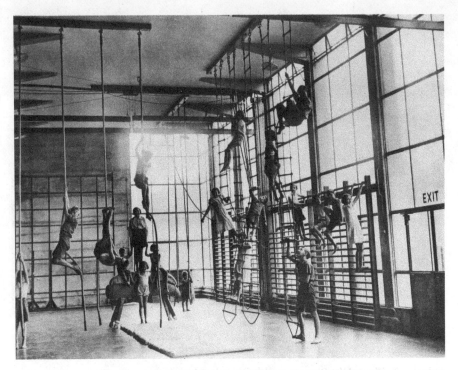

Figure 1.3. Children exercising in the Pioneer Health Centre's gymnasium.
Source: Hulton Archive/Getty images. Photo credit: Fred Ramage/Stringer.

The view that the environment of the hospital or health center could be harnessed for therapeutic ends was not new in the twentieth century. Milieu and occupational therapies had been developed at psychiatric hospitals in Britain, Germany, and the United States in the early decades of the nineteenth century. Following the development of moral treatment at the York Retreat at the end of the eighteenth century, the idea that treating patients humanely, providing them with daily occupations, and having the nursing staff directly engage with them, was widely accepted as a sound approach to treatment.

At Peckham as at many British psychiatric hospitals during the interwar decades, however, environment became even more consequential. For Pearse and Williamson, human activity only reached its "infectious" potential within the context of group interactions. This was a view of life that was fundamentally opposed to Malthus's and Darwin's depictions of the social world as dominated by endless competition for scarce resources. A commitment to dynamic equilibrium rather than competitive struggle drove mid-twentieth-century health experiments at Peckham and beyond. In reframing health and illness as outcomes of the relationship between individuals and their social environment, Pearse and Williamson presented a naturalized, community-centered alternative to the socially "arid" and alienating conditions of urban-industrial, twentieth-century modernity.

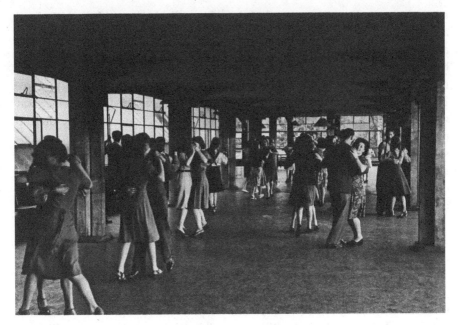

Figure 1.4. A dance class in one of the Pioneer Health Centre's spacious common areas.
Source: Picture Post/Getty images. Photo credit: Kurt Hutton/Stringer.

"Everything We Do Here Is Treatment": The World's First Therapeutic Community

When war broke out in 1939, the Pioneer Health Centre closed its doors and the building was used as a munitions factory.[52] However, experiments with the health-giving impact of democratic environments continued elsewhere during the war. This work was not, however, undertaken under the banner of social biology but within the emerging field of social psychiatry. WWII became a moment of opportunity for developing the wide-ranging applications of social psychological testing and group psychiatric treatment. Psychiatrists made recognized contributions in directing the course of military action. Not only were they involved with officer selection and soldier training at the new battle schools—which became especially important in 1942 when their orientation changed to accommodate a surge in the army's size—but they also produced methods for interrogating prisoners of war and treated thousands of soldiers suffering from neurotic and psychosomatic disorders.[53] They worked in hospitals and in the field, developing new findings and more expedient forms of group-based psychiatric therapy.

Social psychiatry's most emblematic achievement during the war was the creation of the world's first "therapeutic community" at Hollymoor Hospital, Northfield. The hospital, a large Victorian institution on the outskirts of Birmingham where soldiers suffering from neuroses were sent beginning in April 1942, did not initially experience much success in returning men to the front.[54] It was divided into a Medical Ward and a rehabilitative Training Ward, and yet most patients were ultimately discharged from active duty. Given this desperate situation, Majors Wilfred Bion and John Rickman, both psychoanalysts affiliated with the British Psychoanalytical Society, were given responsibility for reforming the Training Ward during the winter of 1942–1943. Bion had achieved positive recognition for his "Leaderless Group test," which was widely used by the War Office Selection Boards (WOSBs) in the months leading up to his posting at Northfield. The test investigated "the quality of the man's relationship with his fellows" by having soldiers to work together to complete a task—for example, building a bridge—while WOSB personnel observed. Men were evaluated on how well they formed relationships with the other team members rather than task completion.

Bion approached the Training Ward primarily as a commanding officer rather than a therapist. He sought to cultivate group morale by treating neurotic disorder as the patients' "common enemy," arguing that "The establishment of morale is of course hardly a prerequisite of treatment; it is treatment." Although Bion and Rickman's approach to group dynamics was modeled on the military unit, patients' freedom of movement was integral to their psychiatric experiment. Using the Training Wing as an opportune space for promoting responsibility in recovering patients, Bion reported that he "found it helpful to visualize the projected organization of the training wing as if it were a framework enclosed within transparent walls":[55]

> Into this space the patient would be admitted at one point, and the activities within that space would be so organized that he could move freely in any direction according to the resultant of his conflicting impulses. His movements, as far as possible, were not to be distorted by outside interference. As a result his behaviour could be trusted to give a fair indication of his effective will and aims, as opposed to the aims he himself proclaimed or the psychiatrist wished him to have.[56]

To encourage unimpeded movement, Bion abolished medical direction on the ward. His "leaderless group" treatment left residents to organize and make collective decisions for the ward without any outside medical guidance. The only input given happened during daily morning parades when the men were assessed and given the opportunity to ask questions. Since Bion's "leaderless group" test was widely used by the WOSBs, his radically democratic approach to treatment at Northfield would not have been unfamiliar to soldiers who spent time on the Training Ward.

Like the Peckham Experiment in its first months, the Northfield Experiment initially fell into disarray. The ward was reportedly "filthy, beds were not made for days, absence without leave and drunkenness increased and the whole hospital staff was alarmed and angry."[57] In Bion's defense, Psychiatrist Lieutenant-Colonel Tom F. Main (who would later claim to have coined the term "therapeutic community") maintained that the disorder began to resolve itself after several weeks as patients slowly grew responsible for themselves and their ward comrades and now formed their own discussion groups and rotas and disciplinary systems. Cleanliness and order, no longer imposed from above, grew inside the ward group.[58]

Despite noticeable improvement in rehabilitating patients, Bion's "leaderless community" experiment was judged unprofessional by his commanding officer, who believed it showed severe lack of regard for hospital staff. The Northfield Experiment was ended in its sixth week, and Bion was abruptly dismissed from the hospital.

Although the "First Northfield Experiment" was declared a failure, a second experiment was initiated the following year. Psychoanalyst Sigmund Henry Foulkes, a key founder of group therapy, was given direction over Northfield's Medical Ward and Major Harold Bridger was put in charge of the Training Ward. Although he lacked a psychiatric background, Bridger was chosen to guide soldiers' rehabilitation because of his extensive experience with psychological testing in the WOSBs. In preparation for his post, he read Innes Pearse's account of the Pioneer Health Centre's work, *The Peckham Experiment: A Study in The Living Structure of Society*. Bridger saw Pearse's book as describing "an unintentional therapeutic community," later remarking that he had been struck by how the center's community had emerged organically out of its member-families' specific needs.[59] This inspired Bridger to focus on creating something similar at Northfield, a "hospital-as-a-whole in the here-and-now."[60]

Inspired by the Pioneer Health Centre's deliberate preference for open space in creating a spontaneous community made up of responsible individuals, Bridger began his work at Northfield by introducing a large open area in the center of the hospital. Given the lack of unused space in a military hospital, he needed to be creative and accomplished this by moving hospital beds more closely together. He then named the open space the "Hospital Club."[61] Bridger, who trained as a psychoanalyst after the war, would later describe the "Hospital Club" as an extension of "the patient's own personality and social gaps within his 'life space.'"[62] He recalled, "everybody used to come along to me, and say, 'when is the club going to start?' And I said, 'when you start it.'"[63] Within a few weeks, patients organized a meeting where they criticized Bridger for wasting precious hospital space in wartime. Elated at this organized collective reaction, he responded that since the "Hospital Club" belonged to them, there was no reason why it could not be used to contribute to the war effort.[64]

Using the club space, rehabilitating patients created several "hobby groups," including a newspaper group, a chess group, a drama group, a carpentry group, a catering group, and a painting group.[65] Within eight months of Bridger's appointment, the meaning of the term "occupational therapy"—which had typically described patients being kept occupied in mundane repetitive work tasks—had been transformed. At Northfield, patient-led initiatives like the hospital newspaper became opportunities for psychiatrists to investigate the psychological dynamics of groups and their impact on individuals, particularly how both shared responsibility and resulting interpersonal tensions affected patients' rehabilitative progress.[66]

While Northfield's staff focused on assessing the therapeutic impact of group therapy and patient-led hobby groups, they also wanted to understand how the psychological dynamics of the entire hospital community influenced not only rehabilitative progress but also staff's mental health. As they saw it, conventional psychiatric hospitals were typically unhelpfully divided into dichotomous groups of "healthy" and "sick." In their view, this "us versus them" social structure dehumanized patients and interfered with treatment. Northfield staff preserved military and professional distinctions, but they sought to make the hospital community more egalitarian by challenging the view that patients were wholly "sick" and staff entirely "healthy." As Tom Main explained:

> This attempt to create an atmosphere of respect for *all* and the examination of *all* difficulties [was] ... a long way from the medical model, whereby disease is skillfully treated in anonymized people under blanket medical compassion and served by a clinically aloof and separate administration.

Everyone at the hospital was seen as existing on a spectrum of mental well-being. Their exact place on this spectrum was affected by the presence of interpersonal tensions at the hospital, not only in staff-patient relations but also in interstaff relationships.

Northfield was not an idiosyncratic exception during the war. Medical staff at the Effort Syndrome Unit at Mill Hill Hospital in north London, under the direction of psychiatrist and therapeutic community pioneer Maxwell Jones, also experimented with social therapies.[67] "Effort syndrome" was a psychosomatic heart condition that was diagnosed frequently enough during WWII to receive its own specialized treatment unit.[68] The use of social therapy techniques at Mill Hill grew out of the reportedly successful use of hospital-wide meetings to provide patients with medical information about their condition and allay anxiety about treatment. These lecture-style meetings quickly turned into highly participatory discussions that inadvertently helped democratize patient-staff relations.[69] As patients became more knowledgeable about their condition, "it soon became evident ... that the discussion group was more than an educational meeting; it was affecting the whole social structure of the ward."[70] Seeing quick improvements in patients' health, Jones introduced additional group therapy techniques, including psychodrama and group occupational therapy. In his view, the Mill Hill wartime experiment showed that democratizing social practices performed a crucial function in restoring mental health.

By the end of the war, a nationwide network of social rehabilitation communities had been organized for Britain's more than thirty thousand repatriating prisoners of war. Mill Hill was chosen as one of the sites for this civil resettlement project. Although the first Civil Resettlement Units (CRUs) were not opened until April 1945, they were several years in the making.[71] As early as autumn 1941, psychiatrists called attention to returning POWs as a major social problem, who by then already numbered close to 100,000.[72] In 1942, repatriated medical officers further confirmed that this was an issue requiring urgent psychiatric intervention. Men returning from Stalag and Oflag showed high rates of sickness, especially psychosomatic disorders. Even many returning soldiers with previously outstanding military records were now embroiled in serious disciplinary issues.

During the same year, army psychiatrists began meeting with groups of returning POWs who either showed symptoms of psychological distress or were determined to be disciplinary problems. Despite having no predisposition to mental illness, the men were judged to require psychiatric treatment because their personalities, "previous level of adjustment and military effectiveness," had not returned to what they had been prior to the war:

> Even when men had been back for 18 months or even longer, serious and persistent difficulties were reported in something like one-third of the men. Such findings pointed strongly to the need for special therapeutic measures.[73]

This was viewed as nothing less than a psychiatric crisis. Reports concerning POWs repatriated after WWI supported psychiatrists' findings, as did those supplied by WWI veterans' wives and family members. Many former soldiers had suffered from psychiatric and psychosomatic afflictions for several years while readjusting to civilian life. In 1943, Wilfred Bion highlighted the psychosocial aspects of the problem, based on his work advising returning officers on finding employment. However, it was not until April 1945 that a Civil Resettlement Planning Headquarters was created to support POWs who were returning to civilian life. Within six months, twenty CRUs were under its direction.

The CRUs primary focus had originally been to improve repatriating POWs' employability by helping create relationships with the Ministry of Labour and local labor exchanges. Residents met regularly with vocational officers who were instructed not to give the appearance of having any psychiatric intent to avoid making returning soldiers feel "sick" or "abnormal." However, in the first few weeks, residents showed more interest in discussing "more intimate matters" than employment issues with doctors and social workers. In addition, the residents showed so many symptoms of emotional and psychosomatic disorder that the CRUs' psychiatrist, Lieutenant-Colonel A.T.M. (Tommy) Wilson (Bridger and Foulkes' colleague at Northfield), introduced therapeutic community methods to guide "resocialization" to civilian life.[74] Group psychotherapy was also incorporated into residents' daily schedules to treat symptoms of anxiety, depression, and psychosomatic complaints. These sessions made it clear that "resocialization" was an overwhelmingly psychological problem:

> Nothing brings out the real difficulties which repatriates face in their resettlement so well as the material they offer in group discussion. No matter what clinical symptom brings a repatriate for consultation—nervousness, insomnia, or inability to mix with people—such symptoms are but the manifest signs of basic psychological difficulties related to "resocialisation." It is instructive to hear a man, who

during the individual interview had complained of irritability or depression, express in the group a most vehement anger and mistrust of authority, and a cynicism and bitterness about life as he has found it upon his return ... He feels that the world has let him down.[75]

Wilson approved of the resettlement units' growing psychiatric focus, explaining that "what at first sight appear to be vocational problems ... only too often prove to be displaced or converted emotional problems."[76] In his view, the CRU was more than a vessel for social therapies; it was itself "a particular technique of social therapy" that made the repatriating former soldier's transition to civilian life possible.[77]

According to Wilson, the CRUs' growing psychological focus was led by residents rather than staff.[78] Like the therapeutic communities developed at Northfield and Mill Hill, the CRUs sought, above all, to enable residents to rediscover their sense of autonomy:

> The programme is planned to encourage initiative, and spontaneous choice is permitted, as far as possible, from the beginning of a man's stay ... there is already evidence from the work of Bion and Rickman (1943) at Northfield that passive non-cooperation with one's community is a painful start from which we emerge with relief, given adequate opportunity.[79]

Rather than the CRUs' administrative and medical staff handing down a set of behavioral rules, they instead indicated that irresponsible behavior would bring the unit to an end. In response, residents performed their own surveillance and did not tolerate either excessive alcohol use or social apathy. Within a few weeks, morale improved, and incidents of drunkenness were significantly scaled back.

The therapeutic community represented a merging of psychiatry with politics from its earliest beginnings during the war. Its psychiatric founders saw it as opposed to authoritarian repression and aggression on the one hand and excessive communalism, social conformity, and state control on the other. Even after the war had ended, the therapeutic community continued to be described by mental health practitioners and observers alike as supporting an anti-authoritarian commitment to democracy. In 1960, sociologist Robert Rapoport—who observed dozens of "therapeutic communities"—stated that despite variations in how they achieved their goals, they were each meant to be, "a place ... [where] everyone [was] expected to make some contribution towards the shared goals of creating a social organization that will have healing properties."[80] Less than a decade after D.W. Winnicott warned that asylum psychiatry was a "localized dictatorship" threatening to unravel Britain's commitment to democracy, Russell Barton compared the neurosis-inducing impact of psychiatric "institutionalization" with the apathetic conformity that marked life under totalitarian rule.[81] During WWII and the decades that followed, psychiatrists merged therapy with an affirmation of democracy's psychological value. Politics were explicitly brought into discussions of mental illness and health.

Nazi Psychology and the Politics of Family Life

Access to German prisoners of war in English camps provided new opportunities for social psychological research into the relationship between political culture and personality development. Early childhood experiences centered on the family played a key role in establishing connections between individual minds and socio-political life. The psychiatrists and social scientists most involved in studying German prisoners of war fused social psychology with a psychoanalytic focus on childhood experiences and relationships. In doing so, they strengthened connections made during the interwar decades between political culture and family life that would endure in post-WWII British mental health initiatives.

In 1947, a sensational study of Rudolf Hess, the Nazi Party's former deputy Führer, by several British and American psychiatrists argued that German family life produced psychiatric illness. *The Case of Rudolf Hess: A Problem in Diagnosis and Forensic Psychiatry* was the product of six years of intensive investigation and the most widely read psychiatric study of a German POW that had ever been produced. Hess had come under psychiatric investigation in 1941, following his crash landing in rural Scotland, ostensibly (according to his telling) on a secret solo mission to negotiate peace with Britain. After parachuting from his airplane into a Scottish village, he was promptly arrested, nursed to health, and placed under psychiatric observation and treatment for psychotic symptoms, including hallucination, delusions of persecution, and amnesia. He attempted suicide twice while under observation, leading to further concern about his mental stability.

The study highlighted Hess's early family relationships. Henry Dicks, Hess's primary psychiatrist, drew particular attention to Hess's distant and unemotional father, setting in motion a disastrous pattern in his interpersonal life. Ever since adolescence, he had "sought out father-surrogates to 'influence' him," ending in full-fledged (albeit temporary) devotion to Adolf Hitler.[82] Although Hess's particular psychopathology and family background were treated as unique to him, Dicks noted their greater prevalence in Nazi Germany in comparison to Britain, stating that "much of his symptomatology, so extremely queer to a British milieu, might be found to differ not very greatly from the norm of Nazi and possibly even German modes of thinking and dealing with reality."[83] Dicks pointed out that Hess's experience of growing up with an emotionally distant, yet domineering, father was not entirely out of sync with German cultural norms; the dominant and unemotional disciplinarian father was a cultural ideal. He thus linked the political values associated with Nazism with the values that were embodied in the excessively patriarchal German family and that German children absorbed as fundamental facts about the world at an early age. Here, we see the idea of "the *Volk*" turned on its head. Countering the Nazi biological view of the nation, Dicks—along with the rest of Hess's team of psychiatrists—gestured toward a neurotic collective German psyche.

Dicks, in collaboration with Edward Shils, followed a similar line of inquiry in a social psychological study of German POWs commissioned by MI19 between 1942 and 1945. Unlike Rudolf Hess, the POWs they interviewed—including fervent Nazi supporters—did not present clear signs of mental illness: "no significant proportion of fanatical Nazis was found to be suffering from gross mental disability in the clinical sense ... It appeared that we were dealing with a group problem, not with individual disease."[84] As a result, Dicks reasoned that new "finer-meshed" techniques of group psychological investigation needed to be applied over the course of the study. To this end, the study divided subjects into groups according to their level of commitment to Nazi ideology and examined the men's relationships with their parents while growing up. Unlike Caroline Playne's earlier study of the German psyche in the 1920s, Dicks and Shils's investigation barely considered historical events surrounding the rise of contemporary German culture.[85] It instead focused on such factors as the subjects' socio-economic backgrounds, their parents' marital status and participation in childrearing, and subjects' identification with their mothers, their fathers, the state, and their romantic partners. Also included in each evaluation was an assessment of signs of sadism, homosexuality, narcissism, anxiety, hypochondria, projection, and feelings of inferiority.[86]

In common with the Hess study, Dicks and Shils found that Nazi valorization of aggressive masculinity coincided with a devaluation of stereotypical feminine traits, including all traces of emotional tenderness in boys' relationships with their mothers. The excessive influence of fathers in families was identified as playing an important part in producing "aggressive," "sadistic," and "inhuman" attitudes, as well as "destructive impulses."[87] Excerpts from interviews with POWs illustrated the ambivalence that the men often felt toward their mothers, not infrequently discussed as contributing to their "underlying femininity" and "pliability and softness":[88]

> PSW: I was my mother's all. But of course it is necessary for Father to have the upper hand, to rescue one from Mother's apron-strings.
> INTERVIEWER: Here in England we send boys to boarding schools for this purpose.
> PSW: That is a great mistake; then a father can't have his boy to shape him to his own liking. If I had a son I would devote myself entirely to his upbringing. With a daughter I could not do that ... of course it would be nice for me if she were very beautiful.
> INTERVIEWER: What made you decide to become an officer?
> PSW: Flying—the fun of it. And, of course, the beauty of educating very young men—to mold their training and their development.
> INTERVIEWER: And what would you have done if you hadn't joined the service?
> PSW: Well, I really like art; interior decorating, etc. My mother is very artistic.[89]

Further elucidating the pathological outcome of this parental ambivalence, Dicks indicated that this young soldier was aggressive to the point of sadism: he was "known to have greatly enjoyed machine-gunning what looked like a garden fête at Eastbourne" and openly "approved of the atrocities against the Czechs and Poles."[90]

In the analysis of his interviews, Dicks drew numerous links between Nazi ideology and the values associated with German private life. Nazi propaganda claiming that Germans required a powerful army because they were "weak and exposed" to surrounding "enemies who envy our greatness" was identified as springing from German sons' relationship to their all-powerful fathers:

> The individual German has felt so small and helpless in this personal relation that he tends to project the situation into his national fate. This is the famous "encirclement fear" which rests largely though not entirely on the impotence feeling implicit first of all in their family life.[91]

Dicks especially highlighted a German fear of outsiders, arguing that the scapegoating of Jewish people stemmed from German peculiarities surrounding the rearing of boys. In Dicks's view, the strong presence of the father, at the expense of respect for the tenderness of a mother's love, caused deep frustrations at the Oedipal level of children's development. He thus vehemently opposed the denigration of women anywhere, maintaining that women were the bearers of peace and stable democracy.

Dicks diagnosed German wartime patriotism as insecure and "fair-weathered" since it was dependent on a widely shared perception of national threat. He contrasted this negatively with Britain's more democratic culture, which he argued was cultivated through family relationships that positively valued tender emotion, especially the loving relationship between mother and child. Dicks pointed out how this basic difference in the quality of British and German patriotism was even apparent to the most perceptive Germans. To demonstrate this, he quoted one POW lamenting that, "The English have a basic unity and love of country, so they can curse as much as they like on the surface. We Germans have the hostility and divisions deep down, so we have to make a parade of our unity and patriotism and cannot tolerate differences of opinion."[92]

This social psychological study of Nazi character was only one of many tasks that the British government had given Dicks responsibility for during and shortly after the war. Employed by MI19, following its creation as a subsection of MI9 in December 1940, Dicks provided psychological support for the Combined Services Detailed Interrogation Centers (CSDICs). Among his many duties at the CSDICs, Dicks advised on interrogation methods, which he held should sometimes involve force, but never extreme measures like torture. He devised different interrogation methods according to German character-types, claiming that the more taciturn, for example, responded best to a calm and humane approach, whereas the rank-and-file Nazi often required the use of force. Believing that Nazis were "characterized by an unconscious over-emphasis of acceptance of paternal authority" and "over-valuation of masculinity," Dicks argued that Nazi prisoners often responded best to interrogation styles that mimicked the behavior of the typical German father figure.[93]

At the end of the war, Dicks was charged with planning, staffing, and helping "to operate a technical unit for the psychological screening of German key personnel and for socio-psychological survey of attitudes, morale, etc., of occupied Germany (British Zone)."[94] Despite this, Dicks's suggestions had little impact on official decisions for ensuring successful denazification. His two main recommendations were focused on elevating women's status in German society and providing support for German churches, both of which he had found correlated negatively with Nazi support. His appeals to the dangers associated with the German cultural denigration of women were met with only a lukewarm response. Members of the War Cabinet criticized Dicks's conclusions as "not terribly convincing," arguing that other male-dominated societies did not show the same level of aggression and delusions of national grandeur. They also brought up an earlier historical example of Elizabethan England, as this was often presumed to have been a society that highly valued women, yet it had not shown any commitment to international peace.[95]

Dicks ultimately judged his wartime work to be largely unsuccessful since it had failed to make much impact on official policy. As he put it, his success was "greater in the academic than the PsW field":

> Persons trained in the relevant disciplines have appreciated my work as a piece of new technique in the study of groups. It had some effect, especially where my personal tuition supplemented paper, as in the training of some interrogation teams. At higher staff levels it aroused interest, but the better entrenched disciplines, as represented by historical or economics scholars, etc., who often filled high places in advisory roles, in many instances dismissed it and probably persuaded policy-makers that they know better. In general, considerable resistance of a nature familiar to psychoanalysts was encountered here as in other fields of effort by depth psychologists in the Forces.[96]

He further lamented that the relatively small number of prisoners sent to England had made it difficult to form conclusive recommendations that might extend beyond the interrogation center. And, moreover, the evidence that he consistently provided for the weakness of German morale had failed to end the war in a timely fashion.

Despite Dicks's own negative evaluation, it should be noted that the War Office took his contributions seriously, even if his conclusions were seen as lacking in sufficient evidence for widespread postwar application. Further, he underestimated the importance of the favorable reception of his work in the creation of British-government-sponsored mental health services after the war. Dicks's emphasis on the family's impact on cultural values was very positively received at the Tavistock Clinic and Institute of Human Relations, where he would continue to develop his psychoanalytic group psychology and its therapeutic applications after the war. As will be discussed in much greater depth in chapter 4, this institutional affiliation and endorsement would play a role in the rapid rise of state provided marriage reconciliation services in the postwar decades.

Conclusion: A Society Rooted in Emotion

During WWII, British psychiatry underwent a transformation that many participants and onlookers alike described as its third, and final, revolution.[97] A new generation of psychiatrists focused on diverse social environments as variously promoting mental health and introducing mental illness in individuals. They also gestured, more broadly, toward a relational paradigm for understanding individual psychological development that was profoundly determined by childhood relationships. Social psychiatrists were confident that this "revolution" in psychiatry had implications extending beyond the practical treatment of mental illness. They saw themselves as uncovering the hidden psychological dynamics governing interpersonal relationships, including their far-reaching impact on wider national (even global) society, and thus on the verge of discoveries that could help introduce vast social and political improvements. Developing methods for both preventing and healing—ultimately eradicating—the psychological underpinnings of authoritarian cultures appeared to be the most promising means for securing liberal democratic values and for eliminating both individual and group "sickness" arising from pathological anti-democratic social milieus. Connecting close personal relationships—including those developed in military units, soldiers' hospital wards, and soldiers' childhood families—to the creation of democratic values, wartime social psychiatrists' work was imbued with profound political consequence.

Whether these wartime social psychiatric developments introduced a "revolution" in British psychiatry is certainly debatable, particularly given the resurgence of biological explanations for mental illness and the psychiatric priority increasingly given to psychopharmacology in the 1960s. However, we need to beware of presuming that a major transformation's success lies only in its lasting endurance and instead consider the contemporary impact and significance of social psychiatry's ascendance during and after WWII. Government recognition of social psychiatrists' wartime successes in treating psychoneurotic illness helped introduce new opportunities for psychiatrists to have their social psychiatric research and new psychosocial therapies funded by Britain's new welfare state and, in the case of treatment, made available to British citizens free of charge.

WWII and its immediate aftermath provided a moment of possibility for rethinking the human costs and benefits of competing forms of socio-political organization. Although Henry Dicks lamented his failure to produce high-level political change at the end of the war due to what he saw as a "lack of respect for psychology" among the War Cabinet, I argue that he was successful in helping introduce an emotionalized view of both authoritarian and democratic societies that linked intimate family relationship dynamics to broader collective values and wellbeing. His success (along with that of other wartime social psychiatrists) can be seen in the wide range of social psychiatric programs introduced in Britain after the war that targeted family relationships to both promote mental health *and* cultivate responsible democratic citizens—including marriage therapy services, an expanded nationwide network of child guidance clinics, in-patient "mother-baby units" in hospitals, and family-based psychiatric therapies. The chapters that follow offer a close look at the government-supported post-WWII mental health initiatives that targeted emotionally "deprived" children, neglectful mothers, and unstable marriages.

As this chapter has shown in its attention to the Pioneer Health Centre in the 1930s, the view that "health" was best cultivated in democratic communities was not entirely new in the 1940s. Near the end of WWII, a contributor to *The Lancet* noted that the understanding of health-supporting, community-based interwar comprehensive health centers like the Pioneer Health Centre offered a visionary example of a dynamic society and a "higher standard of democratic citizenship" when it was most necessary:[98]

> in the midst of social disintegration here there is beginning to appear a nucleus of Society the structure of which is neither "planned" nor "reconstructed" but living ... it seems clear that the British Home Front will not be disbanded without leaving some tangible object of the comradeship and community spirit which has grown up in these changing years.[99]

According to this view, the Pioneer Health Centre had shown that a thriving "healthy" society could not be based in "artificial" planning, a frequent criticism of the post-WWII New Town projects. *The Lancet* contributor saw the Pioneer Health Centre as perfectly exemplifying the ideally organic democratic society of the post-WWII future.

Unlike the "social health" model of democratic community participation developed at the Pioneer Health Centre before the war, however, wartime social psychiatrists' expectations of both mental health *and* good democratic citizenship were informed by a psychologized view of individual human uniqueness and independence balanced against social belonging and interdependence.[100] This psychological view of mentally healthy citizenship would continue to be expressed in social psychiatrists' post-WWII approach to their patients' progressing mental and emotional health. Post-WWII psychiatric initiatives aimed at healing various kinds of family dysfunctions gauged patients' therapeutic success significantly in accordance with their capacity to create and sustain stable and harmonious relationships with family members.

Social psychiatrists' psychosocial view of citizenship had much in common with that of two prominent British mid-twentieth-century welfare state theorists: Richard Titmuss and William Beveridge. Both of these social policy researchers also understood the truly democratic citizen to be a relational being and identified family relationships as playing an important role in nurturing this. They imagined the post-WWII citizen's commitment to responsible democratic citizenship as ideally cultivated within the presumably loving milieu of a male breadwinning, female homemaking family. Beveridge drafted *Social Insurance and the Allied Services* with the assumption that the male-breadwinning, female-homemaking family, rather than the individual British citizen, would constitute the fundamental unit of post-WWII society. He saw married women as making essential contributions to wider society in rearing responsible future citizens.[101] After WWII, Titmuss similarly identified loving nuclear families as both the bedrock for stable democracy and a crucial deterrent against citizens' potential greed in a capitalist society.[102]

This chapter has laid the groundwork for understanding some of the important interwar and wartime roots of the far-reaching social and political value attached to intimate emotional relationships in Britain after WWII. Newly forged interwar and wartime links between health (especially mental health) and interpersonal relationships informed a wide range of state-supported health and social service initiatives that would see the British government invest in citizens' mental and emotional health more than ever before. As Tavistock Clinic Director—and first president of the World Federation for Mental Health—John Rawlings Rees said to members of the National Association for Mental Health in 1946, "Winning the war was a serious matter. Winning the peace is far more difficult."[103] Seen as the primary unit of social *and* emotional life and the chief reproducer of a culture's values, the family was widely looked to as the most promising area for psychiatric study, intervention, and advice in the decades following WWII. If there was hope for a future society committed to peace, it appeared to lie in the outward diffusion of the family's seemingly natural potential for loving intimacy.

Post-WWII British social reconstruction presented new opportunities to intervene in children's development by creating secure loving families, and, in turn, responsible citizens. The next chapter explores the socio-political consequences of the post-WWII preoccupation with the family's central role in producing emotionally healthy children. The rationale behind this aim was well captured in a highly publicized 1946 speech by pediatrician Sir James Spence, urging that the true purpose of the family was to give "the right scope of emotional experience."[104] In his view, one could not overrate its importance for post-WWII reconstruction since, "without emotional health and the happiness and security which goes with it ... there can be no citizenship or other virtues."[105]

2
The Welfare State Begins at Home
"Deprived" Children and Britain's Future after the War

> The wonderful thing about a baby is its promise, not its performance—its promise to perform under certain auspices.
> —Ashley Montagu, *On Being Human*, 1950

> It is apparent that deprived children are as great a source of social infection as are carriers of typhoid and diphtheria.
> —Katherine Simon, review of John Bowlby, *Maternal Care and Mental Health*, 1951

In the autumn of 1939, during the first several months of Britain's wartime evacuation scheme, British newspapers gave voice to the pressing concerns of many of the several thousand citizens who had opened their homes to children moved from London and other urban centers to escape the threat of bombing. Letters from foster parents complained that the billeted children behaved terribly, "befoul[ing] carpets and stairways ... careless of property, rebellious, rude and delinquent."[1] The correspondence expressed a mixture of blame and regret, with some contributors interpreting the children's bad behavior as a sign that the British educational system had failed to civilize the working classes. Sympathy was shown to those individuals and families whose charity had resulted in them experiencing theft and the destruction of their homes and belongings, as well as having to endure billeted children's foul language and outbursts.

By the end of the war, concern for dislocated children had shifted. They were instead seen as innocent victims of the war's disruptive impact on family life.[2] During the summer of 1944 child welfare advocate Marjory Allen, Lady Allen of Hurtwood, wrote a letter to *The Times* exposing the emotional "cruelties" inflicted upon the "many thousands" of children "deprived of a normal home life" in Britain's children's institutions. Public response to Allen's letter was unprecedented. Most agreed that evacuated and institutionalized children's "disorders of behaviour" were "reactions to the distress of domestic disruption," rather than resulting from class-related cultural disparities.[3]

Correspondents now saw the problem as psychological at its core. Child psychologist Susan Isaacs noted that although children's physical needs were being met, they were deprived of basic psychological requirements for healthy development:

> [These children] are given shelter, food and clothing, and some sort of education by the various charitable organizations and authorities, but with regard to many of the psychological needs of normal childhood they remain friendless and neglected. They lack personal affection, spontaneous human relationships, and the opportunity for constructive activities, which most children enjoy in ordinary homes, no matter how poor and simple.[4]

Even contributors lacking formal education in child psychology stressed that residential institutions neglected "the emotional and mental needs of children" because they failed to "keep abreast with modern knowledge of child psychology, and modern standards of child care."[5] The outpouring of correspondence on this topic surpassed that on any other wartime issue. By 1944, concern for uprooted and institutionalized children was focused on the emotional damage caused by the deprivation of "normal home life."[6] Children were no longer condemned for their actions. They were now more likely to be seen as suffering from an emotional disorder.

Like the German POWs encountered in the previous chapter, evacuated children posed a psychological threat to Britain's future. By the end of WWII, the British public had become deeply concerned about the long-term impact of authoritarian environments on emotional development. In the case of British children, who were adult citizens in the making, this initially showed itself as a preoccupation with the damaging effects of residential institutions, which were seen as neither nurturing nor respecting a child's individuality.[7] In line with Dicks and Shils' conclusions about German POWs, *The Times* correspondence revealed that the British public saw children's environments and early experiences as having a lasting impact on who they grew up to become, the jobs they held, the families they created, and the political values that they gravitated toward.[8] Questions remained, however, about precisely how much family disruption caused emotional deprivation. How much separation from their families could children safely endure? Many calls for government-sponsored inquiry published throughout the summer of 1944 asked that emotional deprivation be closely researched, and resolutions promptly enacted nationwide.

Postwar concern for children's future development endowed emotional deprivation research with urgent social relevance. In the decade following WWII, several studies investigating the impact of environment on children's emotional development provided compelling evidence that a loving family—composed of married parents and their children—was the best guarantee of long-term emotional health. These investigations ranged across disciplines and included studies of hospitalized children and adolescents in psychiatric treatment centers, comparative examinations of children's personalities within differing social classes, and anthropological evaluations of the impact of child-rearing styles on cultural norms and values.[9] All concluded that children's environment had a determining impact on their personalities and psychological health as adults, just as Dicks and Shils' study of German POWs had. They all appealed to emotional deprivation as a potentially irreversible outcome, emphasizing permanent lack rather than flexible adjustment to ever-changing circumstances. They therefore focused their proposed solutions on *preventing* deviations from an ideal male-breadwinning, female-homemaking model of loving family life.

In tandem with this post-WWII scientific investment in understanding the full scope and impact of emotional deprivation, Britain's new and expanding welfare state prioritized social policy and services focused on preventing emotional deprivation in children. This chapter tracks how new post-WWII urgency surrounding children's emotional lives fueled efforts to create and preserve stable families and "family-like" environments, including movements to prevent disruptions to continuous maternal care. This included efforts to increase foster care over the use of large group homes; attempts to ensure speedy and permanent child adoption; movements to both increase hospital visiting hours for children and introduce mother-child wards in hospitals to prevent sick children's separation from their mothers; government resistance to state-funded nursery care for working mothers; as well as greater support for child guidance clinics across Britain after WWII. All these state policies and government-supported initiatives sought to promote healthy child development by ensuring that Britain's youngest citizens were guaranteed continuous access to family life.

State interest in children's emotional health may not appear to straightforwardly coincide with the goals of the welfare state, particularly as outlined by its chief architect, economist and Liberal politician William Beveridge. According to Beveridge's 1942 blueprint, the welfare state was intended to eliminate the social "evils" of "Want, Disease, Ignorance, Squalor, and Idleness."[10] I argue, however, that the postwar government's investment in emotional health pursued another crucial and related welfarist purpose, that is, ensuring security in an uncertain world. Supported by scientific studies of children's developmental need for stable and secure close emotional relationships, British postwar social policy sought to protect family love as a bedrock for socio-political stability and security. In the wake of a destabilizing war, the security that Britons desperately longed to recapture was transferred onto families and presented as a psychological state that was most reliably cultivated through a child's intimate relationship with their mother.[11]

Despite the British postwar government's commitment to citizens' security, I argue that social policy focused on preventing emotional deprivation dangerously oversimplified and obscured a range of complex socio-economic realities as problems that were viewed as *actually* emotional when stripped down to their essential causes. The urgent problem of child homelessness was turned into a problem of lovelessness and children's residential institutions inspired alarm because they prevented their young residents from experiencing genuine interpersonal connection. In the wake of the new post-WWII focus on children's emotional lives, the economic protections afforded by middle-class affluence were presented as less consequential than the *feeling* of security that a loving mother could give to her child or a wife to her husband. For many psychiatrists and social planners alike, it was families' emotional defects, rather than the failures of capitalism, that were looked to as the source of inequality and persistent social problems.

New psychological insights heightened the importance and presumed consequences of emotional life. Post-WWII deprivation studies emphasized the value of children's earliest relationships while they diminished the long-term relevance of children's socio-economic circumstances.[12] Earlier attention to deprivation in children, beginning in the late nineteenth century, had focused on malnutrition in working-class urban children and its impact on their growth and cognitive performance. Studies of slum life's effects on child development—notably by social reformers Charles Booth and Margaret McMillan—had stressed the pathological consequences of underfeeding, urban overcrowding, poor ventilation, lack of sunlight, and air pollution.[13] Evidence of deprivation had supported reformers' appeals for public assistance, such as school meals programs, to end the stunting of young bodies and minds. In contrast, postwar psychological appeals to deprivation downplayed the importance of children's material circumstances, focusing instead on the extremely wide-ranging benefits of their access to loving maternal care.

A growing body of scholarship addressing the politics of childhood in post-WWII Britain has illuminated the importance of public concern for children in the creation of an expert-directed welfare state that prioritized social protection for the vulnerable.[14] The aim of ensuring that all British children had access to health and security was immense and required not only substantial state funding but also informed organization. This chapter builds on this expanding body of historical and sociological work, yet more specifically highlights how post-WWII policies and initiatives targeting children's emotional lives helped create a political community that was fundamentally committed to loving intimacy as both a requirement for healthy development and a prerequisite for responsible citizenship. This commitment to the sweeping benefits of loving intimate relationships helped transform post-WWII Britain into an intimate state, that is a political community that prioritized citizens' access to intimacy as a gateway for mental health and good citizenship as intertwined outcomes.

Emotional life became a political priority after WWII as the basis for a psychologized vision of responsible citizenship that was forged in families and implicated all Britons—young and old, male and female. This chapter reveals how emotional health became a new basis for good citizenship—not only helping re-envision what citizenship entailed in terms of social responsibility and active participation, but how it was psychologically forged in loving male-breadwinning, female-homemaking families. Previous scholarship has revealed how psychological insights contributed to not only new post-WWII understandings of "classless" social democracy but also a transformation of the landscapes that British children inhabited (at home, school, and play).[15] In this chapter, I show how a post-WWII British preoccupation with children's emotional vulnerability helped fuel the creation of a welfare state committed to the cultivation and protection of intimacy. Psychological experts played an important supporting role, but this emotionalization of British social and political life involved a broader range of individuals. The ambitious goal of protecting the emotional health of Britain's citizens (including future citizens) relied for its success upon state-led initiatives aimed not only at children but also at mothers and fathers, husbands and wives, and even those beyond the immediate remit of child-producing families. Children were an important initial focal point in the pursuit of postwar security, but the political investment in emotional life—aimed at cultivating good citizenship and thus eliminating all threats to socio-political security—affected everyone, both inside and outside of the idealized stable loving nuclear family.

Troubled Children before WWII

Wartime evacuation helped establish widespread concern for children's need for a stable and loving family. However, in the decade leading up to this, mental health professionals established new connections between psychiatric problems affecting young people and the care they received in their families. As discussed in the previous chapter, the interwar decades saw a rise in medical practitioners' interest in the power of social environments to determine mental and physical health. This rising preoccupation with the impact of environment also marked initiatives focused on troubled children, especially those within the sphere of "child guidance."

Child guidance was imported to Britain from the United States through the Commonwealth Fund, a New York-based foundation launched in 1918 by Anna Harkness, widow of oil baron Stephen Harkness. The fund was primarily focused on juvenile delinquency in its early years and this strongly influenced early child guidance work in both Britain and the United States.[16] Both countries were experiencing a crime wave after WWI, and it was hoped that child guidance would cure young offenders of their law-breaking impulses.[17] By 1923, the crime prevention focus of child guidance had extended from actual offenders to the "pre-delinquent," that is the predominantly working-class child who was presumed to be a criminal-in-the-making due to their poor life circumstances.[18] In response to British interest, in 1926 the Commonwealth Fund granted training in psychiatric social work to twelve British social workers at the New York School of Social Work.[19] The emerging field of psychiatric social work incorporated psychiatric treatment into casework with clients and their families. Training in the United States led, in 1927, to the creation of a British Child Guidance Council. In 1929, the London School of Economics (LSE)—at the behest of its director, William Beveridge—established its own training in psychiatric social work and mental health diploma. Britain's first Child Guidance Clinic was opened in Islington, in north-east London, in 1929. By 1933, there were forty-two such clinics in the United States; Britain would undergo a similar process of rapid development, with over sixty clinics in operation by 1939.[20]

Like their US counterparts, British child guidance clinics targeted "maladjustment." This capacious diagnosis signaled a psychological misalignment between the child and their environment and included symptoms ranging from aggression and criminality to timidity and bedwetting. Since "maladjustment" encompassed such a wide range of problems, a large assessment and treatment net was cast to root it out. Psychologists administered IQ, personality, and other tests; psychiatric social workers visited afflicted children's homes in search of bad home environments; and psychiatrists interviewed the patient and presided over the entire treatment process.

Although a psychiatrist was the de facto head of each clinic, it was psychiatric social workers' interactions with children's families that set the tone for most child guidance work. In the 1930s (especially the latter half of the decade), child guidance professionals' assessment of pathological influences centered on the afflicted child's family life, especially poor parenting—which assumed many forms, from neglectful to overbearing—and parents' dysfunctional relationship.[21] This tendency to focus on the home environment of afflicted children was specific to psychiatric social workers' diagnostic and treatment approach, and likely reflected social workers' long history of work with lower income people living in poor urban neighborhoods. Interwar psychiatrists' psychotherapeutic vision was not nearly as concerned with life experiences. When, for example, John Bowlby, then director of the London Child Guidance Clinic (LCGC), presented a paper on the pathological effects of mother-child separation to the British Psychoanalytical Society (BPS) in 1939, he was denied membership to the organization. Melanie Klein, head of the BPS, maintained that in prioritizing the events that a child lives through rather than their *interpretation* of their experiences, Bowlby had strayed too far from orthodox psychoanalytic understanding.

Although the reasons for children's referral to a clinic—whether by teachers, parents, physicians, or social workers—were diverse, spanning bedwetting and tantrums to minor theft and poor school performance, child guidance treatment focused on the child's home environment. Not only would the patient's parents (typically their mother) be asked to report to a psychiatric social worker on their child's symptoms and progress, but they would also themselves be interviewed and asked to discuss "their problems, difficulties in married life, management of their children, and so on."[22] Children's mothers were also frequently asked to participate in their child's sessions with the psychiatrist, and in some cases, the child's father and siblings would also attend. By the mid-1930s, as historian John Stewart points out, child guidance clinics treated children not as autonomous individuals, but as fully enmeshed in a dysfunctional ecosystem populated by quarreling parents, overbearing mothers, and inattentive fathers. Working to transform the (usually working-class) afflicted child's home environment, the child guidance team treated their young "maladjusted" patients as deeply suggestible surfaces upon which family dynamics were inscribed.

In cases of extreme maladjustment—approximately one tenth of the children seen at child guidance clinics—children were sent to residential schools since their removal from their presumably dysfunctional parenting was seen as essential to their successful treatment. At these residential schools, the child guidance environmentalist ethos was fully put into practice. Charles Burns, director of the Birmingham Child Guidance Clinic, described residential school treatment in this way:

> Treatment consists in the main of the impact made upon the child by the new environment in which he finds himself. This means the community or school as a whole, including the place, the staff, the pets, the lessons, arts and crafts, outings, committees of children, and all manner of things... *everything that happens is educative or the reverse.*[23]

Non-hierarchical democratic environments were believed best for treating severely maladjusted children since they allowed ample space for independence and creative problem-solving and encouraged a sense of responsibility toward the wider community. Psychoanalyst Homer Lane—an early-twentieth-century pioneer in the residential approach to treating children with behavioral problems—maintained that the absence of staff-student hierarchy at his school for delinquent youth encouraged authentic independent expression and liberated the students from the negative influences of their "repressive and condemnatory upbringing."[24]

With its focus on curability during a period of both rising juvenile crime and neurotic illness, the child guidance movement's environmentalist approach to children's mental health problems attracted political support. Local authorities funded more than half of the growing network of child guidance clinics; the Labour Party produced a social policy document on the importance of child guidance;[25] and, in 1939, a state-commissioned report detailing the dire state of Britain's mental health services, amid what was described as a growing national mental health crisis, stressed the need for further government investment in child guidance. The 1939 Report of the Feversham Committee on the state of Britain's mental health services had been compiled over three years in response to reported concerns that as many as 60% of British people suffered from some form of developing neurotic disorder.[26] The report connected this rising mental health crisis to the unique social conditions created by urban industrial capitalism. Alongside concerns about the negative mental impact of socio-economic stressors on adults, the report warned that child guidance professionals had revealed their especially grave consequences for children. Mothers forced by economic necessity to enter the workforce, rising rates of out-of-wedlock births and family breakdown, crowded housing conditions, and urban overpopulation were only some of the problems that the report noted presented obstacles to children's healthy emotional and psychological development.

The Feversham Report set the initial terms for the welfare state's investment in preventative mental health care after the war. Presenting child guidance as one of three major areas to build upon—alongside the National Council for Mental Hygiene and the Mental After Care Association—the committee emphasized the long-term political stakes of children's mental health. Earlier state interest in children had revolved around two key areas: malnutrition and juvenile crime. Growing awareness of malnutrition had led to the passage of the School Meals Act in 1906, arguably Britain's first welfare-state legislation since, unlike the provision of pensions and unemployment insurance, it was not based on workers' contributions to a larger collective fund. This assertion of the state's role in protecting vulnerable citizens was controversial, however, since it threatened to undermine parents' responsibility to adequately feed their children (as the National Society for the Prevention of Cruelty to Children argued). The 1906 Act led to uneven results, and state commitment to feeding malnourished children especially fell by the wayside in the wake of massive economic depression in the 1930s. State interest in juvenile crime, however, produced real changes following the passage of the 1908 Children Act as special juvenile courts were created alongside reform schools focused on rehabilitation.[27] During the interwar decades, various amendments ushered in a curative approach to eliminating juvenile crime, and young offenders increasingly received psychiatric treatment. As Harry Hendrick points out, interest in the child as a potential victim was complicated by children's particular form of victimhood posing a threat to the nation.[28] Lawbreaking juveniles were not seen as entirely responsible for their crimes, and their lack of responsibility—premised on their presumed inability to act as rational agents—made them *even greater* threats to social order.

After WWII, the British welfare government assumed greater responsibility for helping "cure" troubled children. The 1944 Education Act officially recognized "maladjustment" as a disability requiring treatment in the form of special education and therefore a responsibility of the welfare state.[29] Described as "an emotional or psychological disorder,"[30] it was listed alongside blindness, deafness, and "mental deficiency," but unlike these other disabilities, it was considered curable.[31] Child guidance would thus be absorbed into the welfare state after the war as part of British schools' provision of health services and, by 1955, there were more than three hundred clinics in Britain (up significantly from the sixty clinics in operation on the eve of WWII).

During post-WWII reconstruction, concern for children's family environments would move far beyond the spheres of child guidance clinics and education aimed at helping the "maladjusted." The child guidance view concerning the deep (and potentially irreversible) impact of children's home environments on their healthy psychological development pervaded many areas of post-WWII social reconstruction, from child fostering to hospital visiting policies. The notion that children's emotional and psychological vulnerability constituted a social threat that the British government needed to protect against became an even more pressing issue in the wake of the wartime experience of evacuation and discovery of the pervasiveness of emotional deprivation (the subject of the next section). Whereas the signs of (predominantly working-class) "maladjustment" were obvious enough to require interventions like special education programs, "deprivation"—thought to be the immediate underlying cause of "maladjustment"—was expressed in myriad and more subtle ways and seemed to affect children from a much wider range of socioeconomic backgrounds. The consequences for Britain's future seemed even more worrying.

WWII and Deprived Children

In the weeks following publication of Marjory Allen's letter in *The Times*, on July 15, 1944, the emotional fate of children "deprived of a normal home life" was revealed to be a preeminent public concern. No single wartime issue would evoke such a reaction. Published responses to Allen's letter mobilized recent psychological findings to argue against the continued use of residential children's institutions. Foster parent Mrs. Birch Reynardson wrote that several formerly institutionalized children who were under her care showed "something still missing, something 'incomplete' about their personalities."[32] The director of one of Britain's largest foundations lamented institutionalized children's "warped ... outlook on life," bad table manners, and untidy clothes connected to their having lived "their lives as members of a large crowd."[33] Most correspondents agreed that children needed "affectionate relationships" as much as, if not more than, "food, shelter, and cleanliness."[34]

The concerns that permeated *The Times* correspondence were fueled by British wartime psychological observations of evacuation's effects on children. Never had so many children, of such a wide range of backgrounds, been removed from their families and placed either in residential institutions or with temporary foster families.[35] Scholarship demonstrating the positive public response in the same period in France to the removal of working-class children from their families to attend summer camps underscores the particularity of British attentiveness to emotional disturbance. For child psychologists and the public alike, the many troubling behaviors exhibited by the 734,883 British children evacuated during WWII presented irrefutable evidence of the overwhelmingly negative effects of children's "deprivation of normal family life." It did not take long for signs of psychological distress to be noticed following children's placement with rural families in the fall of 1939. Amy St. Loe Strachey, a founding member of the British child guidance movement, quickly recognized adjustment anxiety in several of the eight children she had taken in during the first months of the war. On the first morning following their arrival at her home in Surrey, evidence of bedwetting made their trauma clearly visible. She reported that, upon their arrival, there had been "only one case of tears. But the emotional disturbance was there, for when morning came it was found that a proportion of the children had wetted their beds."[36] She proceeded to consider the hidden nature of their severe anxiety:

> Had they been on guard all day, and was it only in the relaxation of sleep that the immense disturbance and dislocation of their lives had manifested itself? I ought to have seen below the surface, for in talking over at the front door whether it was possible to put up eight children without a helper, in a house prepared for six, a little hand was put into mine and two anxious dark eyes looked up into my face... The dream of eager, active children is to have great adventures. But behind all the excitement and bustle in this adventure there lurked something sinister.

It threatened that "secure basis of home" on which the stability of all child life depends, and it promised to last for so long—for always perhaps.[37]

Strachey noted that bedwetting became a topic in "almost every house" outside the large towns. This difficult-to-ignore fact helped awaken British women to the challenge of providing effective childcare: "the care of a child is not a matter of slaps and kisses, but presents real, hard problems which are not to be solved by rule of thumb— that the words 'good' and 'naughty' do not really count for much."[38] In Strachey's view, the old parenting wisdom that saw punishment as a solution to bad behavior eroded during the war years as "gradually the seed of psychological ideas [was] sown and slowly germinate[d] in the minds of the village mothers."[39]

Evacuation provided a unique—however unfortunate—opportunity for psychological observation of the impact of family disruption. Viennese child psychologist Katherine Wolf condemned the wartime safety measure as "a cruel psychological experiment on a large scale."[40] Emphasizing the important prospects for research, however, Susan Isaacs pointed out that interwar studies of children treated at child guidance clinics had offered an incomplete view of the origins of behavioral disturbances. Case histories, including details about family backgrounds, often described children's disturbances in ways that were unique to them.[41] In contrast to this disorganized picture of the delinquent mind, the patterns noticed in the anxious behavior of evacuated children—including bedwetting, nail biting, aggressive outbursts, and stealing—showed far more consistency.

Researchers' conclusions were strikingly similar. All were emphatic that stable family life was essential to healthy child development. Studies produced by a range of experts, including Anna Freud and Dorothy Burlingham, Susan Isaacs, Donald Winnicott, John Bowlby, and many others involved in wartime child guidance work, unfailingly stressed that family stability needed to be protected—even in extremely trying circumstances—rather than resorting to even the most well-run children's institution.[42] Freud and Burlingham's study of children housed in their residential nurseries in North London concluded that the healthy socialization that took place within families was fueled by the unique emotional charge of the parent-child relationship. Isaacs's edited *Cambridge Evacuation Survey* similarly emphasized that loving family relationships were an essential psychological need, concluding that evacuation had failed—as seen in the mass return to London after only a few months—because organizers had overlooked "the crucial importance ... of the feelings of parents and children towards and about each other."[43] The study stressed the important lessons of the war in demonstrating families' emotional ties to be stronger than the instinct for physical survival.[44] However diverse their professional backgrounds, researchers focused on disruptions to home life above all other war-related experiences as having devastating effects on children's emotional development.

Responses to Allen's 1944 letter showed that concern for children's healthy mental and emotional development had spread far beyond child guidance clinics. Even correspondents who challenged Allen's concerns about children's institutions gave consideration to their impact on children's long-term development (although often from a "habit training" perspective). For example, John Keep, Chairman of Kingsdown Orphanage, insisted that residential institutions were vastly superior in "the training of the children physically, mentally and morally ... than in the majority of homes from which they come," despite their frequent staffing challenges.[45] Others, like Reverend Arthur West, director of Mill House, argued for the benefits of children's institutions over foster homes in terms of long-term "equipment for citizenship and happy adjustment to the community" by focusing on foster parents' economic motives and reports of foster-parent abuse.[46]

While some defended the developmental benefits of children's homes, most presented them as psychologically damaging. Correspondents routinely underscored the importance of prioritizing children's unique personalities and talents when stressing the comparative benefits of foster homes. Enid Moberly Bell, head of an all-girls school in west London, argued that unlike the "unnatural conditions" of an institution where the "individual child is lost," in a foster family "the child is in a small society, among brothers and sisters, each of whom is of unique importance, and has some definite contribution to make to home life."[47] Contributors routinely emphasized the absence of close care relationships in children's institutions as a barrier to healthy development: first, because of their large and impersonal size and second, because staff so often lacked psychological training.

In response to demands for further research into deprivation, the Nuffield Provincial Hospitals Trust granted funds to the Provisional National Council of Mental Health—renamed the National Association of Mental Health (NAMH) after WWII—to examine the "social adaptation of children and young persons brought up in institutions."[48] The trust, founded in 1939 to bring more efficient integration to Britain's health services, had rejected this very proposal for research in April 1943, but changed its position following the publicity that Lady Allen's letter brought to the issue. Deputy director of the Bristol Child Guidance Clinic, Dr. Frank Bodman, led the inquiry, which compared the "social maturity" of institutionalized children to that of children reared in their family homes. He interviewed nineteen girls and thirty-two boys from twelve different institutions who had spent at least three consecutive years of their life in a children's home. His findings confirmed his expectations.[49] Bodman concluded that, "The children brought up in institutions were less mature socially than those in the control group," explaining that they were less familiar with events going on in the world and less able to function independently of caregivers. Formerly institutionalized children, he noted, were also less likely to sustain friendships in the long term, show an interest in developing romantic relationships, and work in their desired occupation.

Concern for children's susceptibility to social development delays also motivated calls for public inquiry into the problem of homeless and institutionalized children in Britain. In 1946, the Committee on the Care of Children, led by Newnham College principal Myra Curtis, investigated the provision of care for "children deprived of a normal home life" in England and Wales. The committee found that the numbers of children housed in public and voluntary institutions far exceeded Allen's rough assessment: 16,895 children were being maintained by public-assistance authorities and 33,500 children lived in homes provided by voluntary organizations.[50] This number included children who were poor, homeless, and orphaned, and "mentally deficient" children in the care of public health authorities and voluntary organizations. To determine the real size and scope of the problem, committee members visited 451 institutions of various kinds throughout the country. The Curtis Committee's major recommendation—that a single government department be formed to assume responsibility for children "deprived of a normal home life"—was not new.[51] The report was notable, however, for bridging the concerns about emotionally deprived children expressed in *The Times* in 1944 to those concerns for preventing emotional deprivation in children that became a core feature of postwar social reconstruction.

The Report of the Care of Children Committee, which detailed the disturbing scale of the problem of children "deprived of a normal home life," led to the passing of the Children Act on July 5, 1948. Alongside the National Assistance Act and the National Insurance Act, this constituted one of the three major pillars of the British welfare state. Coinciding with the abolition of the Poor Law, which had made provisions for homeless and deserted children, the 1948 Children Act entrusted the Home Office with sole responsibility for the care of homeless and deprived children. It presented children's residential institutions as harmful to psychological development and gave priority to fostering. At the heart of both the Curtis Report and the 1948 Children Act was the guiding idea that unless emotional deprivation was addressed, a number of growing social problems—including juvenile crime, mental illness, out-of-wedlock births, and divorce—would continue to worsen.

Wartime attention to the plight of "deprived" children not only helped transform how child development experts thought about emotional life, it also made childhood an important area of government concern. In the years following WWII, evacuation was widely seen as having confirmed the universality and long-term seriousness of children's emotional needs. Whereas the more limited problem of "maladjustment" would continue to preoccupy educational authorities and child health professionals after the war, emotional "deprivation" pointed toward far greater possibilities for psychological injury and arrested development. The troubling figure of the emotionally vulnerable child was at the center of a new and wide-ranging ethos of prevention that was understood to be crucial for Britain's socio-political *and* psychiatric future.

The Emotional Welfare State

The 1948 Children Act heralded the British government's commitment to ensuring that homeless children were reared in environments closely approximating their own biological family unit. This was to ensure they would be as little "handicapped" as possible by emotional deprivation. The act did much more than extend the parameters of the 1933 Children and Young Persons Act, which had introduced legal protections surrounding child labor and the sale of tobacco and alcohol to children and increased the age of criminal responsibility. Addressing the end of the Poor Law—and accompanying fate of the 27,000 children under the care of local authorities after the war—the 1948 Children Act made the state responsible for the care of all children lacking an adequate home life, whether their parents were living or not. It signaled that *all* children—of all backgrounds and life circumstances—had the right to grow up in a stable family setting. In its commitment to enabling all children to have access to an environment optimal for emotional health, the 1948 Act anticipated the postwar emergence of children's rights, which was supported by the principle that children had the right to a healthy development. More than a decade before the United Nations made a formal declaration concerning children's rights, the British welfare state made healthy child development a formal political priority.

The 1948 Act explicitly mandated against the use of residential institutions unless an acceptable foster home was unavailable. The Curtis Committee had reported in 1946 that they had found children in foster homes to be happier and better adjusted than children in residential institutions:

> We found in the children, in foster-homes we visited, almost complete freedom from the sense of deprivation which we have described among children in Homes. On the whole our judgment is that there is probably a greater risk of acute unhappiness in a foster-home (owing to difficulties of supervision), but that a happy foster-home is happier than life as generally lived in a large community.[52]

Following the Curtis Report's recommendations, the act authorized that all children in local authorities' care would be maintained in small "cottage homes" only "where it is not practicable or desirable for the time being to make arrangements for boarding out."[53] The act acknowledged the shortage of foster homes to meet demand in the immediate post-WWII years, which prevented residential institutions from becoming entirely obsolete. Stressing that all foster homes needed to be approved by the local authority and regularly inspected by children's officers, the act made it local governments' duty to "exercise their powers with respect to [each child in care] so as to further his best interests, and to afford him opportunity for the proper development of his character and abilities."[54]

Finding married couples willing to foster children was only part of the problem of transferring children in care from institutions to foster homes. The caution written into the act regarding the choice and inspection of foster homes responded to the highly publicized 1945 murder of twelve-year-old Denis O'Neill by his foster father. In the wake of O'Neill's death and ensuing discovery that social workers had seldom visited his foster parents following his placement with them, stricter foster parent approval and visiting protocols were put in place. Despite this, media reports of foster child abuse in the years that followed regularly exposed social workers' ongoing lack of follow up with foster families.

In addition to continuing problems of physical abuse, neglect, and malnutrition in foster homes, emotional problems became an increasing focus of concern. Just over a decade after Denis O'Neill was killed, the local children's officer in Bath removed fourteen-year-old Mary Ford from the home of her foster parents, the Greenwoods, because Mrs. Greenwood had made repeated threats to Mary that she would be returned to the local children's home as a way of disciplining her: "the continual threats by the Greenwoods of eviction from their home had caused in the girl a most strong sense of insecurity and forged an unnatural linkage of security with, and only with, the Greenwood home."[55] Mary was then placed in a voluntary home where she reportedly made good progress recovering from this emotional abuse. Isaac Pitman, Member of Parliament for Bath, stressed that the best day of Mary's life was when she was placed in the Children's Reception Home in Bristol:

> They said that she had been observed by them, by their staff and by the specialist medical officers, and that all of them had agreed that they had never seen a girl of that age who appeared more deprived of affection, of the ability to receive it or give it, and this, be it noted, from those specializing in receiving children from homes with a bad history of lack of affection; that so soon as any sense of security had been restored Mary became over-demonstrative.[56]

Insisting that even "natural parents can occasionally behave so badly towards their children that the local authority may need to remove the child from the care of the parents," Pitman was adamant that a well-run children's home was preferable to an emotionally abusive foster parent.

Although Britain's children's homes were not immediately closed, the act's influence was quickly felt. Fostering grew as a practice from 1948 onward. While 35% of children in the care of local authorities were in foster care in 1948, in 1964 that proportion had risen to 51%. Already by 1950, 41% of children under state care were placed in foster homes.[57] This was a significant increase compared to the figures reported in 1946—4,900 in total, as compared to the nearly 50,000 being maintained in public assistance and voluntary homes.[58] Prior to 1945, the fostering of children under the Poor Law had been restricted to orphaned and abandoned children (and only then in cases of emergency). The main reason for the change in 1945 was to enable children billeted under the evacuation scheme to remain in private care.[59] It is noteworthy that O'Neill's death had not led to a disavowal of fostering and renewed interest in possibilities for institutional reform. Children's homes had had their day, even if this would not fully bear out in practice for another few decades.

The Curtis Report had indicated that in caring for homeless children adoption was the ideal option, however in practice fostering was the more realistic choice for children whose natural parents were still living. Adoption required the consent of the child's biological mother until 1949. A year after the Children Act was passed, however, the 1949 Adoption of Children Act changed adopted children's legal status, more securely embedding them in their adopted families. As legal historian Stephen

Cretney notes, they now appeared "as if born to the adoptive parents as a child of their marriage."[60] They gained rights of inheritance and citizenship and were no longer permitted to marry their adoptive parent. Thus, according to laws regulating kinship, property, and political membership, they were now the same as non-adopted children. Adopted children's more secure status also corresponded with changes in biological mothers' role in transferring children to adoptive families. Whereas prior to 1949 (that is, since adoption was legalized in 1926) mothers had needed to give their consent to have their child adopted to a particular family, after 1949 decisions surrounding the particularities of an adoption were decided by courts. Consent was presumed implicitly given by any "reasonable parent" who properly regarded their child's welfare.[61] A child could now be adopted by people whose identity was not known to the biological mother, and any attempt to insert herself further into the adoption process could be viewed as evidence that she was not capable of prioritizing the child's needs. The court's role as decision-maker additionally severed the biological mother's ability to establish any connection with the child at a later point.

The absence of publicly funded daycare for working mothers in the decades after WWII similarly showed the British government's reluctance to allow children any interruption in their continuity of parental care. As Denise Riley has shown, the initial impetus behind the closure of day nurseries at the end of WWII followed, in part, from public health concerns about the spread of infection.[62] However, their continued closure in the 1950s and 1960s, in the wake of improved health provision through the NHS, was more closely connected to the increasingly pervasive sense that children (especially those under five) needed to be cared for by their mothers at all times. Children's emotional health, and not only their physical health, would be protected in this new world.

The welfare state's commitment to ensuring that all children had access to stable families and received continuous care from a maternal figure was, in part, fueled by expert recommendations. Among the witnesses examined by the Curtis Committee were Susan Isaacs, John Bowlby, Donald Winnicott, and Clare Britton, who directed a course for training psychiatric social workers at LSE. While psychiatrists Bowlby and Winnicott made less of an impression, Britton presented concrete evidence from casework that persuaded committee members of children's deep emotional vulnerability. In general, however, child psychological findings confirming the importance of family life for healthy emotional development were apparent throughout the report. The priority given to child development expertise could be seen not only in the report's framing but the in the committee's practical recommendations as well. They urged that children's officers—those state officials who had direct personal responsibility for children—have both a warm and affectionate personality *and* professional training in social science.

Although the input of child psychological experts was important, postwar legal reforms surrounding child welfare were intended to stand as practical measures for preventing emotional deprivation in children. Unlike psychological treatment, this was more focused on managing—or, more specifically, emotionalizing—the spaces that children inhabited. Guided by the recommendations of child development professionals, the state, in order to ensure that all British children indeed had the right to healthy emotional development, needed to take a directive role in guaranteeing that children were reared in a family (or "family-like") environment. The state's preference for foster care over residential institutions was intended to provide as many children as possible access to family life; adopted children were more stably rooted in their adoptive families in the hope that they would experience not only the financial and legal but also the emotional benefits of family belonging; and the abandonment of nursery care prevented work-related interruptions to maternal care (as far as the state could truly prevent this from happening).

This preoccupation with children's emotional care after WWII also gave rise to scrutiny of two-parent middle-class families by the early 1950s. Bath member of parliament (MP) Isaac Pitman's insistence upon the emotional damage that could also be done to a child by their "natural parents" had, by 1959, been proposed for more than a decade in inquiries into children's emotional deprivation. Discussions of child neglect in Parliament focused on the difficulty of identifying cases of neglect in their early stages and debating whether removing those children from their parents was ultimately unavoidable or whether it was possible to establish better ways of offering families preventive help. MPs worried that the growing number of reports of child neglect to the National Society for the Prevention of Cruelty to Children (NSPCC) were only the tip of the iceberg and discussed the possibility of creating a better system of either checking in on families or cross-compiling data—from schools, hospitals, and social services—so that problems might be more quickly discovered. It was not only poor families that were singled out—government ministers were quick to note that less visible, but perhaps equally acute, problems were suffered by children deprived of appropriate care in affluent homes. Emotional deprivation research—the subject of the next section—would make these seemingly privileged children's problems a major source of concern in the 1950s.

Child Development Research Guides Social Reform

The earliest psychiatric studies of emotional deprivation focused on children in residential institutional care, particularly orphanages, hospitals, and sanatoria. Since the plight of the child "deprived" of adequate emotional care in their own home was believed to differ only in intensity (rather than kind) to that of children living in residential institutions, children undergoing short-term hospitalization were seen as promising subjects for understanding the impact of family disruption on children's mental health. The Austrian American psychoanalyst René Spitz had popularized direct observation of hospitalized children as a method for studying deprivation in the late 1930s. Following Spitz, British child psychiatrist John Bowlby and his collaborator psychiatric social worker James Robertson observed children in hospital wards in the late 1940s. Bowlby chose the separation of the young child from their mother as his focal point not because he presumed that separation was a very common occurrence, but because it:

> was an event that had happened or had not happened and was therefore easier to document than the more subtle influences of parental and familial interaction; [it] was an event that could have serious ill effects on a child's personality development; [it] appeared to be a field in which preventive measures might be possible.[63]

Separation experiences, Bowlby later remarked, were an exaggerated version of what many children routinely experienced within their families when they were not given adequate parental attention. They often resulted in "neurosis," "instability of character," and, in the worst cases, a complete inability "to make relationships."[64]

Bowlby's research into the causes of emotional disorders experienced by "normal" (rather than "maladjusted") children brought him to the attention of the World Health Organization (WHO) in 1951. Ronald Hargreaves, WHO chief officer of mental health and affiliate of the Tavistock Clinic (where Bowlby headed the children's department from 1946), appointed Bowlby to head UN-commissioned research on the psychological impact of homelessness on children. After WWII, the massive problem of child homelessness was far more pronounced on the European continent than in Britain. As Tara Zahra notes, UNESCO "estimated that 8 million children in Germany, 6.5 million children in the Soviet Union, and 1.3 million children in France remained homeless in 1946. An estimated 13 million children in Europe had lost one or both parents in the war."[65] Despite this, most research on the psychological effects of family disruption on children was pursued in Britain and the United States. When Bowlby had undertaken the task of examining the psychological impact of child homelessness, he had been asked to consider only those children who were "homeless in their native country."[66] The study thus deliberately excluded the many thousands of war refugees and displaced children.

After only six months of study, Bowlby produced the report that would make him internationally famous. *Maternal Care and Mental Health* was published in 1951 and was the product of several months of discussion with child guidance staff and child psychologists in France, the Netherlands, Sweden, Switzerland, the UK, and the United States. Those sites that had seen the most extreme levels of child homelessness by the end of the war—Germany and the Soviet Union—were not included. Bowlby concluded by stressing the acute psychological dangers of "maternal deprivation": "the infant and young child should experience a warm, intimate and continuous relationship with his mother (or permanent mother substitute) in which both find satisfaction and enjoyment."[67] The absence of this "intimate and continuous relationship," he warned, would bring on potentially irreversible mental health consequences: "when deprived of maternal care, the child's development is almost always retarded—physically, intellectually, and socially ... some children are gravely damaged for life."[68] Bowlby underscored the legitimacy of his bold conclusion by mentioning its broad acceptance by child mental health specialists in each of the countries considered.

Maternal Care and Mental Health was well-received and sold widely. It was published in an abridged form in 1953 as *Child Care and the Growth of Love* and translated into fourteen languages.[69] Aimed at a general readership, it sold over four hundred thousand copies in Britain alone. In presenting the absence of a stable family as a "handicap," Bowlby hoped to introduce a widespread transformation of family practices and higher regard for emotional life. Although the WHO report had been commissioned as a study of child homelessness, Bowlby had concluded that the most pervasive emotional problems stemmed from troubled family relationships. Deprived children often came from seemingly stable families, yet they had not been provided with adequate affection. Adults who had grown up in such homes were unable to satisfy their own children's emotional needs:

> It is evident that in a society where death-rates are low, the rate of employment high, and social welfare schemes adequate, it is emotional instability and the inability of parents to make effective family relationships which are the outstanding cause of children becoming deprived of a normal home life ... the investigator is confronted with a self-perpetuating social circle in which *children who are deprived of a normal home life grow up into parents unable to provide a normal home life for their children.*[70]

The fact that deprivation was transmitted to future generations in a "self-perpetuating social circle," meant that even seemingly ordinary families needed to be scrupulously watched for the less obvious ways that parents failed to meet their children's emotional needs.

Echoing the post-WWII drive to eliminate children's institutions, Bowlby recommended focusing on preventing "family failure" rather than removing children from their parents' care. The only exception to this were unmarried mothers. In his view, unmarried motherhood was a symptom of neurosis and those afflicted were unable to provide their children with adequate emotional care. When it came to poor families, divorced parents, and widowed single parents, his commitment to the integrity of biological families echoed sentiments expressed by the League of Nations in 1938 and the Curtis Committee in 1946.[71] Parents who were challenged by difficult circumstances were seen as providing immeasurably better care for their children than an institution. Bowlby even saw foster parents who were not biologically related to the child as lacking the necessary familial loyalty to properly attend to the child's emotional needs. Instead of removing children from their families, he recommended having entire families be treated by mental health professionals: "In practice, this means not only treating children, but the giving of psychiatric help to parents ... Those who have worked with the parents, especially the mothers, of young children believe that there is no more fruitful mental hygiene work than this."[72] He pressed for an intensive nationwide provision of psychosocial services aimed at stabilizing families, including marriage guidance, child guidance, and parent education.[73]

Although Bowlby's findings shared his contemporaries' concerns for children's vulnerable emotions, and similarly saw the stable and harmonious family as a place of love and emotional safety, he more specifically emphasized that *maternal* care was best for ensuring children's healthy emotional development. By 1951, Bowlby attached supreme importance to the mother-child relationship. His emphasis on maternal care in the WHO study did not serve as shorthand for parental care.

Several months prior to his recruitment by Hargreaves, Bowlby had received funding from the Rockefeller Foundation to investigate the effects of mother-child separation on children undergoing short-term hospitalization. Short-term separation experiences were not uncommon in the early 1950s. In most hospital wards, visiting was restricted to once a week for an hour. In some cases, there was no visiting permitted at all during the child's first month of treatment to ensure that they had acclimated to the hospital before experiencing any disruption to their new routine. By 1951, Bowlby and his team had amassed observations of almost fifty children undergoing short-term institutional care. All the children, without exception, showed signs of distress: they cried, pleaded to be sent home, and were at times aggressive toward staff, toys, and other children. While behaviors varied, the children's reactions were described as most clearly manifested through their relationships, particularly with their mothers. Two-year-old "Mary" was unable to "relate to her mother" after spending seven weeks in hospital without a single visit from her parents. "Stanley" scratched, bit, and kicked his mother in the days following their reunion. "Brenda," who had been regularly visited by her parents while in a sanatorium for fourteen weeks, was "subdued and followed her mother everywhere."[74] She showed such extreme dependence that her mother feared she would never return to her carefree pre-hospitalization self.

In line with the Tavistock Clinic's ethos, "no research without therapy," Bowlby and Robertson wanted their research program to help prevent future children from experiencing the trauma of separation.[75] They sought to uncover precisely why children's separation from their mothers took the emotional toll that it did and whether its effects might vary according to age, social background, and previous family experiences. The desired endpoint was large-scale change in hospital policies and procedures as one avenue for entirely stamping out emotional deprivation. They "hope[d] that, once the facts were recognized, practice would change." However their early efforts to educate hospital staff about emotional deprivation were largely unsuccessful.[76] Nurses and doctors alike criticized the accuracy of Robertson's observations and questioned Bowlby's speculations about emotional damage. In response, in 1951 Robertson and Bowlby produced a film to provide evidence for what they believed hospital staff failed to recognize. Believing that accurate observation had the power to change even the most stubborn minds, the film did not include any commentary. It was intended to be a "strictly scientific document."[77]

The outcome, entitled *A Two-Year-Old Goes to Hospital*, was shown to physicians, psychologists, nurses, and social workers in 1952. Filmed using a hand-held camera and natural light, it captured Laura's stay in hospital, beginning the day prior to her hospitalization and ending with her departure following her recovery from surgery. The film began by spotlighting Laura's robust demeanor prior to hospitalization: "It takes a lot to make Laura cry," her father reported.[78] While in hospital, Laura twice underwent an uncomfortable procedure for rectal anesthesia. She also reported feeling pain after surgery and again when having her stitches removed. She was visited twice by her mother on her own and, on two other occasions, by her father and mother together. During each visit, which was kept short, the nurse was reluctant to allow Laura to leave her cot for fear that she might accidentally tear out her stitches.

Throughout her hospitalization, Robertson observed Laura from six o'clock every morning until it was time for her to sleep in the evening. He became especially interested in how her "apparent calmness" and "cool façade" would sometimes crack to reveal "much concealed feeling."[79] During these moments, she often became aggressive with her doll, or sobbed and demanded to see her mother. In addition to these displays of distress, Laura masturbated, soiled herself, refused to cooperate with nurses' requests, and showed "excessive concern" for other children's pain. Although Laura's response to separation was described as "understated by reason of this child's unusual degree of control," Robertson and Bowlby maintained that she, like all children undergoing separation from their mothers, experienced distinctive stages of psychological distress: first "protest," then "despair," and finally "detachment."[80] Bowlby explained that Laura initially responded to hospitalization with protest: she frequently called out for her mother and pleaded to return home. As time passed, she reconciled herself to her situation and became more withdrawn. Her outbursts became less frequent. Rather than interpreting this as evidence of her settling in, Bowlby argued that what seemed like adjustment were actually signs of incipient maladjustment. Laura was becoming emotionally detached from her mother. Her withdrawal became more pronounced as days passed, and upon leaving the hospital, Bowlby noted that she walked at some distance from her mother on her way out.[81] Having repressed the trauma of her mother's loss, he explained, Laura did not wholeheartedly welcome this long overdue reunion.

Rather than relying on a large research pool, Bowlby and Robertson intensively studied a small sample of children in short-term care in hospitals, sanatoria, and residential nurseries. *A Two-Year-Old Goes to Hospital* was presented as an emblematic illustration of the psychological damage that all children experienced when undergoing maternal separation. Counterintuitively, Bowlby argued that once children appeared to have stopped mourning the loss of their mothers and seemed more willing to remain in hospital, they were suffering more than when they had shown clearer signs of distress. While staff might think that the children had adjusted, they had in fact entered a pathological state of repression. Rather than allowing themselves to feel their frustrated attachment to their mothers, children undergoing separation actively suppressed painful emotions. It was this emotional "split" that, according to

Bowlby, most characterized the psychological condition of the juvenile delinquent and adult criminal.

Bowlby also gathered data relating to the longer-term effects of separation. The most extensive sample came from research on children who had been housed in sanatoria for several years in the 1940s. When they were studied by Bowlby and his research team—including psychologist Mary Ainsworth and psychiatric social workers Mary Boston and Dina Rosenbluth—these formerly institutionalized children were young adults who could reflect on their experiences in the sanatoria and their lives since leaving. He compared these young people to a control group of individuals who had never been separated from their families but were of similar ages and IQs. Bowlby reported that those institutionalized as children had experienced far less success making friends and achieving social goals:[82] 63% were rated "maladjusted" and only 14% were deemed "well adjusted" after the experience of long-term hospitalization.

Biological data from contemporary animal researchers further strengthened Bowlby's claims about the developmental importance of maternal love. Over the course of the 1950s, he became very interested in ethology, the emerging biological sub-discipline that developed evolutionary explanations for instinctive behaviors.[83] In ethology, Bowlby saw promising possibilities for understanding both the potential innateness of social impulses and the emotional damage that followed from separation experiences. When he encountered Konrad Lorenz's theory of imprinting in birds in 1951, he was immediately drawn to the view that instinct was hardwired in all animals and central to early behavioral responses. By 1958, following several years of separation research, Bowlby concluded that maternal attachment in human beings was a primary biological instinct. He argued that this instinct's frustration, especially between the ages of one and five, gave way to (potentially debilitating) anxiety: "The hypothesis advanced is that, whenever an instinctual response system is activated and is unable for any reason to reach termination, a form of anxiety results."[84] Because he saw the need for human relationships as instinctive, he claimed that emotional development could be obstructed if the individual were prevented from connecting with others. Thus, for Bowlby and his adherents, the prevention of mother-child separation was key for healthy development.

For Bowlby and Robertson, having their findings concerning the negative impact of mother-child separation be channeled toward positive psychological ends ultimately meant eliminating all spaces and practices that disrupted family cohesion. They supported male-breadwinning, female-homemaking families as ideal for producing emotionally secure and fully relational adults. As both saw it, the welfare state could play a crucial role in making this family arrangement possible, if priority was given to ensuring that married couples had sufficient economic security to make it not strictly financially necessary for both parents to work. Eliminating economic insecurity was certainly important for enabling one parent—typically the mother—to refrain from paid work. However sickness, disability, childbirth, and imprisonment for criminal offenses continued to present challenges to family stability, in addition to unmarried motherhood, divorce, and widowhood. More targeted social reform was therefore necessary to ensure that all British children experienced uninterrupted parental care.

To this end, Bowlby and Robertson sought to abolish the overuse of in-patient hospitalization and promoted healthcare provisions that allowed people to be treated at home. Although many medical professionals might have seen the hospitalization of sick children for weeks, even months, as acceptable for recovery, and alongside this viewed infrequent family visits as keeping stressful disturbances to a minimum, Bowlby and Robertson campaigned to have all restrictions on parental visits removed. They were largely successful in achieving this aim. By 1958, *A Two-Year-Old Goes to Hospital* had become "a standard 'text' in the training of professional workers and administrators in many parts of the world," and "continue[d] to stimulate community discussion of the needs of young children in hospitals and other institutions."[85] It was submitted as key evidence to the Platt Committee on the Welfare of Children in Hospital, and, having a major impact on the committee's findings, "the Minister made it clear that [unrestricted visiting] was now official policy."[86] Following the national televising of *A Two-Year-Old Goes to Hospital*, the patient advocacy group Mother Care for Children in Hospital was formed in 1961 to persuade hospitals across Britain to adopt more open visiting policies.[87]

Although Bowlby saw unrestricted hospital visiting as necessary for safeguarding children's emotional health, he did not believe it made a significant difference in protecting the fragile emotions of children under age five. For young children, he and Robertson advocated a policy of having mothers accompany their sick children into hospital for the full duration of their stay. A central feature of the campaign to change institutional practices in Britain thus came to include a focus on introducing mother-child units in children's wards in general hospitals.

To gather support for their campaign, Robertson produced a film study in 1958 of one such mother-child unit at Amersham Hospital—entitled *Going to Hospital with Mother*—in which he demonstrated the many benefits of allowing mothers to accompany their children into hospital. At Amersham, one ward had been set aside for mothers accompanying their children since 1953: glass partitions formed cubicles, and each was fitted with a cot for a sick child, a bed for their mother, a sink, a locker, and a chair. *Nursery World* described each cubicle as "a room of their own."[88] In addition to caring for their sick children, the mothers on the children's ward helped with nursing and other hospital chores, thus lightening nurses' workload and enabling them to spend extra time with children whose mothers were unable to reside in hospital. Robertson's film showed the mothers at Amersham helping with one another's children and having tea together during quiet hours. Robertson emphasized parents' widespread approval of Amersham: during the five years of the mother-child unit's existence, half of the sick children admitted who were under five had been accompanied by their mothers.[89]

The film highlighted twenty-month-old Sally's cheerful response to her hospital stay with her mother at her side. The stark contrast between this film's protagonist and sullen Laura did not go unnoticed by viewers:

> Naturally, interest centers on the robust assertive little patient—so different from the sensitive Laura of the first film with her unusual control and silent suffering. Nevertheless, twenty-month-old Sally has plenty of disagreeable and frightening experiences to endure, and the way she meets and deals with them in her mother's arms and recovers from them with Mother by her side, is a heartening revelation of what more may be done in the near future, to make "hospitalization" an event which the average child, even of tender years, may take in his stride.[90]

Unlike Laura, Sally remained a resilient child, who responded to the challenges of hospitalization, surgery, and recovery with relative ease in her mother's care. Her compliance with hospital procedures was presented as possible because she felt secure.

By the late 1950s, Bowlby and Robertson's views on separation had met with widespread support within medical, governmental, and, especially, popular arenas—the BBC and other media outlets (including *The Observer*, *News Chronicle*, *Housewife*, and *Nursery World*) received hundreds of letters in response to the televising of both *A Two-Year-Old Goes to Hospital* and *Going to Hospital with Mother*.[91] In 1958, the British Medical Association Council backed not only unrestricted hospital visiting but the admission of mothers into hospital alongside their sick children, stressing that "Allowing the mothers to remain in hospital with infants and young children and take part in their care should be the rule in all children's departments."[92] The 1959 Platt Report on the welfare of children in hospital stressed popular recognition of the positive impact of the mother-child ward on children's emotional wellbeing, stating that:

> Hospitals that have tried admitting mothers with their children claim that the young child shows less emotional disturbance on his return home, that the experience is beneficial to nurses and mothers and creates a happy atmosphere in the ward ... We think that there is much to be said for the extension of the practice ... The correspondence received by the BBC makes it clear that the practice is gaining popularity with parents.[93]

That same year, *The Observer* announced that Bowlby and Robertson had been right all along: "How seriously and lastingly young children may suffer if separated for even a day or two from their mothers ... has been abundantly proved."[94]

A world in which children's emotional development was truly protected meant a serious scaling back in the use of institutions as places of treatment. In the view of Robertson, Bowlby, and their growing body of supporters, a child never needed to enter hospital for long stays and could ideally have most of their nursing done at home. When considering the most effective place for healing, arguments against the use of hospitals looked to the home as a more authentically therapeutic space. And for those more intensive medical procedures that required young patients to stay in hospital, their mother's presence as a co-resident avoided the potentially serious emotional harm caused by separation.

Bowlby's emphasis on the developmental importance of continuous maternal care intensified remarkably after WWII. In 1939, in his presentation for membership to the British Psychoanalytical Society, Bowlby had proposed that a limited amount of separation was unlikely to harm a child: "Provided breaks are not too long ... there seems no evidence to suppose that the child who is always with his mother is any better off than the child who only sees her for a few hours a day and not at all for odd holiday weeks."[95] The arguments put forward in his WHO report, however, showed that he had abandoned this more moderate position by 1951. Rather than supporting the idea that a mother could take breaks from childcare, and even work outside of the home without causing her young child psychological damage, Bowlby now declared uninterrupted maternal care necessary for preventing the harms associated with "maternal deprivation." He pushed his earlier argument for the necessity of attentive childcare much further, now additionally claiming that mothers played an integral role in their children's immature psyches as surrogates for their egos and superegos until these developed. Bowlby's perception of human beings as fundamentally biologically and psychologically relational directly contributed to his outspoken support for the Labour party and the welfare state. As he saw it, emotional and social development were intersubjective from the earliest moments of life and if properly nurtured, responsible citizenship was guaranteed.

Although the popularization of Bowlby's research did help legitimize the British post-WWII government's commitment to protecting the male-breadwinning, female-homemaking family, prominent social scientists, ethologists, and psychiatrists contested the priority that he placed on maternal care. His most renowned critics in the 1950s disputed the importance that he attributed to periods of disruption in the mother-child relationship. Family psychiatrist J.G. Howells praised Bowlby for "perform[ing] a great and continuing service to child psychiatry by focusing attention on the emotional life of the young child," but criticized him for "confus[ing] separation with privation."[96] In Howells's view, Bowlby's focus on mother-child separation took attention away from the damaging effects of bad parenting. In his view, emotional "privation" more often resulted from children's neglect and bad treatment within—rather than outside of—families. Margaret Mead had initially enthusiastically supported maternal deprivation theory; however, she became very critical after reading accounts of successes with group child rearing in many parts of Africa. In 1954, she urged that maternal deprivation was "a new and subtle form of antifeminism in which men—under the guise of exalting the importance of maternity—are tying women more tightly to their children than has been thought necessary since the invention of bottle feeding and baby carriages."[97] Still others, including American psychologist Harry Harlow, questioned the emphasis that Bowlby placed on the mother-child relationship and argued that fathers could perform as perfectly satisfactory primary caregivers in children's emotional upbringing.[98] Notably, while Bowlby's ideas raised significant controversy for the importance that he attributed to mothers, few took issue with his pronouncement that healthy emotional development fundamentally depended on close loving relationships from infancy onward. Even critics praised Bowlby's contributions in making this widely understood. The key point of controversy was whether the child was best off if they attached primarily to one person (their mother), two (both parents), or several (a wider range of family members and close neighbors). The immediate postwar consensus was that children's early emotional relationships had a lasting impact on the kinds of adults that they grew up to be. This bound the (presumably emotionally oriented) family to society in consequential new ways.

British perceptions of the looming threat of emotional deprivation in children was certainly supported by respected child development experts and child welfare advocates. However popular British media—including films, plays, and novels—also spotlighted the dangers of emotional deprivation for a variety of audiences. The figure of the insecure child, a victim of circumstances they had not chosen, appeared with increasing frequency in the British media after WWII. A 1950 film adaptation of Phyllis Hambledon's 1948 novel *No Difference to Me*, re-titled *No Place for Jennifer*, focused on ten-year-old Jennifer's emotional breakdown following her parents' divorce. The film showed her falling behind at school and crying when overhearing arguments between her estranged parents as she confessed to feeling "torn in two."[99] Jennifer experienced temporary relief when brought to a local child guidance clinic for bi-weekly appointments where, through play therapy, she could express her "mixed up feelings." The film took a dramatic turn when her therapy sessions were ended because of a move, and she ran away to live with a family who offered to take her in. Ultimately, the film showed Jennifer's parents acknowledging that they had caused their daughter's emotional pain and agreeing to allow Jennifer to live with a new family. The final scene focused on Jennifer's euphoric reaction to being accepted into a "real family," where she had not only two devoted parents, but also siblings, to rely on for love and support.

Several other films and plays echoed *No Place for Jennifer*'s warning of divorce's emotional dangers from the child's point of view. The 1953 films *Background* and *Twice Upon a Time* both focused on the negative emotional impact of divorce by showcasing the child's perspective.[100] British child development experts lauded these productions. Hambledon's book was only referenced favorably following its publication. Mary Braybury mentioned David Lean's production of *Oliver Twist* as presenting an accurate representation of the effects of deprivation at the 1956 meeting of the NAMH:

> the children in it are stunted, thin, unhappy, and aghast at the freedom that asks for "more." So it is not just a high-faluting idea of psychologists; it is something recognised by thinking, observing members of the general community, and it is the effect, I would submit, of losing home care, and, when I say "home care," I mean the home in the sense of a place where love and family prevail.[101]

Films featuring emotionally deprived children warned of the dangers of broken homes, of homeless children who had no recourse to foster care, and of mothers' separation from their children following their hospitalization.[102] In doing so, they reflected growing concern for children's emotional wellbeing back to audiences. Playing to audiences' readiness to accept warnings of childhood trauma, melodramatic representations demonstrated the repercussions of emotional life within the context of the reader or spectator's own heightened emotion. Although critics remarked upon the low artistic merit of many of these films, many continued to watch and take in their highly emotional message.

Relationality in Welfare-State Britain

In post-WWII Britain, the prospect of children's vulnerability to emotional harm raised enormous anxiety about the future—both individual futures *and* the future of Britain. This was not the first or only time that children would hold such a dominant place in a collective imagination. As Lee Edelman points out, the futurity embodied by the figure of the child has played a central role in hardening heteronormative values in the modern West, particularly since heterosexuality is presumed to be directed toward child production.[103] While heterosexuality has been invested with hope for the future and good citizenship—with the child standing as a symbol of potential for both—homosexuality has been linked to loss of reproductive potential and the end of humanity.

The vulnerable, potentially deprived, child in post-WWII Britain was, above all, a relational figure. This child was not a self-contained individual who required extensive training for good citizenship to one day result. This was a child who needed a steady supply of their mother's love to develop into an emotionally healthy, well-adjusted adult. Carolyn Steedman points out that childhood became central to understandings of psychological interiority in the nineteenth century. The "interiorised self," she explains, was "understood to be the product of a personal history, [and this] was most clearly expressed in the idea of 'childhood,' and the idea of 'the child.'"[104] In Britain in the mid-twentieth century decades childhood was even more prominently connected to understandings of the primary psychological importance of relationality. This was a view of human sociability that focused not on large groups (such as the neighborhood, workplace, labor union, town, city, or nation). This was an intimate form of sociability that was rooted in deep emotional connection between two (and *only* two) people—a devoted mother and her emotionally fragile child.

In the 1930s, following the era that saw the rise of the psychologized "interiorized self" that Steedman describes, British and American mental health and social work professionals became more concerned about children's vulnerability to their social circumstances. "Maladjustment" had entered the popular lexicon in Britain by the late 1920s as a concept linked to the perceived childhood origins of criminality, alcoholism, prostitution, and unmarried motherhood. Each of these social problems was seen as stemming from early "adjustment" to a pathological social situation and an ensuing failure to "adjust" to the demands of respectable middle-class society.

Given children's presumed vulnerability to lasting harm, alongside their importance for ensuring better days ahead in an era of imperial decline and economic struggle, Britain's new welfare government assumed responsibility for children's healthy emotional development. This chapter reveals connections between emotions and socio-economic life after WWII. Scholarship by Viviana Zelizer, Eva Illouz, and Arlie Hochschild has challenged presumptions of inherent separateness between financial and emotional life by highlighting forms of intimacy that are reliant upon financial transactions, such as paid childcare and prostitution.[105] This chapter builds on this work by demonstrating the emotional underpinnings of the British welfare state. It argues that far from detaching emotion from money, this post-WWII "classless" universalizing project treated financial and emotional security as intertwined. The welfare state's solution to instabilities generated by economic depression and total war brought money and love into closer connection as twin features of the same goal of guaranteeing citizens' security.

Scientific research into emotional deprivation played an important role in supporting the British welfare state's expansive responsibilities toward citizens in the 1950s. Psychological experts and their social reform allies made children's emotional struggles visible and proposed socially transformative solutions to protect children from lasting harm. The Children Act of 1948 prioritized family and "family-like" environments as ideal for healthy child development. This was given further specificity by child development specialists including John Bowlby, James Robertson, Mary Ainsworth, and others. The ideal loving family environment was most strongly marked by a mother-child relationship that was uninterrupted either by paid work and use of day nurseries or extended hospital stays, whether for mothers (including those who had just given birth) or their sick children. Government-led measures were extended over the course of the 1950s in pursuit of creating and stabilizing male-breadwinning, female-homemaking families. This was an ambitious program in which children without families would be provided with close substitutes, and institutional practices that caused harmful parent-child separations would be eliminated. Many of the places where children spent substantial time were scrutinized for their capacity to either add to or take away from their access to intimate relationships.

Bowlby played a crucial role in rationalizing the post-WWII preoccupation with children's emotional vulnerability through his highly publicized research program. The popularity of his theories explaining the origins of juvenile delinquency and worrying consequences of child homelessness revealed the urgency of these issues for the British public (and beyond, as seen in the international scale of the research and audience). "Maternal deprivation" provided a compelling rationale for reforms in hospital policies and for opposition to the use of children's residential institutions. Later, it would help support government opposition to the provision of nurseries for working mothers.[106] The idea that children required continuous maternal care placed the emotional wellbeing of future adult citizens ahead of shorter-term financial goals.

Despite the lack of scientific consensus surrounding Bowlby's findings, the British government remained steadfastly committed to the idea that children were emotionally secure in male-breadwinning, female-homemaking families. Ultimately, Bowlby's conclusions about the primary importance of continuous maternal care resonated with already existing concerns about child development—and the consequences of emotional life experiences more generally—than those of other experts (like Margaret Mead, for example), making "Bowlbyism" a significant cultural and political force. As Edelman has noted, concern for child welfare has pervaded modern Western politics in nuanced, yet all-embracing, ways. Rather than being tied to one partisan political agenda, it has come to shape "the logic within which the political itself must be thought."[107] Widespread anxiety surrounding children's emotions in the 1940s and 1950s was connected to broader fears about the direction of Britain's uncertain future and doubt that even the most benevolent and competently run state could effectively institute positive changes without partnering with British families (the real source of social and political power).

Bowlby had been explicit about the wider political implications of his concern for children's psychological welfare since the late 1930s. Folding a discussion of parenting into an explanation for war, he and his friend economist and Labour MP Evan Durbin established connections between family life, emotional development, and wider socio-political structures. Asking the timely question in 1938 of whether "democracy or socialism or a peasant economy—or any other form of society—makes in itself, for peace,"[108] they proposed that perhaps certain *kinds* of people favored both democracy and liberal values. Thus, peaceful individuals were "not peaceful because they are democratic. *They are peaceful and democratic because they are the kind of people they are.*"[109] As the primary technique for making democratic "kind[s] of people," Durbin and Bowlby proposed that children's "emotional education" in families bore a much closer relationship to socio-political cultures than had previously been understood. In their view, it was the family, rather than government or civil society, that was responsible for creating good citizens.

The belief that family intimacy was the most reliable foundation for social stability was a core tenet of the British welfare state in the decade immediately following WWII. The Children Act 1948 and government provision of family benefits and family healthcare were central features of the welfare state. New reforms to adoption and fostering and resistance to public daycare facilities similarly expressed the government's investment in ensuring the integrity of the male-breadwinning, female-homemaking family as the basic unit of British society.

That mother love was identified by the early 1950s as necessary for children's healthy development infused social politics and institutional practices with a new psychological emphasis on the far-reaching importance of emotional life. It also produced enormous guilt and distress in many women who were forced to shoulder unrealistic new burdens, especially as it was never clear precisely how much love was enough. This is the subject of the next chapter.

3
Problem Mothers

Maternal Neglect, Mental Illness, and the Fragility of Female Maturity

> Being a good wife and mother is a skilled job, bringing its own rewards and satisfactions in a way a repetitive job cannot. The standard of child care and housecraft is much higher for all homes today than it was 50 years ago.
>
> —Women's Liberal Federation, *The Great Partnership*, 1949

> It is ... curious that, in view of the scientific and practical concern given to the disruption of the mother-child pair, the psychological problems of the child should receive almost exclusive emphasis and those of the mother so little.
>
> —Tom Main, "A Fragment on Mothering," 1958

In May 1961, *The Observer* published a three-part exposé entitled "Miserable Married Women," prompted by hundreds of women across the UK confessing their overwhelming dissatisfaction with marriage and motherhood. The series of articles, produced by ITV broadcaster and documentary filmmaker Elaine Grand, responded to more than two hundred sympathetic letters received in the days following a recently aired BBC afternoon television program—"The Housewife at Home: Is She Bored and Lonely?"—in which new mothers shared their personal reactions to motherhood. While many contributors confessed to feeling shame for having wasted their education and early work experience by opting to stay home with their children, the most prominent complaint was "another kind of guilt, stem[ming] from disappointment over their emotional reaction to motherhood."[1] One correspondent, a former teacher, described how she "had been through all the stages that follow even the most contented motherhood: the loneliness, the boredom, the frustration, and the guilt."[2] Another woman, identifying herself as an artist before becoming a mother, stressed that, "The lonely woman is almost without exception the mother of under-school-age children, which means she is absolutely tied."[3] Most confessed to finding round-the-clock childcare not only physically challenging, but also mentally dulling.

The Intimate State. Teri Chettiar, Oxford University Press. © Oxford University Press 2023.
DOI: 10.1093/oso/9780190931209.003.0004

Some expressed real concern for "the possibility of mental illness resulting from their boredom."[4]

> They write: "I would go so far as to say that the stress and strain of managing without proper facilities during children's younger years does infinite harm to the mental health of mothers *and* their families." [and] "I would like to see some figures on the mental disturbance of women who are temperamentally unsuited to an exclusively housebound existence."[5]

Grand was emphatic that, "these letters did not come from neurotics or hysterics," but showed how many young mothers suffered because of unmet hopes that motherhood would be a predominantly joyful experience.[6] It was not enough to simply become a mother to successfully meet motherhood's demands. The women who wrote in revealed how defeating it felt to be unable to muster up the positive emotions they had expected to feel when caring for their children.

It made sense for so many women to experience such despair when motherhood was widely portrayed as overwhelmingly enjoyable during and after WWII. Parenting literature—from guides to breastfeeding to practical advice on raising young children—highlighted pleasure in motherhood. Dr. Merrell Middlemore's bestselling 1941 *The Nursing Couple* emphasized the enjoyment of breastfeeding as necessary for its success, concluding that "if breast feeding is to succeed it is as important for the mother to enjoy her task as it is for her breasts to be fully developed."[7] Renowned child psychologist Donald Woods Winnicott informed mothers in his BBC lectures in the 1940s and 1950s that "the pleasure the mother takes in what she does for the infant" was crucial for effective child-rearing: "No book rules can take the place of this feeling a mother has for her infant's needs, which enables her to make at times an almost exact adaptation to those needs."[8] In her popular 1946 BBC talks, psychiatrist Doris Odlum highlighted the "tremendous joy" that mothers experienced in simply "being needed by their children ... even though it does mean a 24-hour job seven days a week."[9] This perception that women, on the whole, enjoyed caring for their children was also emphasized in popular publications on both sides of the Atlantic. A 1958 article in the US women's magazine *Ladies Home Journal* stressed modern mothers' emotional contentment:

> Whether they work at outside jobs or not, today's young mothers find their greatest satisfaction in home, husband and children. They realize that they are not men, and they don't want to be. Nor would they willingly change places with their husbands if they could. On the whole, they are pretty well satisfied with things are they are—probably about as much so as men.[10]

That a woman might experience any difficulty (or even ambiguity) in devoting herself to her child was not addressed in the vast majority of postwar parenting descriptions.[11] Child rearing gurus, from Winnicott in Britain to Benjamin Spock in the United States, insisted that "ordinary" mother love, which was proclaimed instinctive rather than learned, was the essential foundation for successful child rearing.[12] Parenting experts doled out advice to help new mothers become more attuned to their natural maternal impulses and did not address the possibility that expectations surrounding "natural" motherhood might require a conscious management of emotion, and even possibly involve the acquisition of new emotional skills. As Arlie Hochschild and others have emphasized, care work—whether paid or unpaid, as in the case of uncompensated childcare—requires the deliberate cultivation of feeling toward the person being cared for.[13] Care work constitutes "emotion action," or "emotion work," rather than "mere being."[14] That is, it is not an automatic response to the presence of a vulnerable person in need of care. Hochschild argues that the view that maternal emotions are straightforwardly given is prevalent in societies ambivalent about care, where such activities are relegated to the private world of home and family.[15] Instead, those prized emotional attitudes in childcare, such as selfless devotion and stoic self-sacrifice, are achieved by managing other emotional reactions, including anger, worry, and detachment since these have been spotlighted as harmful to children's healthy emotional development. Far from acknowledging the possible ties between emotion and work, postwar child-rearing gurus presented the emotions associated with effective childrearing as naturally effortless.

The idea that a mother's caring for a child might constitute work is typically associated with second-wave feminists' criticisms of the male-breadwinning, female-homemaking nuclear family and the real and unacknowledged labor burdens that this socio-sexual division of labor placed on women.[16] Although connections between childcare, emotion, and work were little pursued in the 1940s and 1950s, the possibility that childcare relied upon deliberately cultivating an emotional facility for loving relationality was discussed in seemingly unlikely places in Britain after WWII. The newly created in-patient family psychiatry units and other rehabilitative spaces that sought to reform mothers who failed to care adequately for their children saw their primary aim as inculcating their female residents with the emotional capacity to rear psychologically healthy future citizens. In other words, there is a longer and more complicated history to the notion that self-sacrificial maternal love is neither a straightforward product of a woman's biological nature nor an inevitable cornerstone of the mother-child relationship.[17]

Postwar child development specialists' speculations about the impact of "maternal deprivation" on children rarely considered the mother's experience so as to understand why a child might be "deprived" of her attention in the first place. In 1961, when the BBC and *The Observer* investigated the suffering experienced by many middle-class mothers, women's diverse and often complicated responses to motherhood were still left out of most women's magazines and parenting literature. In medical and psychological arenas, maternal dissatisfaction was interpreted as a symptom of neurotic disorder ranging from low-lying depression to severe anxiety. The diversity of women's responses to the demands of motherhood kept psychiatrists occupied as the numbers of female sufferers of anxiety and depression—many of whom were mothers of young children—significantly outstripped their male counterparts in the decades after WWII. When Mick Jagger declared valium "mother's little helper," in the winter of 1965, most of the growing supply of tranquilizing and anti-depressant medications were being prescribed to women, many married and middle-class.[18]

This chapter examines the increasingly medicalized postwar problem of the "bad" mother, who figured as variously detached and overbearing. During the same moment that prominent social reformers, social workers, and psychiatrists were focused on ensuring that children receive attentive care to prevent emotional deprivation, a small, but not insignificant, number of lobbyists and experts—including feminist Eva Hubback of the Women's Group on Public Welfare and Thomas F. Main, medical director of the Cassel Hospital for Functional Nervous Disorders—were attempting to solve child neglect by beginning not with the "deprived" child but with the distressed mother. They insisted that she suffered as much as, if not more than, her child and needed help, whether in the form of social assistance or psychological therapy. Their initiatives made the experiences of overburdened, dissatisfied, and apathetic mothers newly visible. Despite this, this chapter shows that they did not challenge the widespread belief that motherhood was a naturally satisfying emotional experience. Instead, psychiatric and social reform initiatives focusing on rehabilitating troubled mothers prioritized the cultivation of intimate relationships between mothers and their children in instances where these were seen as wanting. They treated nurturing emotions as fundamentally connected to a woman's adult psychosocial role—one that emerged from healthy feminine psychological maturity—rather than a form of skilled work, for which she should be justly compensated.

At the heart of this chapter are expert-driven postwar initiatives developed to cultivate positive maternal emotion in cases where a woman's capacity to form a loving relationship with her child (or children) had been seriously impaired. Parent education literature and advice columns in women's magazines filled gaps in many women's understanding of their duties and innate capacities as mothers. However, in more critical instances of maternal failure, such as diagnosed cases of post-partum mental illness (in Britain typically referred to as "puerperal psychosis" until the late 1970s) and women convicted of child neglect, more hands-on measures were needed to rehabilitate mothers to become capable of effectively loving their children. When given "the good start" of their mother's love, the person that developed was not only physically healthy and emotionally well-adjusted; they were, as Donald Winnicott described it, both "independent *and* society-minded adult individuals."[19]

This chapter examines the emerging idea in the 1940s and 1950s that mother love would flourish only under certain circumstances by examining the specialized therapeutic and rehabilitative sites designed for making positive maternal emotion possible. Exploring initiatives aimed at resolving maternal failure, this chapter provides a lens to see how motherhood came to be conceived by some as an overwhelmingly difficult emotional undertaking in the decades after WWII. Although this vision of motherhood did not invoke the language of emotional work or labor, it presented attentive motherhood as arrived at through conscious practiced effort. Some went so far as to claim that a great number of women might be unable to undertake the enormous responsibility of childcare without considerable assistance, whether in the form of family allowances, social work, or accessible mental health services.

In examining postwar responses to mothers' perceived failures, this chapter explores the many—sometimes contradictory—means through which a mother's love for her child was cultivated when a woman's life circumstances had ostensibly interfered with nature taking its course. In doing so, it uncovers the complicated consequences of the postwar prizing of mother love as a natural feature of female adulthood when set against growing evidence that the conditions under which girls grew to adulthood and their circumstances as mothers might have crucial roles to play. Services geared toward rehabilitating mothers were underwritten by a desire for social reform. They promised not only to help individual women better cope with pregnancy, birth, and childcare but also guarantee a more stable and secure future for all citizens.

Poverty and the Problem of Maternal Neglect

Over the course of many months spanning 1946 into 1947, the Women's Group on Public Welfare conducted a study of women imprisoned for child cruelty and neglect to understand why women convicted of such offences had so egregiously failed to perform their maternal responsibilities. The group—created during the war to promote the welfare of women and children—had previously published *Our Towns: A Close Up*, a widely read 1943 study of the negative impact of poverty, unemployment, and bad housing on women and children.[20] In 1946, in the wake of the Curtis Report's publication, they turned their attention to those women that the Curtis Committee had declared irredeemably deviant, inquiring into their life circumstances and seeking to understand how their capacity to care for their children had been so gravely impaired. What, they asked, were the specific "influences which lead to behaviour so contrary to natural instinct as for parents to ill-treat or neglect their children?"[21] Their objective was to understand the problem of neglect "so that appropriate intervention and treatment may be provided."[22] Their report was meant to serve as a follow-up to the problems that the Curtis Report had identified.

Questionnaires were distributed to women imprisoned for child neglect at Holloway prison asking what might have prevented them from committing their crimes. Twelve women answered, and from this small sample the group concluded that financial stressors were to blame. The women described a "difficult to break" cycle that began with financial mismanagement, was followed by poverty, malnutrition, and ill-health, and ended in total apathy.[23] The picture that emerged was of a woman who had never entirely stopped feeling love for her children. But lack of help with her relentless daily responsibilities had worn her down and made her unable to provide adequate care:

We are left with the impression not of willful, cruel, reprehensible mothers (though these do exist), but of women struggling, with inadequate equipment, mental and material, to deal with problems which would tax even those highly endowed.[24]

The committee's chair, social reformer and birth control advocate Eva Hubback, maintained that a voluntary organization like the NSPCC could not prevent children from being neglected in their own homes. Only the state had adequate resources for this enormous task.[25] Hubback argued that although no fewer than one hundred thousand children had been dealt with by the NSPCC in 1948, a number that "almost equal[ed] the number of Curtis children,"[26] this number would be much larger "if a higher standard of child care were demanded by the law in accordance with present day knowledge of a child's emotional needs."[27]

Although the group focused on financial burdens, the report did not propose large-scale socio-economic restructuring under the aegis of the new welfare state. Their preferred solution instead lay with state-funded social services that would prevent mothers from "breaking down."[28] In Hubback's view, child neglect could be prevented by expanding Britain's health services, providing rehabilitative centers for overtaxed mothers, and having social workers focus on helping families at risk. The aim was early education of young women for motherhood, making health services more widely accessible, and having social workers assist mothers in managing childcare burdens before problems arose.[29]

The targeting of mothers—rather than parents—as the recipients of the proposed provisions was deliberate. This is especially striking since the Women's Group for Public Welfare noted that those families that struggled most were headed by widowed fathers. Despite this, researchers "remarked again and again that the father's deficiencies were not the determining factor" in child neglect. Rather, they looked to the "incapable mother," since it was mothers rather than fathers who were presumed to be "the coping stone of the [family] structure."[30] On the whole, the group characterized child neglect as a problem that was primarily emotional in nature, even if economic factors were emphasized as playing an initiating role. Since mothers were described as providing the emotional "'temper' to the household"—with fathers influencing only "the economic situation of the family"—it was mothers who were seen as most directly responsible for both preventing and perpetuating neglect.[31]

Targeting a struggling mother's life circumstances was presented as the best, even if costly, approach to resolving the emotional causes of neglect. Both the Women's Group on Public Welfare and a 1956 report published jointly by the British Medical Association (BMA) and the Magistrates' Association commented favorably on an existing residential option, the Brentwood Recuperation Centre for Mothers and Children in Cheshire, in both treating child neglect and preventing its future occurrence. At Brentwood, the first residential home for "problem mothers," fourteen women, accompanied by their children under the age of eight, shared house chores and child-rearing responsibilities. The center's aim was to ease overburdened mothers' workload by having them live in a community setting for one to four months, where they were supported by paid staff. At the same time, the space was meant to cultivate respect (even desire) for a well-ordered and hygienic home:

> It will be education, but never obviously so; it will provide opportunities of learning by observation and participation rather than by precept, about how to run a house and cook and look after children and how to do simple mending and dressmaking. It will provide the opportunities for the building up of health, physical and mental, which a period of relaxation in a happy, well ordered atmosphere can supply ... It will achieve much of its purpose because it demonstrates a standard of life, not remote and unattainable, yet higher than the problem families are accustomed to, and shows it to be a purposeful and happy one and therefore desirable.[32]

It is noteworthy that the women who spent time recuperating at Brentwood in the years following WWII emphasized poor health, poverty, and bad housing as the major issues contributing to their need for rehabilitative care.[33] Extended exposure to Brentwood's hygienic surroundings not only provided an ideal backdrop for rest, but residents were also meant to specifically take in the positive impact that a tidy well-managed home had on family happiness. It was intended, above all, to enable its residents to form "happy" relationships with their children:

> Many of the case histories indicate a deprived and unhappy childhood. We try to give them a home in the fullest sense—a place where there is order and cleanliness and where it is easy to give and to receive affection ... To help to create a happy relationship between mother and child is the ultimate purpose of Brentwood's work.[34]

The BMA committee recognized this particular benefit in residential treatment to which both mothers and their children were admitted. Their report presented the "ideal solution" to child cruelty and neglect as one in which "the whole family could be sent for a period of re-education."[35] By 1959, this was the approach that Brentwood was taking, with husbands spending weekends there with their wives and children, "join[ing] in the life of the household and help[ing] in washing dishes and cleaning rooms."[36] In addition, staff would discuss "relevant family problems" with willing couples.[37] Physician Mary Sheridan's 1956 study of close to one hundred mothers charged with child neglect affirmed that the children in such residential centers improved rapidly as their mothers learned how to run a clean and well-functioning household through example.[38]

Both Brentwood and the studies that recommended its use focused on the emotional factors underlying neglect and presented poverty as a circumstance that negatively impacted some women because of the emotional strain that it caused. Although all early postwar studies of child neglect were focused on rehabilitating mothers—particularly if they were married and had a stable home to return to—none of the researchers focused on measures directed at the family's lack of financial means.

Instead, low-income mothers were seen as needing supplementary education and health services to both learn how to cope with their trying circumstances and be provided opportunities for rest when their lives became exceptionally difficult. The underlying problem was seen as a relational one—whether poor relationships with their own mothers in childhood or strained relationships with their husbands.[39]

It is important to note that a mother-child rehabilitation center like Brentwood was favored by those focusing on maternal neglect since it offered temporary shelter from the slums where "problem families" often lived but did not address the complex question of how impoverished urban neighborhoods might be improved. Although these studies broke the silence surrounding maternal neglect—by refusing to dismiss it as a problem for the prison or the psychiatric hospital—they failed to address the problem of poverty and instead focused on emotions and women's capacity to parent effectively despite their challenging circumstances. They argued that it was a mother's emotional stores that needed replenishing and not her financial resources. Britain's welfare state was presented as a provider of services that would reinvigorate maternal love rather than offer low-income families more adequate financial means and greater economic security.

Maternal Neglect as a Psychological Problem

If, in a general sense, the problem of child neglect lay with the impoverished mother whose circumstances had rendered her incapable of adequately loving her child, then how to explain child neglect in middle-class families? J.B. Priestley flagged this question in his preface to the Women's Group on Public Welfare's 1948 report, urging that middle-class child neglect was both likely more prevalent than people assumed and required a different explanation since middle-class mothers typically did not lack education or financial support, mismanage their finances, or suffer from bad nutrition and poor health. Middle-class women's apathy toward their children was an altogether different kind of problem.

Many medical professionals interpreted middle-class women's problems in caring for their children—ranging from a complete lack of interest in motherhood to excessive maternal control—as possible signs of mental illness in the decades after WWII. Women complaining to their physicians that they found infant care to be exceedingly challenging led to suggestions that depression and anxiety following childbirth resulted from the life-transforming experience of having a child, whether it was the mother's first or her sixth. Most physicians, however, denied any direct connection between mental affliction and childbirth; they instead argued that mental illness had merely been triggered when the stress of childbirth inflamed an underlying condition.

The status of post-partum mental illness was subject to polarizing medical dispute in Britain and the United States until the 1990s.[40] However, when British physicians first began to consider it a psychiatric event linked to motherhood, treatment involved a psychotherapeutic aspect. This stands in contrast to the current view that

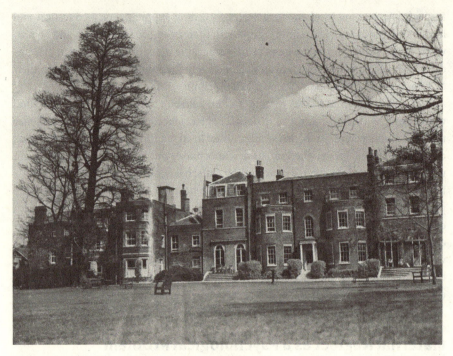

Figure 3.1. Cassel Hospital exterior and grounds.
Source: Mulberry Archive. Reproduced by permission of the Cassel Hospital Charitable Trust.

post-partum mental illness is primarily a physical problem requiring antidepressant medications and hormone therapies (and, in some cases, counseling). The most cutting-edge post-WWII treatment instead focused on the mother and her infant together in a psychiatric hospital setting. The first psychiatric hospital to develop a "mother-baby unit" to treat the mother-child relationship was the Cassel Hospital for Functional Nervous Disorders in Richmond, an affluent suburb in southwest London.

The Cassel had been transformed into one of the world's first "therapeutic communities" after the war under the medical directorship of psychoanalyst and former army psychiatrist Thomas Forrest Main and was brought under the aegis of the NHS in 1948. That same year, mothers and their young children began to be admitted to the hospital together. Staff at the Cassel—a large team that included psychosocial nurses, psychiatrists, occupational therapists, and psychiatric social workers—tailored all aspects of the hospital's daily operations to confront every social and psychological obstacle to loving maternal care. Their treatment of the mother-child pair focused on the emotional difficulties that women experienced when engaged in full-time care of their children.

The Cassel employed therapeutic community techniques for mental treatment, an approach that had evolved after the war alongside the growing use of voluntary mental

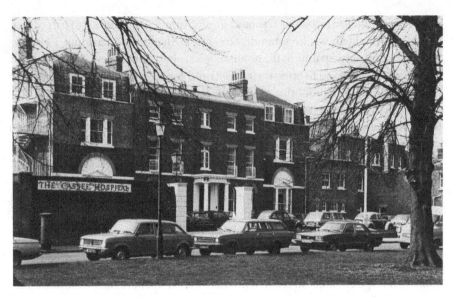

Figure 3.2. Cassel Hospital, street view.
Source: Mulberry Archive. Reproduced by permission of the Cassel Hospital Charitable Trust.

hospital confinement and sought to restore responsibility to the patient as a core feature of therapy. As Tom Main put it, the passive "sick role" was replaced by patients actively participating in restoring their health.[41] The therapeutic community's approach was seen as suited to the growing body of neurotic patients who belonged to the expanding upper working- and middle-classes, educated, and, to a greater extent than previous generations of patients, psychiatrically literate and self-aware.[42] The Cassel abolished the hierarchical relationship that had long existed between staff and patients and made residents' participation in running the hospital's daily operations part of their therapeutic regimen. Staff focused on restoring full humanity to their mentally ill patients. As they saw it, the "sick role" that residents assumed at conventional psychiatric hospitals robbed them of the fullness of their pre-admission identities. It also replicated the dehumanizing power relations that were at the heart of authoritarian regimes, to which Britain's new generation of democracy-championing psychiatrists were very sensitive.

The Cassel had a long history, over several decades, of developing psychotherapeutic treatments, but it was only under Main's direction that the hospital was transformed into a therapeutic community—a term that Main reportedly coined in 1946—and integrated into Britain's NHS.[43] Main had been central to developing the world's first therapeutic community at Northfield Military Hospital in Birmingham during the war. Unlike Northfield, however, two-thirds of the Cassel's patients were female—mainly working- and middle-class women between the ages of twenty-one and thirty-five. This reflected the fact that women were the fastest growing segment of the population afflicted with psychiatric disorders. Just as male patients at Northfield had been encouraged to assume responsibility for running the hospital as part of their treatment—maintaining the grounds, working in the kitchen, creating a hospital newsletter, and participating in the hospital's governing committees—female patients at the Cassel were asked to bring their infants and young children with them to avoid evading the responsibilities that were at the heart of their pre-admission lives. The reason behind this practice was the idea that women, like male residents of therapeutic communities, should retain an uninterrupted connection to their work and social identities. Reversing the increasingly prominent impetus to move mental care into the community, when it came to the treatment of mothers, the Cassel brought the patient's most immediate community into the hospital.

Although most of the Cassel's patients were married mothers of young children, at the outset of Main's medical direction in 1946, hospital staff did not view their symptoms as a reaction to childcare. In 1948, when the first baby was admitted to the hospital with his mother, it was at her request. Main honored this for two reasons. First, since he believed that patients needed to retain an active connection with their pre-admission responsibilities to recover, mothers should not have their childcare duties interrupted. Second, both his association with James Spence at medical school and his wartime work with John Bowlby and Anna Freud had made him very familiar with recent child psychiatric claims that children experienced lasting harm when separated from their mothers. When he admitted the first baby to the hospital with his mother, Main was "interested in the penalties of separating mother and child as they related, first, to the child's physical and emotional health, and, second, and hardly at all, to the woman's confidence in her future capacities as a mother."[44] It was not until the early 1950s, following several years of female patients being admitted with their babies, that staff began to view motherhood as a psychologically meaningful experience.[45] Although some female patients welcomed the option of bringing their young children with them into hospital, many more rejected this proposal when presented to them. They felt that they could not bear to be around their children and feared that they might harm them if they continued to be their main caregivers. It was this strong reaction against bringing children into hospital that convinced Main of its psychological importance. By 1954, mothers' acceptance as patients became conditional upon their willingness to bring their children under age five into hospital with them.

The staff's change in outlook at the Cassel was connected to a transformed psychological understanding of motherhood. In the years following Main's decision to admit the young children of female patients, it was taken as a matter of course that mothering was a form of work, akin to practicing a trade or profession. By 1955, this would change as staff began to treat motherhood not as a collection of work tasks, but as a defining stage in a woman's psychological development. Following from this, post-partum mental illness—or mental illness experienced by any woman with young children—was seen as bearing a special relationship to the mothering *role*. The experience of motherhood, as Main increasingly saw it, represented a major shift in a woman's life as she was forced to renounce her child-like "daughter role" for the adult "mother role." The relationship that she forged with her children was crucial to the success of this major transition: both mother and child were seen as undergoing this developmental milestone together.

While Bowlby had pointed to the absence of a stable maternal presence during the first years of a child's life as the basis for much mental illness in adults, Cassel staff instead sought to understand the psychological conditions that made a mother unable to bond with her child. Main came to understand "mothering" as "a feat of feminine maturity often precariously arrived at."[46] At the same moment that the BMA was declaring the *emotional* neglect of children a form of cruelty and sociologists Viola Klein and Alva Myrdal were affirming that child-rearing was connected to women's natural adult role, Cassel staff were helping women to arrive at the psychological maturity that they believed was necessary for a mother to form loving relationships with her young children. For Main, being a capable mother was a core feature of self-realized adulthood in women, a view that feminist sociologist Ann Oakley would criticize two decades later, underscoring the harmful limits that women experienced through mainstream psychology's insistence that motherhood was women's "sole true means of self-realization."[47] At the Cassel, there was nothing inevitable about feminine psychological maturity. In direct opposition to the claims of contemporary child rearing experts that love flowed naturally from women's maternal instinct, Cassel staff saw women's capacity to love and nurture their children as the outcome of a long and sometimes arduous developmental process. It did not straightforwardly accompany physical maturity.

Addressing the psychological difficulties of motherhood, Main focused on the incompatibility that many patients experienced between their sexuality and the British ideal of asexual motherhood. This introduced a deep guilt that, Main argued, made it impossible for some women to function as both a wife and mother, and could even bring on childlike regression:

> [It] centers on womanhood being burdensome ... She is unable to enjoy and advance in feminine achievement as a sexual woman and as a mother, to take and give pleasure in her strength of body, her vagina, her breasts and nipples, her milk, her limbs, her warmth, and her adult powers of loving. Enjoyment and activity of those aspects of her body are banned to her, along with pride in herself as a wife who can make her husband sexually happy or as a mother who produces a lusty and passionate child ... Where there is massive guilt the very marriage and the maternity themselves have to be quite wrecked and a much greater degree of suffering must ensue, together with a full renunciation of all pleasures of adulthood, and a return to childlike innocence and obedience.[48]

The clinical features of this regression included an inability to look after her home, husband, or child. For example, Mrs. D., who felt "anything but loving" toward her baby also disowned her husband and "expressed a determination never to return home."[49] Her rejection of motherhood was connected to a larger rejection of marriage and home, all key features of female adulthood.

In some cases, maternal rejection stemmed less from feelings of feminine inadequacy and more from deep-seated masculine identification. This was the case for "Mrs. Wilson," described as "a female Don Juan," who openly pursued extra-marital affairs and was very controlling of her sons. Whatever the primary reason for a woman's struggles with motherhood, it was always interpreted as a "retreat from adult life."[50] In its most extreme form, the afflicted woman regressed to a "state of anxious, childlike helplessness."[51] Behaving like a traditional psychiatric patient, she sought to be cared for, fed, and sheltered from the world. At the heart of a woman's inability to care for her children was her failure to mature emotionally; this was therefore of enormous importance for understanding "maternal deprivation."

Main challenged widely held beliefs about the biological inevitability of the maternal instinct present in modern parenting literature. He argued that there was something fundamentally awry in British families, and British culture more generally, that interfered with many women's adjustment to this seemingly natural feminine role. The British idealization of mothers as providers of uninterrupted devotional care was, in his view, a fantasy that stemmed from grown-up children's retrospective wishes about their own childhoods. Cultural expectations of mothers were created, absorbed, and reproduced by people who were dissatisfied with their own childhood experiences:

> The common concept of mothering is one of slavish devotion, selfless love and infinite patience. Whether any mother reaches such an ideal may be speculated upon by anyone who cares to remember his own childhood, but certainly the standards the child sets for his mother are very high ... Such standards for mothers remain latent within all of us, and show themselves in distress and urgency when, in the course of our work, we become involved with a disturbed mother-child relationship. All the more does a young mother feel the presence of these ideals, and if she is neurotic it is likely that her dealings with her children will be especially urgent and distressing.[52]

Main diagnosed twentieth-century British culture as problematically child-centered. He argued that it was especially troubling that scientists—as individuals who should stand apart from culture—tended to identify with the child's perspective, rather than the mother's, in their investigations:

> We who are grown-up children tend to use a frame of reference in which she [the mother] is the background of the child's life; it is uncommon for her to be taken as the initial figure for study, with the child as merely part of *her* background ... it is also important for science that we should grant equal attention to the question of what mothering means to mothers and study their behaviour not for the child's sake only ... but that we may learn something of maternal parenthood as a step in the psychological development of women.[53]

Prevalent inattention to the realities of motherhood only added to the difficulties that many women faced as mothers. The challenges associated with pregnancy, childbirth, and breastfeeding complicated things even further. In Main's view, female adulthood was taxing in ways that male adulthood was not: "The *curse* of womanhood and femininity" was for some women "a painful lot, and the states of depression that follow childbirth, lactation, or weaning may be of psychotic magnitude."[54] He saw pregnancy and childbirth as inherently distressing events, and this, in combination with the culturally created guilt that British women experienced when trying to reconcile their sexuality and motherhood, was to prove too much for many women to bear.

Rehabilitating Mothers at the Cassel Hospital

Despite Main's insistence on empathy toward mothers, the therapeutic community that he developed at the Cassel focused on producing loving mothers and wives under the guise of rehabilitation. The hospital's therapeutic perspective was predominantly child-centered, despite Main's criticism of the cultural expectation that mother love was a panacea for all contemporary ills, personal and social alike.

Patients who were mothers were expected to retain full responsibility for childcare. To achieve this, the care duties traditionally performed by psychiatric nurses were massively scaled back. Nurse Matron Doreen Weddell described the psychosocial approach to nursing as supported by a non-infantilizing view of the patient as "an adult, a citizen, with diminished capacities perhaps, yet nevertheless a responsible person, who had something to contribute to, as well as expectations of, society."[55] In the mother-child unit, nurses were trained to avoid succumbing to their "natural" inclination to take over childcare.[56] Rather than assisting with patients' children, nurses' duties were instead focused on ensuring that patients did not renounce their familial responsibilities.

Although psychosocial nurses were primarily meant to observe and offer guidance, in practice their duties were difficult to perform. Nurses had to make substantial effort to monitor mother-child interactions since patients kept their children away from staff scrutiny. Patients encouraged their children to take long naps and play quietly in their rooms. They would also often prepare and eat their meals in their private quarters. In response, a nursery was created so that staff could more easily observe children playing without parental interference. They soon came to see style of play as an expression of the children's troubled relationships with their mothers. For example, in the nursery, Mrs. Wilson's sons were observed bullying the other children and Main presumed they were re-enacting her rough treatment of them. The nursery was also seen as crucial for children's healing since it offered them a space where they could adjust to both changes in their mother's mental state and in their relationship with her.

Case studies show that maternal distress assumed many forms at the Cassel, from depression to anxiety to mild psychosis. Some patients were admitted immediately following childbirth and others arrived a few years after their last child was born. Despite this variability, the goal in the mother-child unit was to cultivate a maternal style that was nurturing yet supportive of children's unique individuality. Much like a psychosocial nurse's approach to her patients, the emotionally mature mother respected her children's developing need for independence.

When the twice-married, thirty-six-year-old Mrs. Wilson was admitted for treatment of disabling anxiety, the two youngest of her seven children—two-year-old Jimmy and four-year old Peter—accompanied her.[57] Mrs. Wilson was struggling to care for her children; she had lost interest in her marriage and had pursued several extra-marital relationships in the preceding months. When she first arrived at the Cassel, her appearance was remarked upon as both heavily made up and disturbingly masculine. She was described as resembling a "male comedian dressed as a woman."[58] Her masculine likeness went beyond physical appearance; her marital unfaithfulness and domineering treatment of her male children were framed as rejections of her femininity. Her first marriage had failed following an extra-marital relationship, and she continued to pursue other sexual relationships in her second marriage. Nurses described her as a "female Don Juan" who desired to be "an active, seductive son."[59] Because she controlled so much of her sons' behavior, Cassel staff believed that Mrs. Wilson competed with her male children and took "any sign of initiative and spontaneous behaviour from the boys" as a threat to her own "masculine" aspirations.[60]

Mrs. Wilson's progress in therapy centered on new awareness surrounding her envy of men and troubled relationship with her mother, whom she believed had resented her because she had wanted a son.[61] Once the psychological root of her problem had been identified, her stay in the therapeutic community helped Mrs. Wilson embrace her femininity. Cassel staff understood emotional maturity to be forged through acceptance of adult roles within a heteronormative child-producing family, and so Mrs. Wilson's therapy was focused on her relationships with her husband and children. She was guided to adopt a flexible, yet gently nurturing, approach to caring for her sons, and eventually accepted monogamy as a foundational condition of her marriage. All parts of her life that did not relate to family were left out of her case report since it was assumed they held little relevance for her recovery.

Mrs. Smith exhibited very different symptoms when she was admitted to the Cassel. She had had a "weird psychotic personality" ever since "a depressive breakdown" following her daughter Mary's birth three years earlier. She had undergone electro-convulsive therapy (ECT) for post-partum depression, but this had been unsuccessful in spurring recovery. Although she too had experienced feeling rejected by her mother—because her mother had wanted her to grow up to become a professional dancer—she did not react to this by embracing masculine behaviors, but instead by overly identifying with her mother. Hospital staff found this particularly alarming as Mrs. Smith would mimic her mother as she had been during the late stages of Parkinson's disease. The rest of Mrs. Smith's time was spent focused on her three-year-old daughter, which put great demands on her. Hospital staff viewed this as a re-enactment of her dysfunctional relationship with her own mother.[62] Therapeutic progress began with her realization that she had not moved on from her childhood relationship with her mother. She then gradually learned to parent Mary without smothering her and entered a renewed sexual relationship with her husband, who, by the time of her admission, had given up on the marriage.

Like many of the Cassel patients, Mrs. Wilson and Mrs. Smith had been admitted for in-patient treatment as a last resort. And, although their problems were markedly different, their struggles caring for their children were the focus of treatment. In both cases, dysfunctional parenting was seen as stemming from pathological relationships that they had experienced with their own mothers as children.[63] They were caught in a cycle of immaturity. Cassel staff lamented that this crucial common experience had been overlooked by previous physicians, all of whom had been insensitive to the lasting damage that resulted from troubled mother-daughter relationships:

> The main task for a new mother is the re-negotiation of the mothering which she herself had. If this was successful, she can tend her baby and fulfil its needs. If this cannot happen, usually because there were flaws in her own mothering, breakdown occurs. Universally, women turn to their mothers in the puerperium.[64]

At the Cassel, motherhood was seen as a universal psychological experience. Although patients who were admitted alongside their children had diverse life histories, they all struggled to perform what was seen as their most essential adult task, that is forming loving relationships with their children in which they stood as a stable nurturing adult rather than another erratic and dependent child.

The very existence of post-partum mental illness was contested in the decades after the war. Although Cassel staff would treat post-partum mental illness as bearing a special relationship to childbirth and motherhood, this was only beginning to gain acceptance in psychiatric circles. Most British psychiatrists saw a predisposition to mental illness as the primary cause and considered other stress-related factors, like sleep loss and hormonal shifts, as triggers for post-partum mental breakdown. As R.E. Hemphill noted in the *BMJ* in 1952, physicians typically agreed that "no form of psychiatric illness occurring in pregnancy or the puerperium is a specific clinical entity":

> The general opinion seems to be that the ordinary stress and strains of pregnancy, operating in predisposed individuals, produce non-specific mental illnesses which are indistinguishable from other mental reactions.[65]

One *BMJ* contributor declared as late as 1966 that "no good evidence has been found for regarding puerperal psychosis as distinct from psychosis outside the puerperium."[66] Mary E. Martin, assistant medical director of St. Patrick's Hospital in

Dublin, was particularly outspoken in her opposition to medical arguments speculating that post-partum mental illnesses might constitute a special type. She was concerned about the implications of childbirth being seen as making women vulnerable to mental affliction. Adamant that ECT always proved an effective treatment, she maintained that the birth of a new child was psychiatrically significant *only* because it could cause stress.[67]

The mother-baby unit played an important role in the discovery of the psychological burdens of motherhood. Martin's concern for normalizing childbirth—emptying it of any special psychological importance—also meant that she did not see value in the psychosocial treatment of a mother and baby together as a "unit," and strongly discouraged this therapeutic approach. She singled it out as especially ineffective since it presumed the mother-child relationship bore a unique connection to women's (and never men's) mental state.

That Hemphill and Martin felt they needed to argue against the existence of post-partum mental illness had much to do with growing medical interest in the mother-baby unit as a form of treatment. By the mid-1960s, several psychiatric hospitals—including Banstead, Shenley, and Stratheden Hospitals—were experimenting with mother-baby units and reporting on their effectiveness in treating post-partum mental illness. In addition to administering psychotropic drugs and ECT in some cases, psychiatrists in mother-baby units experimented with psychotherapy and psychosocial nursing (of the kind pioneered at the Cassel). When staff at Shenley Hospital published a decade-long study of their mother-baby unit in 1968, they affirmed that psychosocial treatment had significantly improved relationships between mothers and their children:

> The present study confirms ... that by offering them graduated responsibility in a supportive setting ... it is possible to get a satisfactory result in terms of the mother-child relationship in a high proportion of cases (89% in the present series) at time of discharge. As a result of our experience we believe that the procedures described constitute an advance in the treatment of puerperal mental illness.[68]

It was further argued that the presence of babies in the psychiatric hospital positively brought out maternal qualities in unmarried female patients, and published results always mentioned that children were not adversely affected by living in a psychiatric community for limited periods of time.

The patient's relationship with her husband was also implicated in her mental illness. Since Main saw the basis for post-partum mental illness as a conflict between sexuality and motherhood, he brought not only the mother-child relationship under greater scrutiny but also the husband-wife relationship. By the late 1950s husbands began to be admitted to the hospital, not simply as auxiliary nurses—as their role in the hospital was initially seen—but as part of the psychosocial field within which their wives' neuroses had developed:

> We found that admitting a mother with her baby compelled us all to face the major root troubles of mothering... we could no longer evade the patient's daily difficulties of mothering and her deep problems of maturation. If the husband's own neurosis played into his wife's, he too could be treated while in contact with her. Such work cannot occur in out-patient clinics and is a specific hospital contribution to therapeutic technique.[69]

Similar to the first joint admission of a mother and her young son, when the practice of admitting patients' husbands began in 1957, it was in response to a husband's resistance to being separated from his wife and baby. He requested admission to the hospital with them, and Main accepted. In the years that followed, husbands were admitted as full members of the hospital community along with their wives and children: they came to be seen as an equal member of a single "mental treatment unit." They participated in childcare and hospital management duties, ate meals with their families, and spent leisure time with their wives on the hospital grounds and in Richmond's nearby parks and shops. Patient-run nurseries were organized to not only ease the burden of childcare but also help toward improving married couples' relationships. The prototype of the mentally healthy family continued to circulate around the figure of the nurturing mother, but rather than merely attempting to repair her relationships to her children, the hospital increasingly came to focus equally on restoring her connection to her husband. Marital harmony came to be seen as a key marker of psychological maturity. The male-breadwinning nuclear family thus became essential not only for early childhood emotional development but also for the healthy completion of emotional development in adulthood. As the *Evening News* reported, "In the view of Dr. Tom Main, 'a lot of healing takes place in a double bed.'"[70] Main's view that the emotional and sexual integrity of the marital relationship impacted spouses' mental health culminated in the 1963 opening of an outpatient "Marital Clinic." Marital dysfunction—thought to be widespread after WWII—came to be treated as its own therapeutic specialty at the Cassel under Main's directorship.

Cassel staff prioritized protecting the fragile spousal and parent-child relationships being rehabilitated at the hospital. In other words, the Cassel's psychosocial objective of creating a fully interdependent community had its limits. Close patient friendships were frequently worried about as threatening to dilute family bonds and confuse patients' primary allegiances. The hospital community was described by patients and staff alike as similar to an "extended family" in both anxious and encouraging tones. Families were given separate accommodation to prevent them from merging with the rest of the hospital community. Domestic privacy, seen as the nuclear family's emotional backbone, was nurtured, and evenings were devoted to family time. Married couples were encouraged to participate in the hospital's social life during the day but expected to spend time together away from the rest of the community once the day had ended. Responding to the perceived vulnerability of marital and family relationships, in the 1950s and 1960s Cassel staff steadily pushed the therapeutic community enterprise further into patients' intimate lives, determining who they ate with, spent their evenings with, and slept with. Spending time with one's family was seen as both therapeutic and a sign that patients were recovering. The ability to act like a family was both a barometer and the constitutive basis for mental health.

The Politics of Childcare in Welfare-State Britain

Residential spaces devoted to maternal rehabilitation like the Brentwood Centre and the Cassel Hospital's mother-child unit operated on the notion that capable mothers were created through the positive influences of the democratic community and the well-managed middle-class home. However, in the decades following WWII British women far more frequently encountered the message that life circumstances were largely irrelevant when it came to effective childcare, with experts urging women to tune into their natural maternal instincts. Dr. Spock counseled his female readers to forget the experts and follow their innate ability to intuit their infant's every need. In Britain, Winnicott advised mothers not to worry about losing interest in politics and employment and instead happily immerse themselves in the important activities that came with motherhood. His central piece of advice was for mothers to enjoy themselves:

> So here you are with all your eggs in one basket. What are you going to do about it? Well, enjoy yourself! Enjoy being thought important. Enjoy letting other people look after the world while you are producing a new one of its members. Enjoy being turned-in and almost in love with yourself, the baby is so nearly part of you. Enjoy the way in which your man feels responsible for the welfare of you and your baby. Enjoy finding out new things about yourself... Enjoy all sorts of womanly feelings that you cannot even start to explain to a man. Particularly, I know you will enjoy the signs that gradually appear that the baby is a person, and that you are recognized as a person by the baby.[71]

Women on both sides of the Atlantic were repeatedly told that childcare came naturally. Arnold Gesell described a mother's ability to care for her child as a "natural aptitude";[72] psychoanalyst Therese Benedek maintained that "mothering behavior" was tied to normal brain functioning.[73] Not only was there no special training or knowledge required, but since it was also fundamentally pleasurable, its relationship to the onerous paid work involved in "look[ing] after the world" was tenuous indeed.[74]

Cassel staff saw their work as having a beneficial socio-political impact in the shaping of Britain's future citizens. They sought to end maternal deprivation and all other forms of harmful parenting—from the neglectful to the smothering—not only to help female patients become mentally healthy, but also to ensure emotional wellbeing in future generations. For example, Doreen Weddell explicitly promoted family-based therapy at the Cassel as contributing to British social wellbeing. "The relationships of one family," she argued, "set a pattern for a community."[75] Viewing political culture as a direct extension of the psychological dynamics of family life, Weddell urged that, "Experiences of the members of a family in respect of authority, obedience, rebellion, controls, freedom, cooperation, domination, leadership, etc. are reflected in community responses to family-like situations."[76] The Cassel's experiments with democratic therapeutic community and rehabilitating families in crisis was supported by a new, specifically post-WWII, psychological understanding of healthy motherhood. More than anyone else, mothers, given their presumed capacity to love steadfastly, were seen as setting the tone for all relationships. In bringing the family and emotional development to the foreground of socio-political thinking when considering the Cassel's broader impact, Cassel staff enlarged conventional understandings of politics.

Cassel staff were not unique in spotlighting the crucial political work that housewives and mothers performed after WWII. In their joint 1956 report, the BMA and the Magistrates Association similarly stressed the far-reaching benefits of "sound family life, where such virtues as unselfishness, self-discipline and caring for others flourish" as "a major factor in developing responsible citizens."[77] Mothers, the report emphasized, were best suited to help cultivate such values. Mothers were also recognized as performing important political work toward securing Britain's future as a global power in early plans for the welfare state. As early as 1942, William Beveridge acknowledged mothers' "vital work" in postwar reconstruction in ensuring not only "the adequate continuance of the British race" but also "of British *ideals* in the world."[78] Given the crucial role that mothers played in safeguarding British values during an uncertain moment regarding Britain's continuing global influence, Beveridge insisted upon women's equality within their marriages. He was adamant that housewives' "vital unpaid service" as an "occupation" should not render them dependent on their working husbands, but rather "partners sharing benefit and pension."[79] He emphasized that his proposed welfare state would recognize housewives' needs: "the real needs of widowhood and separation, for maternity in grant and benefit, for children's allowances, and for medical treatment both of the housewife and of the children for whose care she has special responsibility."[80] Following Beveridge's 1942 emphasis on married mothers performing socially necessary work, in 1948 he mentioned Brentwood as a vital service since it offered married women the rest that was essential to optimal job performance: "a housewife and mother may at times be as much in need of rehabilitation to do her job as a crash-shocked airman or injured workman."[81]

Despite Beveridge's insistence on mothers' crucial socio-political contributions, Britain's welfare state did not offer housewives provisions that were sufficient for many married women to afford not to engage in paid work.[82] Moreover, married women's role as dependent was confirmed in many aspects of Britain's postwar provisions, including policies affecting wages, unemployment, pensions, and marital property.[83] A large portion of government lobbying by women's organizations after WWII was focused on elevating housewives' legal status and bringing formal recognition of the social value of their work in the home as equivalent (if not more robust) to that performed by working husbands.[84] Groups like the Married Women's Association (MWA) and the National Federation of Women's Institutes (WI) campaigned to have British marriage laws reformed so that housewives would legally own half of their marital property and income. The MWA's "Charter for Wives," drawn up by physician and Labour MP Edith Summerskill, announced that:

> The time has arrived when society should recognize that the woman who bears and rears children and works in the home is making a contribution of inestimable value to the State... she should be entitled to a legal share in the family income.[85]

Additionally, the MWA demanded that housewives receive their own pensions, independent of their husband's contributions, and access to separate unemployment insurance for security against their husband's potential unemployment. In campaigns to have the marriage law reformed to end housewives' financial dependence on their husbands, lobbyists emphasized housewives' work as a crucial benefit to the nation. In a letter to Summerskill in 1942, Beveridge agreed with the MWA's arguments highlighting the importance of women's work within their families, but stated that he ultimately believed that organizing the emerging welfare state to reflect married women's many contributions to the nation as individuals—rather than as an integral part of their family unit—would upend longstanding British property laws.[86] When, in 1964, property laws were finally updated to reflect spouses' equal ownership of all marital property and income, it was in keeping with the notion that housewives worked and were therefore entitled to income.[87] Summerskill was clear that the rationale was one of equal contributions in terms of services put into the household rather than presuming that marriage, by nature, entailed joint ownership.

Social psychiatrists, designers of the welfare state, and groups campaigning to introduce legal recognition of the social value of housewives' work were only some of the more prominent voices highlighting the urgent necessity for women's contributions to postwar social reconstruction. They presented a "community-based model of politics" that was, as Krista Cowman puts it, "feminized if not feminist."[88] Alongside this emphasis on the benefits of women's unpaid work in the home, mother love was assigned supreme value in providing safe shelter in an otherwise uncaring world. Commercial advertisements capitalized on images of the happy mother and child. Not only were baby food, formula, and diapers advertised as supporting children's happiness and wellbeing, but the loving mother-child relationship was used to sell a wide range of products, from food and household medicines to the latest household technologies. In popular representations of contented domesticity, leisure hours were depicted as much more than recompense for hard work. They also offered a warning against the perils of overwork. Images of mother and child communicated that the real value of life was not greater purchasing power but the enjoyment of a loving family.

The British cultural ideal of the harmonious male-breadwinning, female-homemaking family with mother always at home and father spending evenings and

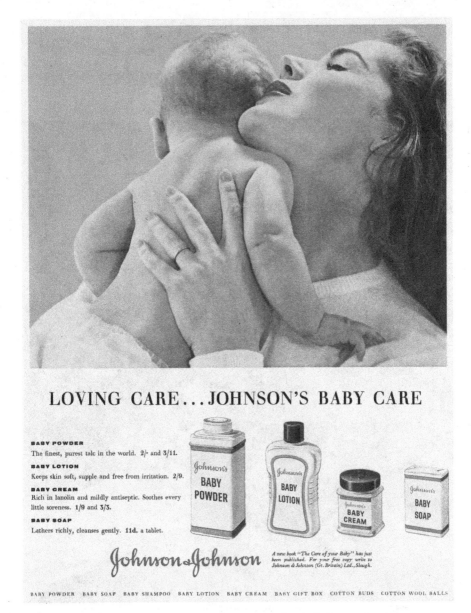

Figure 3.3. 1957 UK advertisement for Johnson & Johnson baby care products.
Source: Neil Baylis/Alamy Stock.

weekends with his family existed in a world where overwork and excessive consumption were seen as corrupt values. In response to increasing post-WWII affluence, the intimate love embodied by the nuclear family ideal was presented as an antidote to the materialistic aspirations of an acquisitive society. Mother love became more necessary than ever before. James Spence, leading pediatrician and Tom Main's mentor

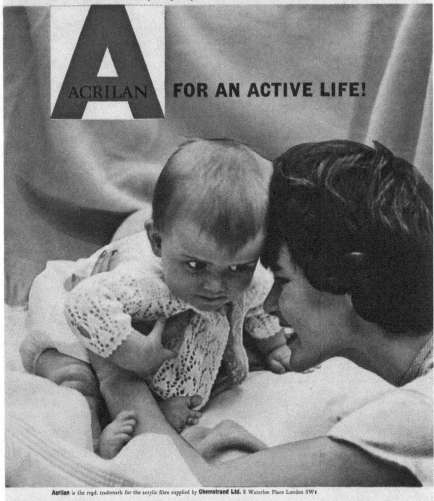

Figure 3.4. 1958 UK Acrilan blanket advertisement.
Source: Hera Vintage Ads/Alamy Stock Photo.

as an undergraduate student, warned that motherhood was under attack in societies with spiraling material ambitions. As families became more expensive to maintain, married women were forced into the workplace. Similarly, sociologist Talcott Parsons presented housewives as increasingly necessary in materialistic cultures since the

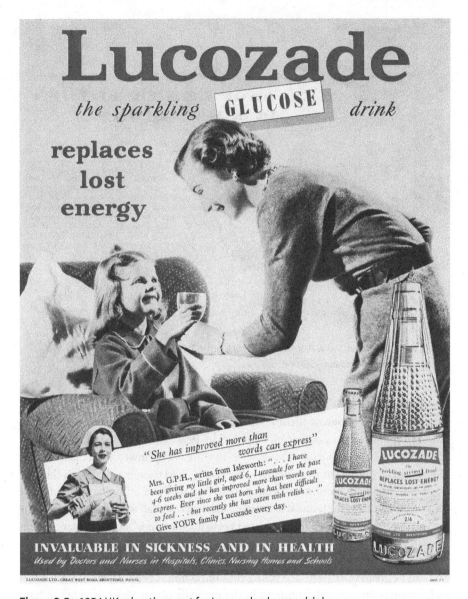

Figure 3.5. 1954 UK advertisement for Lucozade glucose drink.
Source: Neil Baylis/Alamy Stock Photo.

housewife cultivated empathy within her family, in his view the highest value of a civilized society.[89] The perception that motherhood was under threat was often linked to alarm over rising consumption in the post-WWII decades.

On both sides of the Atlantic, children's perceived need for a steady supply of maternal love was at the heart of debates over mothers in the workforce, laments over the impact of suburban alienation on family life, and demands for greater subsidies

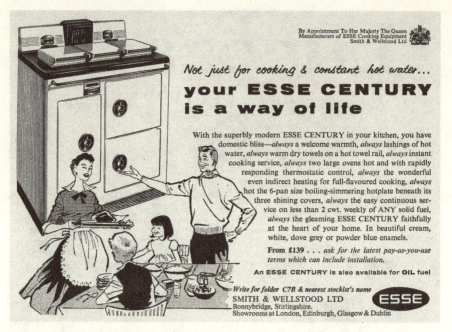

Figure 3.6. 1958 UK Esse water heater advertisement.
Source: Hera Vintage Ads/Alamy Stock Photo.

to enable women to devote themselves to full-time childcare. In a frank discussion of working mothers in *Ladies Home Journal* in 1958, US Secretary of Labor James Mitchell warned readers against forgetting "that the very primary, fundamental basis of a free society is the family structure—the home—and the most vital job is there."[90] A national survey of hundreds of young American mothers' attitudes toward female employment outside the home had revealed that just over half would work outside the home if they could and 22% had answered yes to the question, "have you ever thought you'd like to be a man?"[91] John Bowlby and psychoanalyst Florida Scott-Maxwell lamented the results, agreeing that there was something fundamentally wrong with a woman's desire to work if she had young children at home. Scott-Maxwell argued that such women—increasingly common in the previous twenty years—tended to have worked before marriage and had developed a pronounced "masculine side mak[ing] them restless and bored in their homes."[92] When addressing working-class families whose financial burdens made both spouses' employment necessary, contributors to the discussion looked positively on women who chose the more "feminine" option of night shifts. Assuming that interruptions in childcare were kept to a minimum during daytime hours, they described the mother who worked round-the-clock as doing it "gladly because it is selfless, it is sacrifice, which is what women have always stood for."[93] Scott-Maxwell advised that the solution to the problem of working mothers lay in fostering a broader appreciation of feminine values in US society:

The feminine has always been under a shadow. America has grown great by stressing the masculine—the things people do here! The activity—the accomplishments! The very thrust of your marvelous skyscrapers! But these wonders have their dangerous side and it almost seems that an American man cannot feel sure of his strength if he does not push the feminine behind him, or above him, where he worships it with false sentiment.[94]

Bowlby targeted working women as themselves the source of the problem and argued that for social attitudes to change in Britain and the United States, "career women" needed to stop "look[ing] down on women who stay home."[95]

Social scientists similarly called attention to the lack of full-time maternal care in post-WWII Britain as a problem that especially implicated middle-class families. A range of studies focusing on working-class urban neighborhoods argued that the spirit of devoted motherhood was alive and well among the lower strata of British society. Child psychologists John and Elizabeth Newson's cross-class study of infant care in urban communities revealed that a working-class mother still "expect[ed] to find her major satisfaction in being the indispensable provider and minister to the needs of her husband and children," and was valued in her community as "our Mam."[96] By contrast, the Newsons pointed out, the middle-class wife's value lay with her contributions to her husband's success in his career. It was this that accounted for her frequent dissatisfaction:

> [She is] supposed to be a social asset to her husband, helping him to entertain his friends and associates and generally sharing in all his social activities. The arrival of young children inevitably restricts her horizons rather drastically ... Her dissatisfactions with the role of "Mummy" can well be seen in the floods of letters from discontented young mothers, usually of better-than-average education, which periodically fill the women's pages of newspapers such as the *Guardian* and the *Observer*."[97]

Explaining the rise in the phenomenon of the "miserable married woman" as resulting from middle-class obsessions with career at the expense of family, the Newsons saw some hope in the fact that large segments of the British population continued to value maternal care highly. Sociologists Peter Willmott and Michael Young similarly found many fewer unhappy young mothers in the working-class borough of Bethnal Green, which they compared to a working-class housing estate in Greenleigh in their 1955 study. In the housing estate, far from her community of origin, the young mother was "hard put to avoid the loneliness and exasperation of being confined day in, day out, in her one-person workplace."[98] In the established community of Bethnal Green, where mothers typically lived near their own mothers, maternal dissatisfaction was nowhere to be found.[99]

During the same mid-1950s moment that Main was discovering motherhood to be a challenging psychological *role* rather than a potentially onerous collection of *work* tasks, social scientists were similarly finding that mothers were often rewarded with a high social status for performing a valued role within their immediate communities. Unlike Beveridge, who had compared married housewives' work to the paid work that their husbands performed, social scientists investigating changes in British family life in the post-WWII decades—including Elizabeth Bott, Alva Myrdal, Viola Klein, and John and Elizabeth Newson—appealed to the concept of roles to make their arguments about married mothers' vital contributions to social reconstruction and reform. An important difference was stressed here between work and social roles. According to Wilmott and Young, the contributions that men made to the economy were different in kind to those that women made in maintaining community relationships—kinship networks produced the social realities that men and women inhabited.

Social scientists unfailingly noted that the social role that married women had traditionally inhabited was undergoing enormous transformation in urban settings. With the breakdown of extended families following young people's migration to housing estates, couples more than ever depended upon one another for emotional support. Bott noted that the roles that husbands and wives played in their families had become less differentiated. Cassel staff were familiar with these studies of British families. Psychotherapist Peter Lomas lamented that the women in Bott's "loose-knit" families made up most female patients treated at the Cassel for post-partum mental illness:

> In keeping with Bott's predictions there was no well-defined differentiation of roles between husband and wife. Within such a family structure deviations from a conventional masculine-feminine relationship are more likely to appear. The most obvious deviation to be seen was a lack of femininity on the part of the wife.[100]

In 1950s British family studies and family therapy literature alike, the dissolution of gender-differentiated roles in families was presented as an outcome of late-industrial capitalism. Despite this, sociologists Willmott and Young like psychotherapists Main and Lomas did not see this trend as the only possible outcome of modern industrialized societies and advocated for change along community-based lines.

In the wake of longer life expectancies and an earlier average age of marriage in the early 1950s, sociologists Viola Klein and Alva Myrdal appealed to the logic of social roles rather than work in presenting a solution that respected both women's perceived suitability to childcare and the increasing economic need for women to engage in paid work. Their objective, in arguing that women had "*two* roles" to perform over the course of their lifetime, was to make the case that motherhood constituted *only one* phase of a woman's life rather than its totality.[101] Although Edith Summerskill and other housewives' rights lobbyists claimed that housewives performed essential work worthy of greater remuneration, they mentioned children's emotional care as socially valuable but did not include it as a work task alongside home-making, cooking, cleaning, and managing household finances. Myrdal and Klein, however, mentioned childcare's emotional aspects as the main reason that a woman needed to leave the workforce when her children were young. However, in presenting childcare as a predominantly emotional undertaking, they avoided terminology related to work, which pervaded housewife organizations' demands, and instead appealed to the apolitical language of roles. They argued that the modern woman had "two roles" to perform—one at home with her children and the other in the workforce. The timing of each was determined by her stage of life. Once her children were attending school, it was time for her to advance to the next life stage and return to paid work. Several reasons were given for this, financial *and* psychological. Not only was it increasingly necessary for both husband and wife to be gainfully employed to afford the costs of modern living but work itself had taken on important psychological meaning: it not only allowed one to make ends meet, it also enabled self-expression.

Like the insistence by Cassel staff that married women exchanged the "daughter role" for the "mother role" when they had children, Myrdal and Klein's "two roles" spoke to a family-centered conception of female adulthood, albeit a more expansive version that was separated into three phases: study, motherhood, and work. Women living their lives in the correct sequence made key contributions to national wellbeing. Here, the work that Beveridge and housewife organizations insisted married women performed had its meaning transformed. Rather than placing women's work in the home on the same level as men's paid work outside the home, women's contributions were presented as overwhelmingly emotional in nature. They were both vital to the good of the community and women's own healthy maturity.

Studies of British families and family therapy initiatives like the one launched at the Cassel similarly distinguished between emotional care and work performed for financial compensation. Recent scholarship, however, reveals how heightened expectations surrounding childcare in the second half of the twentieth century entailed the acquisition of new emotional skills. Sociologists Jean Duncombe and Dennis Marsden point out that scholars' focus on domestic work has led them to overlook the emotional work that goes into child-rearing and the care of family members. They argue that this is crucial to investigate as it is women far more often than men who assume responsibility for the many emotional aspects of family life: "the gender division of labour results in a gender division of emotion."[102] Although not all scholars agree that equivalencies can be drawn between emotional care work and paid work, they do not disagree that care requires conscious practiced effort to perform. For example, sociologist Kathleen Lynch argues that love labor is non-commodifiable because genuine emotional care cannot, by its very nature, be manufactured in exchange for money. However, she notes that it "involves at different times and to different degrees, emotional work, mental work, cognitive skills and physical work," and thus truly constitutes labor:

> Without such labouring, feelings of love or care for others can simply involve rhetorical functionings, words and talk that are declaratory in nature but lack substance in practice or action.[103]

At the Cassel, female patients' recovery coincided with their performance of love labor within their families—with *both* their children *and* their husbands. For example, Mrs. Wilson's recovery involved her relinquishing a controlling parenting style and adopting a more accepting attitude toward her children. The hope was that a more supportive relationship would make her boys feel secure expressing their individuality and developing masculinity. Mrs. Smith's "disturbed" behavior ceased as she began to cherish her daughter's unique interests and re-established her sexual relationship with her husband.

At the Cassel, just as in Klein and Myrdal's study, none of the effort aimed at generating intimacy between mothers and children and wives and husbands was described as work. However, although it was not considered work to create and maintain stable emotional relationships within one's family does not mean it was not seen as an important contribution to public life. The Cassel's approach to motherhood was consciously intended to introduce a revolutionary transformation both in the treatment of childbearing women in the decades after WWII and in understandings of democratic community.

Cassel staff's preoccupation with motherhood may have appeared to correspond with broader concerns about modern transformations in childbearing and childcare—surrounding, for example, hospital deliveries and formula feeding—and its movement away from the family home. However, Main's attention to the psychological "burdens of motherhood" was less attached to worries about departures from "nature" than concerned—along with Bowlby and other attachment theorists—with illuminating the central psychological importance of the mother-child relationship as the bedrock for national wellbeing.

The therapeutic initiatives discussed in this chapter sought to bring greater visibility to the frequently arduous nature of childcare and laud mothers' enormous contributions to public welfare. However, their desire to have motherhood seen as a role rather than a collection of work-like activities evaded the politics of work, social benefit, and labor exploitation. At the same time as Cassel psychiatrists presented stay-at-home mothers as the bedrock of harmonious community life, they rendered the childless working woman a selfish—antisocial—being. Stressing the emotional care aspects of motherhood and undermining connections between care and work was meant to emphasize motherhood's social urgency (with the assumption that seeing care as a form of work would cheapen it). Motherhood was thus re-inscribed with a sense of inevitability in fertile women's lives, which made not having children a very difficult option to choose.

Conclusion

The Cassel became a major site for training psychiatrists, psychotherapists, and psychosocial nurses in the 1950s and 1960s. Several Cassel nurses went on to have influential careers and shape the direction of psychiatric healthcare offered through the NHS.[104] The Cassel was often described in both the medical and popular press as a progressive site to be emulated. Although it was a costly endeavor, the admission of children to a psychiatric hospital for adults, alongside their mentally afflicted mothers, generated a positive public reaction and was greeted as a hopeful direction in psychiatric treatment at a moment when the Victorian custodial institution had come under widespread attack. In November 1958, the *Daily Mail* favorably reported that, "The whole idea of this novel treatment is to provide almost a replica of normal home life ... They cook, clean and wash. They discuss and decide."[105] What struck journalists who visited the Cassel most was the hospital's domestic feel. A reporter from *The Evening News* stressed the beauty of the hospital and its grounds, as well as its home-like feel, while the *Woman's Mirror* commented that high recovery rates reflected the hospital's "homely atmosphere": "I found it easy to understand how a patient ... comes to recover. Her life is exactly the same as usual, except that she gets extra help to cope with it."[106] Far from what one would expect of a psychiatric institution, Cassel staff sought to create an environment that embodied what home life was ideally supposed to be: mothers spent most of their time with their young children and fathers went to work, returning to the hospital for family time on evenings and weekends.

While acknowledging the apparent strangeness of a family-centered psychiatric regime, several reporters emphasized that the idea for this type of treatment resembled how illness was dealt with in less industrialized cultures. *Daily Mail* reporter Olga Franklin cited Main criticizing the increasing lack of regard for family life in post-WWII Britain. In Japan, conversely, where the family was deeply valued, "the whole family go to hospital when one is sick: even the in-laws who are sometimes the cause of the trouble."[107] The piece concluded by mentioning growing medical support for the Cassel's family-based approach to the therapeutic community: "[Main's] experiment is now being discussed by the medical profession. Two hospitals have already announced they want to copy."[108]

At sites like the Cassel Hospital and Brentwood Rehabilitation Centre, the assumption of joyful motherhood that pervaded popular parenting literature was affirmed. At the same time, both challenged the idea that effective motherhood was a direct outcome of biological instinct and physical maturity. Maternal neglect was shown to be more frequent than expected. Main went even further than this, declaring capable motherhood across the social classes to be a "feat of feminine maturity." If mother love required the right circumstances to flourish, then appeals could be made for changing women's social conditions. Main criticized British culture for its expectation of maternal asexuality; Eva Hubback condemned the state for its lack of social and health services to support overburdened mothers. At the Cassel, the prevention of post-partum mental illness was seen as requiring marital happiness, family planning, more realistic expectations of mothers, and state support in the form of family allowances and health and social services.

Housewife organizations also strived to improve the conditions surrounding motherhood. They prefaced their claims for greater recognition and financial support with appeals—resembling Main's—to the family-centered culture of a truly civilized modern state. The supported mother could more easily provide appropriate care for her children. The ability to love one's children effectively depended on a range of factors: access to meaningful paid work in middle-age according to Myrdal and Klein, sufficient family allowances according to Summerskill, exposure to the hygienic norms of middle-class family life according to Brentwood staff, a harmonious and sexually fulfilled marriage according to Main.

Exposing the limits of 1950s instinct-based assumptions about maternal love ended up creating more possibilities for maternal dissatisfaction to be expressed. Women had new language to explain how their lives spent significantly at home led to loneliness and resentment toward their children. Others could now express how their focus on housework and childcare presented a barrier to self-realization and prevented them from enjoying their children. Few put the blame on motherhood itself. It was the conditions that surrounded it—an inattentive husband, insufficient finances, the lack of variety in work centered on the home—that interfered with a woman's ability to care for her children. Thus, claims of ineffective motherhood could become the basis for new demands for structural change.

The idea, however, that women needed to become mothers to complete their psychological development as fully mature and self-realized adults was dangerous. The notion that women needed their children as much as their children needed them became a feature of discussions of state-funded family planning—especially fertility treatments for childless couples—as well as the promotion of early adoption and debates surrounding the legalization and state funding of artificial insemination for childless couples. Although Britain's mostly male Parliamentarians were disturbed by the prospect of husbands supporting children who were not biologically related to them, many nonetheless expressed sympathy for childless women who wanted to be mothers but experienced involuntary infertility. Some, however, focused on possible connections between childlessness and psychological pathology, thus making such a woman unfit for motherhood:

> The question arises whether the type of woman whose "child hunger" cannot be assuaged is suited to conceive a child by A.I.D. [artificial insemination by donor] ... With some women, the frustration caused by childlessness may by itself become pathological, or it may be merely an accompaniment of a more widespread breakdown of the personality.[109]

If a woman expressed a strong desire to have children after infertility had been identified, adoption was presented as preventing her from developing a "personality disorder." It should be noted, however that adoption was only seen as healing childless *married* women's psychological torment. The notion that women needed to be mothers was stressed only in relation to married women. Similarly, spaces at Brentwood were reserved for married women who were seen as likely to improve as mothers because they had marriages and homes to return to. The psychological burdens experienced by unmarried women giving up their children for adoption were rarely discussed.

Ultimately, projects to rehabilitate neglectful and mentally ill mothers were part of a middle-class domestic civilizing mission that functioned in part to clarify married women's social role. They were underwritten by the view that mothers' contributions were not only not work but because they remained free of financial motive—and were governed by an irrepressible desire to love—remained uncorrupted by the modern world. If dysfunctional mothers could be rehabilitated to care for their children effectively, there was hope for everyone to be healed by their love, mothers and (grown-up) children alike.

4

"More than a Contract"

Marriage Welfare Services and the Politics of Intimacy

> No marriage is entirely materialistic; emotional qualities enter into it so very deeply that I think it would be wrong to try to make marriage no more than a contract.
> —Dr. Eustace Chesser, Evidence Presented to Royal Commission on Divorce, 1952

> My husband sometimes says to me, "You have made me a better character," and for me that is the heart of our marriage.
> —Honor Thomson, *Good Housekeeping*, November 1954

At the International Congress on Mental Health held in London in August 1948, Edward Griffith, popular sex education author and founding member of the National Marriage Guidance Council, lamented the widespread decline in the value that British men and women accorded marriage and family life. He noted that one in four British brides became pregnant before marriage and that abortions, out-of-wedlock births, and sexually transmitted diseases were all "on the increase."[1] Most distressing, was the sharp rise in the divorce rate: "In this country in 1900 there were 500 divorce and separation cases; this year there will be at least 50,000."[2] Griffith linked the resolution of Britain's alarming "divorce epidemic" to broader challenges of mental illness prevention and the state-directed reorganization of Britain's health services. He urged that the nationwide expansion of Britain's new marriage counseling services offered the most promising means for stabilizing British marriages.[3]

In the years immediately following WWII, government-commissioned inquiries echoed Griffith's assessment and declared an urgent need for state intervention. However, panic surrounding marriage breakdown was not tied to anxieties about Britain's dwindling population size, which had been a prominent source of worry during the interwar decades. The British birth rate had finally surpassed replacement level in 1947, and concern was now focused on the psychological health of the growing number of people reared outside of the presumably loving milieu of the nuclear family. In the popular press, divorce was connected to a host of distressing social problems: youth crime had steadily risen since the war's end (following a drop during the war); a prominent study of Britain's mental health services warned that a "great army" of citizens suffered from neurotic illness;[4] and an alarming increase in the number of sexual crimes alongside the growing visibility of homosexuality in cities were repeatedly linked to family breakdown.

Postwar British marriage welfare initiatives almost always relied upon depth psychology to both understand and "cure" dysfunctional marriages.[5] Government committee researchers and legislators reported being impressed with recent insights into the psychodynamic underpinnings of intimate relationships, and by 1949 government funding was aimed at incorporating depth psychology into marriage reconciliation workers' training. Within a decade, most British marriage counselors understood their work as fundamentally targeting the unconscious dynamics of intimate relationships, regardless of whether they were primarily trained as a social worker, a general physician, a psychiatrist, or a volunteer counselor at a local marriage guidance center. The appeal of specialized psychological techniques for marriage reconciliation only intensified in the decades that followed. Services grew in number, government grants and private donations increased alongside the cost of running the expanded services, and public demand rose each year. The scale of this expansion was significant—while the number of couples who underwent marriage counseling in 1946 was in the hundreds, in 1968 the National Marriage Guidance Council saw more than thirty thousand clients and the Family Welfare Association had been approached about more than one hundred thousand marital problems.[6]

These postwar developments raise several questions: Why did the government actively integrate marriage counseling and therapy services into Britain's new welfare state? How were these psychosocial services seen as contributing to the broader welfare-state project of eliminating "want, disease, ignorance, squalor, and idleness" (in conformity with William Beveridge's plan for Britain's post-WWII government)? How did they contribute to making Britain a (relatively) "classless" democratic society (following the reasoning of welfare-state theorist T.H. Marshall)?[7] Moreover, given their growing popularity, how did these services' treatment of marriage as first and foremost an emotional relationship contribute to changing expectations of marriage during decades when personal satisfaction in love relationships became increasingly valued across the social classes?[8]

This chapter explores how adult citizens' emotional lives emerged as a central object of political concern in Britain after WWII and how intimate relationships became the subject of legal reform and new expectations of emotional fulfillment in the decades that followed. The previous two chapters showed how children's emotional and relational lives were invested with enormous political importance after WWII (and, following from this, mothers' emotional health in some quarters). This chapter demonstrates how the post-WWII political priority attributed to intimate emotional relationships also strongly impacted adult men and women as married (or if not already married, one-day married) people.

To this end, it presents two related narrative threads. First, I argue that state support for a network of marriage welfare services was integral to the wider welfare-state project of eliminating deep class divides. Britain's new marriage welfare service affirmed the universal importance of emotional relationships as a key determining fact of citizens' lives at a moment when the government claimed to have largely solved the acute interwar problem of socio-economic inequality. Second, I argue that the treatment of marriage as a fundamentally emotional relationship by marriage counselors and therapists helped shape an epochal shift in popular attitudes toward marriage. There was a widespread appropriation of psychological concepts in the movement to liberalize the divorce law in the 1960s; divorce reformers also promoted marriage services as a humane and scientifically grounded alternative to a restrictive divorce law. Divorce reform advocates were overwhelmingly concerned that the laws impacting private life align with citizens' natural emotional needs. The psychological "discovery" of the wide-ranging importance of emotional relationships for healthy human development framed the new emotionally oriented political landscape—focused on the private world of the family—that emerged in Britain during the decades following WWII.

Examining how citizens' intimate relationships were politicized as they increasingly became objects of therapeutic intervention, this chapter builds on scholarship revealing the close relationship between twentieth-century developments in the human sciences and the politics of democratic citizenship.[9] This literature has shed new light on how a diverse range of modern psychological and psychiatric agendas have aspired to also function as political theory and, in some cases, have shaped public health, family, education, and labor policies. I similarly explore how Britain's marriage services were embedded within discussions about Britain's future, in exchanges between pioneering marriage therapists as well as in debates within the halls of Parliament. In doing so, this chapter highlights the centrality of intimate relationships to new connections drawn between healthy human development and responsible citizenship in Britain in the middle decades of the twentieth century.

This chapter problematizes claims advanced in several recent histories of modern British sex, marriage, and love that the rising value attributed to the emotional aspects of romantic relationships in the post-1945 decades was driven by an unshackling of individual desire from the bonds of public duty.[10] This chapter does not hold to this view of emotions straightforwardly driving historical change and instead examines precisely *what* post-WWII Britons came to believe constituted desirable emotional relationships and *how* they judged the difference between viable and failed marriages. British marriage services—which did not necessarily view emotional satisfaction as achievable by large numbers of people—provided clarifying language for understanding the difficulties of monogamous heterosexual married life, as well as for apprehending marriage's social importance. As Eva Illouz has pointed out, the emotionalization of romantic relationships went hand in hand with their rationalization.[11] Marriage became a laboratory for making emotionally fulfilled selves and thus retained political value in the 1960s despite growing support for liberalizing Britain's divorce law and apparent distancing of marriage from public life. Divorce reformers believed that prioritizing access to more personally fulfilling emotional life would help stabilize families. Far from liberating emotional life, however, they presented new constraints. Emotional satisfaction, and not merely permanent marriage, became imperative. As several scholars have noted, this is a state of being that remains elusive to most and connected to a very limited conception of freedom.[12]

Britain's marriage welfare service played a crucial role in cultivating a fundamentally emotional purpose for marriage—making it "more than a contract"—and promoting a new understanding of the wide-ranging consequences of emotional fulfillment in the immediate postwar decades. Far from simply keeping couples out of the divorce court, marriage experts helped alter perceptions of what marriage meant and what it should ultimately involve: much more than a biological and social unit for procreation, stable marriage was reconceived as a necessary psychological platform to produce psychologically mature and emotionally satisfied selves. While marriage counselors and therapists only ever came into direct contact with a few hundred thousand men and women in the decades after WWII, their work was nonetheless crucial for providing a compelling language and set of concepts that elevated the stable lifelong marriage to a position of social and emotional cure-all in the public imagination.

Rationalizing Intimacy: Sex Advice and the Interwar Roots of Marriage Therapy

The British public was first introduced to strategies for marriage improvement during the interwar decades, partly in response to anxieties surrounding Britain's falling birth rate. Unlike postwar marriage reconciliation services, which focused on emotional conflicts, interwar marriage improvement initiatives primarily targeted problems in married couples' sexual lives. Concerned physicians, sexologists, and birth control advocates—including Marie Stopes, Helena Wright, and Edward Griffith—identified widespread ignorance about the precise mechanics of sexual pleasure as the leading cause of marital unhappiness (and ensuing population decline) and published extensively on sexual matters. These new self-styled marriage experts all insisted that mutual sexual enjoyment resulted from instruction rather than improvisation.[13] Stopes's own first marriage, as she confessed in her controversial 1918 bestseller *Married Love*, was never consummated, and she claimed that sexual ignorance had caused her to pay the "terrible price" of a failed marriage.[14]

Sex manuals frankly explained widely misunderstood differences between male and female sexuality and focused especially on educating readers on how women experienced sexual enjoyment. For sex education authors, husbands' and wives' shared experience of sexual pleasure was not only a physical benefit but the foundation for a deep and lasting emotional connection between spouses. Stopes maintained that mutual orgasm was "extremely important" for enhancing spouses' emotional relationship and occurred regularly between the "perfectly adjusted" husband and wife.[15] Edward Griffith also stressed mutual orgasm as having not merely procreative value but also serving to "revivify" each spouse's "whole personality" and bring partners together in an ego-transcending union.[16] Griffith went so far as to insist that mutual sexual fulfillment was also training for good citizenship; in his view, the ability to establish a deep emotional bond with another person prepared the individual to participate fully in community-oriented pursuits.[17]

Despite its controversial content, British sex advice literature attracted a large readership. Stopes's *Married Love* had sold more than half a million copies by 1925;[18] Griffith's *Modern Marriage and Birth Control* went through nineteen editions between 1935 and 1946 and established him as a preeminent medical expert in the treatment of sexual problems;[19] Helena Wright's *The Sex Factor in Marriage* sold over one million copies, and immediately became a bestseller when it was published in 1930.[20] As there was clear public demand for knowledge about sex and marriage, several physicians (including Griffith and Wright), psychiatrists, and clergymen introduced sex education lectures to youth organizations and secondary schools,[21] launched birth control clinics, created a centralized National Birth Control Council in 1930, and formed a subcommittee specializing in preparation for marriage through the British Social Hygiene Council in 1931.

For sex educators, birth control advocates, and pioneers of marriage preparation courses, harmonious marriage was seen as having important consequences for the health of adult men and women and their future children alike. Stopes argued that unhappy marriages were responsible for a range of nervous illnesses. Griffith pointed to their negative impact on women's fertility.[22] Dr. Jessie Margaret Murray, in her preface to *Married Love*, argued that marriage problems had a profoundly damaging effect on young children's personalities.[23] Like child psychologist Ethel Dukes, Murray saw marital harmony as important in preventing "maladjustment" in children. The cultivation of loving marriages thus became a central focus of an expansive updated eugenics in the 1930s that targeted not only Britons' reproductive practices for their impact on population health, but also the environments in which children were reared.[24] Sex educators and marriage reformers' eugenic convictions merged a commitment to educating the public about marriage's emotional virtues with the goal of expanding popular—and expert—understandings of the meaning of health to include intertwined physical, environmental, and moral aspects. To introduce the radical changes that sex and marriage reformers believed were necessary for measurable improvements to national health, they coupled the dissemination of marriage advice literature with public lectures and new specialized advisory services where married couples could receive expert guidance.

It was in this spirit that the Marriage Guidance Council (MGC) was launched in 1938 with a small grant of £200 from the Eugenics Society. The MGC—which was mainly composed of progressive physicians and clergymen—promoted a comprehensive medico-moral view of marriage that highlighted marital harmony's positive impact on population health.[25] They promoted the benefits of premarital medical examinations (to determine compatibility and eugenic "fitness") and birth control for spacing children and emphasized the *dual* purpose of sex in both producing healthy children and establishing a lifelong emotional relationship between spouses.[26] Approaching their goal pedagogically, marriage guidance pioneers initially focused on circulating educational material and providing public lectures on healthy marriage. During the first course of lectures held in London in the autumn of 1938, attendance ranged between 150 and 250, "mainly young office workers, shop assistants, etc., with a sprinkling of students."[27] The MGC's first report optimistically commented that, "the group as a whole was obviously keenly interested in marriage and sex problems and was considering them in a thoughtful and serious manner," so much so that many stayed after the meetings had ended to ask follow-up questions.[28]

This commitment to the transformative power of education was challenged by surges in the divorce rate during the war, and many reformers felt their efforts to improve British marriages had failed. The MGC was thus updated in 1942 to confront the more immediate problems that married couples faced—not only those forced separations and insecurities introduced by the war, but also the range of everyday problems that couples experienced in peacetime. Perhaps fittingly, given the larger context of international conflict, members transformed the MGC to focus more directly on resolving marital conflict, whether sparked by poor sexual relations, cramped housing, financial worries, or troubles with in-laws. The MGC's new secretary (and former Methodist minister) David Mace was most responsible for introducing this new emphasis. He was adamant that couples' access to medical and psychological consultants was necessary to overturn Britain's escalating "marriage crisis." Mace noted that whereas dissatisfied spouses may have once turned to a spiritual advisor or an older relative for counsel,

> The man who is ill today ... wants the judgement of a trained scientist, and is prepared to pay to get it. In his personal problems, likewise ... He has read enough popular psychology to know that his condition may admit of some deeper and more technical explanation, and he wants an authoritative verdict.[29]

With donations received from their expanding membership, the MGC opened its first marriage advisory center in a small, rented office in London in June 1943.[30] Mace advertised widely, and by November the advisory center had seen 250 cases.[31] A year later he proudly reported that that number had grown to eight hundred.[32]

The MGC's updated focus on emotional conflicts in marriage was the result of almost two years of intense negotiation between its founding members. Mace and Griffith had initially proposed separate, and distinctly different, plans for the future of marriage guidance in 1941. Despite their shared commitment to marriage improvement as the foundation for social reconstruction, the two clashed over the methods they believed a marriage service should employ toward the goal of marital stability. Mace's idea was that the MGC should be "roughly a movement parallel to that which has established the Child Guidance Clinics throughout the country."[33] His vision for a nationwide network of marriage guidance clinics where couples could get access to professional help for resolving marriage problems was rooted in the transatlantic mental hygiene movement that had been imported to Britain from the United States in the late 1920s. Griffith's plan was of a very different order. He drew up a detailed proposal for an Institute for Marriage and Parenthood that he was optimistic could be established at one of London's hospitals. Primarily medical in inspiration, Griffith's proposed institute was "directed towards the encouragement of parenthood; the strengthening of the family unit and the raising of the quality and numbers of the population."[34] Griffith's proposal would certainly have resonated with the interwar founders of the marriage guidance movement, many of whom were also members of the Eugenics Society. However, Mace's concern for the emotional difficulties of marriage was met with far greater enthusiasm at the height of the war when long separations between husbands and wives coupled with women's entry into the workforce were widely seen as having put a strain on an unprecedented number of British marriages.

Despite its humble beginnings, the marriage guidance movement expanded rapidly. By April 1946, marriage guidance councils had been established in more than one hundred towns and cities in Britain.[35] This rapid growth, alongside the probation service's expanded duties, which now included a new focus on matrimonial conciliation, in addition to the launching of marriage therapy services at the Family Discussion Bureau in 1948 and the Tavistock Clinic's Marital Unit in 1949, both reflected and cultivated demand for specialized services for improving British marriages. Unlike interwar marriage improvement efforts, most of these post-WWII initiatives cast doubt on the efficacy of educational approaches to marriage improvement, claiming that relationship problems were rooted in unconscious conflicts that had their origins in spouses' early childhood experiences. Their resolution was argued to lie beyond the scope of rationality.

Why, during this moment of postwar reconstruction and recuperation, did an interest in the psychology of relationships dominate British marriage services? The answer is certainly connected to postwar optimism surrounding the reach of scientific progress and the appeal of the promised efficacy of scientific solutions for solving personal problems. A science of marriage appeared especially possible after WWII as psychiatrists had demonstrated during the war that depth psychology had a broad range of uses. More importantly, Britain's psychologically oriented national marriage welfare service appeared consistent with the democratic values of postwar era. Not only did men and women increasingly seek out expert-directed marriage services that were aimed at resolving conflicts, the British government regarded the provision of such services as appropriately non-coercive and geared toward cultivating clients' capacity to make autonomous decisions. Although emotions had featured positively in experts' discussions of sexual and marital reform before WWII, it was only after the war that a couple's shared emotional life, as opposed to their sexual relationship, became a key basis for conceiving of the social consequences of marriage.

Targeting Emotional Life through a State-Sponsored Marriage Welfare Service

Immediately following WWII there was yet another sharp rise in the divorce rate—this time an unprecedented doubling of the number of breakups during the war. Fueling alarm surrounding the post-WWII "divorce epidemic" were reports that the incidence of extramarital births had more than doubled over the course of the war, while the married birth rate had itself dropped significantly.[36] The wartime rise in extramarital sexual encounters, alongside the birth rate remaining below replacement level, contributed to panic that Britain was in a state of precipitous decline. To many observers, moral standards appeared to be eroding, and it seemed that wartime conditions were not to blame since a comparable increase in extramarital births and divorces had not occurred during or after WWI.

State-appointed committees charged with investigating the rise in divorce petitions concluded that the state needed to be more active in protecting families from further disintegration. This was seen as urgent in the wake of the church's perceived failure to make a strong imprint on the marriage guidance movement before the war.[37] Following six months of investigation, the 1947 Committee on Procedure in Matrimonial Causes—led by high court judge Lord Alfred Thompson Denning—urged the government to provide substantial support for a nationwide "marriage welfare service" focused on matrimonial reconciliation. Their report stressed that, "[t]he reconciliation of estranged parties to marriages is of the utmost importance to the State as well as to the parties and their children. It is indeed so important that the State itself should do all it can to assist reconciliation."[38] Although committee members emphasized that British marriage services should be state funded, they were adamant that the state needed to avoid any appearance of coercion in providing couples with marriage advice. The decision to stay married needed to come from clients themselves.[39]

The prospect of state intervention in citizens' private lives seemed dangerously close to the practices of the authoritarian regimes that the new postwar welfare government was consciously avoiding emulating. As a result, Parliament decided to provide funding for already existing marriage services—including the National Marriage Guidance Council (NMGC), the recently launched Catholic Marriage Advisory Council (CMAC), and the Family Welfare Association (FWA)—rather than create a centralized government service. They explicitly wanted to provide a "marriage welfare service *sponsored* by the State, though *not* a State institution."[40]

Government researchers' support for a nationwide marriage welfare service was fueled by recent psychiatric discoveries highlighting the negative impact of family disruption on children's emotional development. As discussed in chapter 2, family instability was presented as the underlying psychological cause of a wide array of social problems, including juvenile crime, neurosis, illegitimacy, and divorce.[41] Government committees mobilized these psychological findings to argue for Britain's pressing need for a marriage welfare service. Members of the Denning Committee were "much impressed by the evidence of experienced workers in this field that the basic causes of marriage failure are to be found in false ideas and unsound emotional attitudes developed before marriage, in youth and even in childhood."[42] Similarly, the 1948 Committee on Grants for the Development of Marriage Guidance, chaired by child welfare advocate Sidney Harris, discussed marriage's psychological impact on children in their report. The committee noted that since "it is widely accepted that successful marriage relationships can generally only be achieved by persons of sound and balanced character ... The welfare of the family is profoundly affected by the behaviour of parents to one another, and the impression left on the minds of the children may influence their attitude to the community and to their own future marriages."[43]

Government researchers' preoccupation with the psychological impact of the social environment was also informed by other wartime developments in British psychiatry. In response to reportedly successful experiments with group therapy in rehabilitating neurotic soldiers, psychological methods for officer selection, and studies of German POWs that isolated the origins of Nazi ideology in authoritarian family dynamics, several prominent British psychiatrists criticized biological approaches to mental life as crudely reductive. They focused instead on the psychologically transformative effects of the social environment as the foundation for healthy mental and emotional development.[44] As discussed in the first chapter, the emergence of the democratic "therapeutic community" was perhaps the most emblematic example of the psychosocial turn within postwar British psychiatry.[45] However, an even more pervasive marker was the growing focus on mental illness prevention that targeted eliminating authoritarian and "affectionless" influences within families.

In 1949 the Home Office alerted the NMGC and the probation service that marriage counselors needed to undergo psychological training and that the government would assume responsibility for funding such programs.[46] The Harris Committee recommended that all marriage reconciliation work adhere to expert-informed methods, since "[a]ll the good qualities that a counsellor should possess ... may not carry him very far without special instruction in the nature of the problems he will have to face."[47] Although the Harris Committee did not specify the precise content of the suggested training, the professional rigor of two recently launched marriage therapy initiatives impressed government officials with their theoretically sophisticated and seemingly objective approach to treating marital conflict. The FWA had created the Family Discussion Bureau (FDB) in 1948 as a social work initiative specializing in marital problems. Several months later, the Tavistock Clinic—one of Britain's leading centers for psychoanalytic therapy, research, and training—created a marriage therapy unit under the leadership of Henry Dicks. Unlike the NMGC's empirical style of counseling, these psychotherapeutic initiatives were committed to developing clinical techniques that would universalize the treatment of problem marriages by approaching intimate relationships as new kinds of therapeutic objects. As

Dicks crisply put it, instead of treating two separate afflicted individuals, "the marriage became the patient."[48]

The postwar turn toward treating relationships, rather than individuals, as the object of therapy had grown out of wartime experiences. Dicks saw the creation of the Tavistock Marital Unit as an opportunity to put into practice his wartime research on the origins of Nazi ideology in childhood family dynamics: "The War of 1939–45 sharpened our awareness ... that the quality of marital life was a crucial factor in moulding the personalities of children, and thus the psycho-social climate of the future."[49] Drawing from a different set of experiences, the FDB's first secretary, caseworker Enid Eichholtz (later Balint), credited the origins of FDB's psychodynamic orientation to her wartime work with the Citizens' Advice Bureau. At the bureau, she had discovered that the dislocated families she helped find housing were most interested in talking about "their personal experiences and relationships."[50] She later described becoming "convinced that behind many practical problems were relationship problems—more specifically marital problems—and that these were surprisingly difficult to resolve."[51] In setting up the FDB, Eichholtz prioritized bringing the most up-to-date psychological knowledge and techniques to bear on marriage problems. She had a deep appreciation for Freud and had recently begun training in psychoanalysis at the British Psychoanalytical Society under John Rickman. In developing social workers' training at the FDB, Eichholtz established close relationships with psychiatric staff at the Tavistock Clinic, several of whom—including Bowlby, Dicks, and her future husband Michael Balint—were sympathetic to her commitment to merging social work with psychotherapy.[52]

The early innovators of marriage therapy were inspired by object relations psychoanalysis, an approach that Austrian émigrées Melanie Klein and Anna Freud and Scottish psychiatrists Ronald Fairbairn and Ian Suttie developed in Britain in the 1920s and 1930s. Basing many of their conclusions on clinical observations of infants and young children, object relations theorists deviated from orthodox Freudians in identifying human drives as motivated not by sexual desire but by a desire to develop relationships with other human beings. They argued that normal psychological development proceeded through interpersonal relationships—first with the individual's mother, later their father, siblings, friends, teachers, colleagues, and, finally, their spouses.

For marriage therapists at the FDB and the Tavistock, relationships were the object of therapy; clients were guided to view themselves as fundamentally relational and shaped by the relationships they established, beginning in early childhood and continuing on into adulthood. Although clients most often approached marriage therapy as an opportunity to have complaints about their spouses heard, in therapy they were guided to see themselves as equally implicated in creating their marital problems. For example, at the FDB a "tomboyish" young woman who complained of her husband's sexual rejection was told that she was unconsciously choosing to relive her adolescent experience of having a mother who behaved coldly toward her and who frequently criticized her disinterest in dresses and makeup.[53] At the Tavistock, the wife of an adulterous husband was discovered to have had a father who was "very much wrapped up" in her mother and had found her own presence "a nuisance."[54] She was helped to see that her marriage was a return to this early childhood moment when she had felt she needed to compete for her father's attention.

As clients discovered their shared responsibility in creating their marital conflicts, improvements in each partner's behavior were understood to support beneficial developments in the other. For example, over the course of several months of therapy at the FDB in the early 1950s, the "flirtatious" Mrs. Greenwood delighted in her formerly "weak and childlike" husband becoming "more manly and independent." By the end of therapy, she expressed relief that "he no longer seemed like a child."[55] In turn, she found herself "able to respond to him more cooperatively, both in a mutually satisfying sexual relationship" and in running a more efficient household.[56] Stressing the reciprocal feedback effect that improvements in one partner brought about in the other, marriage therapists emphasized that through therapy "vicious circles of intolerance and resentment" gave way to "a beneficent spiral in which more positive behavior on both sides evoked a warmer response."[57] Their hope was that couples would seek help soon after the recurring nature of their conflict had become clear to them. If it were left too long, then even the most experienced therapist might not be able to help a couple undo the psychological damage incurred by their neurotic relationship, and divorce would become inevitable.[58]

Prompted by the Home Office decision in 1949 that all services offering marriage counseling adopt a consistent professional approach, the FDB and Tavistock expanded their training programs. Within a decade, probation officers, family planning physicians, and counselors at marriage guidance clinics were receiving training in their psychotherapeutic techniques.[59] Since marriage welfare services were provided free of charge, an exceptionally diverse range of people became acquainted with the language and goals of marriage therapy. Clients at Britain's marriage welfare services included everyone from working-class divorce petitioners who approached the probation service as a requirement for legal aid to upper-middle-class couples who were referred to the FDB by a family physician because they were having trouble conceiving a child.

The cross-class universality of marriage problems in Britain was consistently emphasized in discussions of funding for marriage services. MPs arguing in Parliament in favor of increased funding for marriage welfare services unfailingly pointed to the proportional rise in the divorce rate across the social classes beginning in 1949, when legal aid was made available for divorce petitions. They argued that since divorce was no longer only available to the well-to-do, solutions needed to be directed at the entire population.[60] The goals of marriage welfare work at all British marriage services were similarly framed in terms of national—as well as personal—improvement. Marriage counselors and therapists alike emphasized that a depth psychological approach was appropriate for clients of all backgrounds. Dicks affirmed this following his work with the probation service in 1949, where he had found "no essential class-difference in the dynamics of marital interaction."[61] Probation officer

Joan King similarly stressed that a psychotherapeutic approach to marital conflict was effective in helping working-class couples to "look below the surface" of their marriage.[62] However, one (ostensibly minor) class-based difference was consistently mentioned by both King and Dicks: that working-class clients often required a more openly didactic approach in therapy than educated middle-class couples. Both practitioners cautioned that counselors needed to "use simpler words" and "be prepared to play more overt parental roles" at the same time as they should expect and "accept cruder transference-manifestations."[63]

Despite the appeal of psychoanalytic marriage reconciliation techniques at services across Britain, the NMGC was initially resistant. This may seem surprising since the organization had since 1946 envisioned "counseling"—a term that David Mace had imported from the United States—as a "skilled job" that helped clients develop new, conscious awareness of the emotional underpinnings of their marital conflicts. Mace described the learning process during the first months of marriage guidance work as propelled by clients' failure to grasp the true nature of their problems:

> In some cases the nature of the trouble appeared to be quite clear from the outset. One obviously needed a doctor, another a psychologist, another a social worker. But more often the situation was far from clear, and superficial judgments often fell wide of the mark. *We soon learned, for instance, to put little trust in the opinions of the people themselves*, as to whether their trouble was medical, or legal, or spiritual. *They were as often wrong as right in their verdict!*[64]

Unable to trust that clients accurately understood the real basis for their conflict, Mace devised interview methods to "diagnose" marital problems. This introductory interview quickly expanded into a counseling session as he "came to realize that most of these interviews required a full hour to be effective."[65] Mace was insistent that marriage counseling sessions should be different than consultations with experts. Aimed at "the deep emotional tensions at the heart of [a] relationship," which Mace claimed were the "real cause of conflict," counselors sought to help couples understand their emotional dynamic.[66] Unlike the psychotherapeutic model of marriage work developed at the FDB, at the NMGC counseling was seen as resting only in small part on the counselor's knowledge of the basic principles of clinical psychology. More central to the NMGC's model of expertise was counselors' direct experience of marriage.[67] Mace consistently emphasized that his happy and fulfilling marriage to Vera—his wife and collaborator in marriage counseling and marriage enrichment initiatives—was far more important than his familiarity with psychology in preparing him to help couples resolve their conflicts and improve their marriages.[68] In line with the NMGC's privileging of personal experience, divorced men and women were not accepted as marriage counselors until the early 1970s, several years after the laws surrounding divorce had been relaxed.

Although the NMGC remained committed to its experiential approach to expertise, by the mid-1950s its leadership was increasingly interested in incorporating more specialized psychotherapeutic techniques. Not only was the government-appointed marriage training board pressuring the NMGC to professionalize its lay counselors through more thorough training in psychology, but clients were also increasingly demanding that their spouses' personality "defects" be transformed through marriage counseling—in their view this was the only way to save their marriage. Training officer John Wallis emphasized the challenge that this presented since personality problems were far more difficult to resolve than complaints about sex, housing, or in-laws. In the NMGC's first official history, Wallis explained that he and his colleagues saw this shift in clients' expressions of marital dissatisfaction as calling for a more rigorous application of psychological methods.

A psychological understanding of marriage was also adopted at family services that did not explicitly make marriage reconciliation part of its work. By the early 1960s, the Family Planning Association (FPA) had begun to integrate marriage therapy into its work as part of clinic physicians' updated duties, since "marital difficulties" were believed to be "often part and parcel of the desire or request for birth control."[69] A 1963 report emphasized that, "Every clinic doctor should be perceptive to emotional aspects of sexuality which cause unstated anxieties in many clinic users ... [and] also be able to spot and know what may be done about more serious disturbances deserving the name of 'marital difficulties.'"[70] The selection of clinic physicians thus increasingly prioritized their "interest in psychological medicine, awareness of the emotional aspects of sexuality, [and] appreciation of psychosexual symptoms in neurosis and personality disorder."[71] This was a timely shift of focus given that the FPA's client base was increasingly middle-class and thus likely to be at least casually familiar with psychotherapy.

By the mid-1950s, the orientation of marriage counselors and therapists had expanded beyond earlier interwar preoccupations with sexual problems to encompass a much broader, and more nebulous, range of interpersonal issues. Emotional conflict had replaced sexual ignorance as the most pervasive threat to family stability and become the focus of marriage improvement work. While sexual dissatisfaction remained a major area of concern for marriage counselors, it came to be treated as one (of many) symptoms of a dysfunctional emotional relationship. Although they served a diverse clientele, marriage therapists and counselors treated all intimate relationships as emotionally the same. The shared approach of most British marriage services revealed a growing consensus that emotional factors were at the heart of all marital problems and that these required special techniques to resolve.

Marriage therapists justified their requests for government funding by arguing that in Britain's more affluent postwar society emotional problems had risen to the forefront of citizens' everyday concerns, surpassing the economic unease affecting most strata of society during the interwar decades. Appealing to the middle-class myth of universal postwar prosperity helped make marriage welfare services seem essential, while it also aligned these initiatives with the postwar government's mission to eliminate vast social inequalities. The postwar government aimed to create a largely classless society through universal welfare, and this objective was supported by marriage therapists' claims about the universality of citizens' emotional need for marriage and family. Furthermore, in line with the British government's disdain for coercion, a psychological rather than an overtly didactic approach appeared to be the most promising method for nurturing (rather than enforcing) the public's positive regard for marriage. It was in this spirit that Tavistock director J.D. Sutherland underscored the unsuitability of teaching for reaching the goal of resolving marriage problems, urging that "the traditional methods of exhortation and advice are of little or no value in emotional conflicts" or in emotional life more broadly.[72]

Marriage Therapy and the Cultivation of Relational Selfhood

When Marie Stopes and Helena Wright first began gathering information from their correspondents about their unhappy marriages, the letters they received primarily focused on sexual dissatisfaction. Stopes herself had experienced living through a profoundly unsatisfying sexual relationship with her first husband and explained this as having been fueled by sexual ignorance, resulting in mutual resentment, escalating levels of conflict, and a deep sense of shame. A second problem area that Stopes and Wright's correspondents consistently mentioned was fear of unwanted pregnancy. These letters also frequently pleaded for information about reliable methods of contraception and asked about both the safety and morality of their use.

By the mid-1950s, as growing numbers of couples turned to marriage reconciliation services, counselors reported that clients focused on a different form of marital dissatisfaction, one framed within the language of "personality." The NMGC's records for 1952–1954 show that spouses most often complained of one or more undesirable personality traits in their partner. Marriage guidance counselors adopted the capacious category of "personal defect" to describe the focus of approximately 45% of clients' complaints, which encompassed "a range of different factors such as emotional immaturity, selfishness, financial incompetence and being unduly interested in persons of the opposite sex."[73] Descriptions of spouses' "defects" far surpassed the frequency of mentions of "difficulties in intercourse and anxieties about contraception."[74]

NMGC clients' decreasing focus on sexual problems mirrored developments at other British marriage services. The Catholic Marriage Advisory Center similarly reported that clients' complaints were most often expressed as emotional (rather than sexual) dissatisfaction. They wanted to see changes in their spouses' personalities. Catholic opposition to contraception certainly helps explain the greater likelihood of Catholic clients focusing on personality problems rather than sexual problems, especially since sexual issues mentioned elsewhere often related to the stress of potentially producing unwanted children. However, the FDB and the Tavistock Marital Unit similarly reported that clients tended to focus most on perceived shortcomings in their partners' personalities. Personality problems were often described in terms of spouses' inability to embody conventional masculine and feminine behaviors and fulfill the responsibilities typically expected of the breadwinner and the homemaker in a middle-class marriage. At an early point in therapy, spouses often communicated a desire to see the other change in some fundamental way.

Jan Goldstein has helpfully introduced the term "self-talk" to describe how people talk about themselves as specific kinds of individuals to fashion a meaningful (and socially rewarded) life.[75] In cultures where "self-talk" is prevalent, she argues, there is more at stake in what the self can—and presumably should—be. Goldstein tracks changes in the form that "self-talk" takes in nineteenth-century France to uncover the widespread sociopolitical importance of a volitional self in the decades prior to Freud's cultural ascendance in many parts of Europe.[76] Attention to "self-talk" in mid-twentieth-century British marriage reconciliation work, however, offers a viewpoint into the high value attributed to a far more relational and interdependent model of the self—a self that was achieved in its most perfect form through marriage. Marriage therapy came to function as much more than a means for ending conflict; it became a platform for making fully mature and highly socially attuned selves. Through marriage therapy, the pursuit of marital harmony came to be closely bound up in narratives and experiences of a form of social selfhood that was consistent with liberated self-expression. Moreover, despite the growing preoccupation with the achievement of "self-realization" through marriage, expectations of strict gender-differentiation in marital roles remained largely unchallenged. Although the self-talk encountered in the case reports of marriage therapists and counselors was often prompted by marriage welfare workers, who also supplied the appropriate vocabulary and conceptual framework, clients did often (even if reluctantly) come to see themselves as formed through a series of intimate relationships stemming back to early childhood, with their marriage to their spouse constituting the pinnacle of this lengthy process of self-development.

The rationale for the state's provision of financial support for marriage welfare services was largely focused on protecting children's healthy emotional development. By 1960, good parenting was seen as one of the many positive outcomes of a well-functioning, emotionally fulfilling marriage at Britain's marriage welfare services, since this crucial adult relationship was seen as the gateway for making fully mature men and women. As a result, marriage counselors and therapists were far less focused on simply keeping couples together as they had become unsatisfied with merely restoring equilibrium to dysfunctional relationships. They saw these relationships as existing only for the satisfaction of each partner's "neurotic" needs. Viewing the "growth of personality" as central to "preventive mental health work," they instead sought to guide their clients toward mutual personal development.[77] This was explicitly stated in the first report of the Institute of Marital Studies in 1968 (as the FDB was re-named that year to signal its focus on marriage):

> we are particularly concerned with the use people make of marriage as a vehicle for developing maturity ... Successful work with marriages enables people to

be richer as individuals in their own right, and therefore to contribute to a richer partnership.[78]

In a similar spirit Tom Main, director of the Cassel Marital Clinic, explained that marriage provided a necessary platform for personal development, which proceeded relationally: "within the marital relationship the self-realization of each partner is achieved through the other by the steady reality testing of the partner against the fantasies derived from earlier conflicts."[79] Lily Pincus emphasized that marriage formed the psychological core of the family since it made possible both "the self-realization of husband and wife, and the social development of their children."[80] Marriage was likened to the mother-child relationship in counselors' training literature to emphasize its developmental importance, and the aim of counseling was increasingly described in the 1960s as not only keeping marriages stable but helping couples make use of "the potentialities for growth and self-realization which are inherent in the marital union."[81] At the height of Britain's "sexual revolution," marriage therapists viewed marriage as having the capacity to make spouses (and their children) both "richer" and "poorer" selves depending on the strength of their relationship.

Although clients generally approached their marriage therapist or counselor with complaints about their partner, over the course of therapy, they were guided to understand their spouse's shortcomings as reinforced by their own insufficiencies as a partner. As the focus of conversation shifted from complaints to an examination of each individual's life history and the role that each played in supporting their partner's problematic behavior, both were shown to equally suffer from personality "deplenishment" resulting from their troubled relationship. For example, in February 1962, Mr. Adams, a twenty-six-year-old mechanic in an aircraft factory, was referred by his general practitioner to the newly launched Marital Clinic at the Cassel Hospital for treatment because he was "unable to achieve satisfactory intercourse with his wife and could not maintain an erection."[82] His marriage of three years had yet to be consummated, and his physician suggested that—although the problem apparently appeared to lie with Mr. Adams alone—marriage therapy was more likely to prove helpful than any other medical or psychological intervention. During their first joint therapy session, Mrs. Adams reported to their therapist, psychiatrist Jean Pasmore, that the problems in their marriage lay exclusively with her husband. According to her account, he was a "useless" man who could not maintain steady employment and "so childish" that he could not spell correctly and spent most evenings playing with model trains. Pasmore found that although she was sympathetic to Mrs. Adams's complaints—finding Mr. Adams to appear dimwitted and dull even though he showed above normal intelligence on an IQ test—she saw Mrs. Adams's "henpecking" and contemptuous attitude as greatly intensifying the "icy atmosphere" between the two.

Therapy focused on uncovering the ways that both spouses' earlier relationship experiences were being repeated in their marriage. In Mr. Adams's case, he had had a "useless" father and domineering mother, and his choice of the overbearing Mrs.

Adams as a spouse had reinforced his own tendency to behave as "uselessly" as his father had. Mrs. Adams's father had died soon after she was born, and this was thought to explain her assumption of more outwardly "masculine" behaviors in her marriage. In therapy she revealed that she lay on top of her husband when attempting sexual intercourse, corrected his speech, wrote all his letters on his behalf, arranged all their holidays, and informed her husband of what opinions to hold. To move toward greater harmony in their relationship, Mrs. Adams was guided to renounce her "dominating behavior," and Mr. Adams was shown that he had to face up to his identification with his "immature" father and become more of a "useful" and "aggressive" man himself.[83] As each became aware of the childhood experiences that underpinned their immaturity, they were transformed both as individuals and as a couple. Mr. Adams experienced new freedom to express his unconsciously suppressed "masculine" aggressive traits (which he reportedly enjoyed) and began looking for work and a new home for himself and his wife. In turn, Mrs. Adams found herself capable of assuming the role of supportive wife: "in her new legitimacy of herself and her femininity, she could love [her husband] for being himself and a man."[84] The couple was described as having discovered a new closeness and ease in their interactions because of these fundamental changes. Therapeutic success was declared when Mrs. Adams became pregnant—a development that, importantly, both appeared to embrace.[85]

In practical terms, clients' personal development was most often gauged according to the degree to which they accepted and enacted conventionally expected feminine and masculine spousal roles. The Cassel Marital Clinic was not unique in this regard; Lily Pincus emphasized that at the FDB, "confusion about sexual roles" was one of the "fundamental themes in marriage problems" encountered in all of their cases.[86] For example, Mr. Robinson, who first made contact with the FDB in 1962, was initially noted to have had the demeanor of a "shamefaced boy," but through regular meetings with his caseworker steadily came to accept his "role as a man":

> Mrs. A. encouraged him to be an adult man in the casework situation, and to see her less as one of the organizing and controlling women whom he had felt his mother and his wife to be. With Mrs. A. he experienced a relationship in which his masculinity was acknowledged ... This experience seemed to give him sufficient confidence to begin to seek ... a more positive expression of his masculine drive.[87]

Mr. and Mrs. Cooper experienced a similar transformation over the course of eighteen months of therapy at the FDB. By the end, Mr. Cooper appeared "surer of himself, a man of some standing," and Mrs. Cooper "look[ed] very much a mother now, someone to be respected and reckoned with."[88] With past traumas uncovered and explored, spouses could more adequately fulfill the requirements of marriage: husbands became capable of taking financial responsibility for the household while their wives became willing to take on the emotional responsibilities of childcare. Spouses' heightened "self-realization"—language used in the bureau's pamphlets and reports—was assessed through their confident expression of the normative markers of adult masculinity and femininity. Therapeutic progress was measured in terms of spouses' apparently joyful enactment of appropriate masculine or feminine spousal roles and readiness "to move forward into full adulthood and parenthood."[89]

The commitment to gender-differentiated marital roles was not solely the projection of marriage welfare workers. Case reports indicate that clients—at least those who underwent a full course of therapy—frequently adopted behaviors and attitudes that their counselors and therapists described as signs of progress in their healing. At the FDB, Mrs. Carter's caseworker had only praise for her beginning to dress in a more feminine manner, wear makeup, and perm her hair.[90] Mrs. Carter in turn expressed gratitude to her caseworker for encouragement in taking on this difficult challenge. At his local marriage guidance council, Mr. Danvers found the necessary support in therapy to accept new challenges at work and move up the corporate ladder.[91] Case files reveal that in many instances clients made use of the therapeutic relationship to address their unfulfilled desire to be a different—more conventionally masculine or feminine—kind of self.

The idea that recent developments in psychology could be directed toward helping women to become the more feminine self they had always wanted to be can also be seen in social scientific studies of marriage at this time. Drusilla Beyfus's studies of contemporary attitudes and practices vis-à-vis marriage reveal disappointment that courtship rituals had changed—they had been de-romanticized, she argued, as a result of being democratized—such that young girls and women felt that they had to find new avenues for cultivating femininity.[92] Women who found themselves at a loss when attempting to "learn" how to become appropriately feminine adult women greeted relationship advice columns, marriage preparation courses, and reconciliation services with enthusiasm.

During the first two decades following the war, Britain's marriage welfare services deepened their exploration of psychotherapeutic techniques, and many clients were drawn to their increasingly overt psychotherapeutic commitments, even if this was driven by their belief that a more clinical psychological approach would "fix" their damaged spouse. Even the NMGC adopted psychoanalytic techniques in 1968 when an FDB-trained caseworker joined the counseling staff at their London office and introduced her colleagues to joint psychotherapy.[93] Although by the end of the 1960s marriage reconciliation workers had largely abandoned their earlier use of language like mutual "adjustment" and "self-sacrifice," in favor of a self-improvement "personal growth" model, marriage counselors and therapists continued to associate spouses' performance of differentiated gender roles with therapeutic progress. Clients who underwent a full course of therapy appear to have accepted the terms of the therapeutic encounter, even if with some hesitation toward their therapist's interpretation of their marital struggles. Their "improvement" as a married couple was displayed through their adoption of the behaviors expected of them.

The relational model of the self that postwar marriage therapists cultivated in the middle decades of the twentieth century was rooted in a commitment to the social and psychological benefits of gender complementarity. Therapists and their clients affirmed rather than undercut gender-differentiated roles and identities within the intimate space of the interview room. While therapists' case reports offer glimpses into clients' changing expectations of marriage in the decades following WWII, they also reveal how desire for change was carefully managed within the therapeutic encounter. Although therapists avowedly did not hold to a biological view of many of the perceived differences between men and women, they created new natural associations between gender-differentiated family labor and marital happiness. At Britain's marriage welfare services, monogamous heterosexual love was endowed with new social and psychological importance through its associations with developmental health.

The insights of marriage therapists reverberated beyond the clinic. In the media and Parliament alike, discussions of divorce reform in the 1960s increasingly relied upon depth psychology when explaining marriage breakdown, and public conversations showed increasing concern for the impact of a failing marriage on spouses' emotional wellbeing. Supporters of divorce reform argued that incurably dysfunctional relationships needed to be publicly acknowledged as irreversibly "broken down" and spouses given freedom to seek out more suitable love relationships. Reformers maintained that legal recognition was not sufficient to constitute a marriage as real; its true foundation lay in the emotional relationship that spouses either nurtured or neglected.

Divorce reformers' newly appropriated psychological understanding of marital dysfunction was one important outcome of marriage therapists' engagement with the public not only through radio programs, marriage advice columns, and popular sex and marriage education literature, but also through their participation in contemporary government and church-led inquiries into marriage and divorce.[94] However, despite their deliberate attempts to shape public opinion and bring about a deeper valuation of lifelong commitment to marriage, marriage therapists could not control how their message was received. Marriage therapists' psychological language and concepts permeated British culture but were absorbed in unexpected ways as British men and women contemplated what marriage meant to them and reconsidered how many unmet expectations and how much dissatisfaction they were willing to endure.

Bringing the Law into Conformity with Love in 1960s Britain

Marriage therapists' observations about the emotional nature and purpose of love relationships were not entirely new after the war. Arguments urging the importance of emotional satisfaction in marriage had found a sympathetic audience within the growing movement for divorce reform in the 1930s and even successfully provoked changes to the Matrimonial Causes Act in 1937. Alan Herbert's 1934 novel *Holy Deadlock* was instrumental in gaining public support for the view that marriage was essentially an emotional, rather than an economic or legal, relationship. Having left his career as a lawyer, Herbert wrote *Holy Deadlock* as a meditation on the moral conundrum that Britain's offense-based divorce law introduced. It told the moving story of a childless couple that had grown apart—through no fault of either spouse—after many years of marriage. While neither husband nor wife wished to pursue an extramarital relationship, both desperately wanted to divorce in order that they might seek out a more satisfying marriage.[95] However, the only way that an unhappy couple could obtain a divorce was if one spouse (but never both) committed adultery, or at least persuaded a judge to believe that this had happened. *Holy Deadlock* elicited enough public outrage to push the Matrimonial Causes Bill through the House of Commons in 1937.

Although Herbert made a persuasive case against the offense model, the 1937 Act merely eased the conditions and waiting period for divorces sought on certain limited grounds (such as women seeking to divorce adulterous husbands and divorce petitions proceeding from desertion). The basic framework of the offense model was kept intact, and divorce continued to only be granted if one party could prove that they were the innocent victim of an unjust injury by their spouse. It was only at the end of the 1960s that the offence-based model for divorce would be abolished. Marriage therapy, which had become increasingly popular, provided a persuasive and scientifically grounded framework for articulating the damaging psychological stakes of a bad marriage, providing the movement for divorce reform with more compelling ammunition.

The massive disorder that WWII brought to British family life fueled the perceived need to replace the offense model with divorce by mutual consent. Arguments in favor of liberalizing the divorce law now broadened to focus on the misery of not only unhappy spouses but also children—such as the social stigma that children born of relationships between married men and their mistresses faced. An article published in *The Guardian* in 1950 highlighted the many debilitating injuries that children of the "upwards of 300,000 couples more or less permanently separated and unable to re-marry" were forced to experience.[96] Underscoring the inexorable breakdown of an increasing number of families, the British news media was awash with arguments that once marriages had ceased to exist in anything but name, the law needed to stop preventing new, legitimate unions from being formed and their children from being legally recognized.

By the early 1960s, arguments in favor of liberalizing divorce increasingly reflected concern for spouses' mental and emotional wellbeing. Commentators on marriage and divorce in national newspapers emphasized the unending despair—even resulting in neurosis—caused by unhappy marriage. Many noted that as men spent more hours at work, rarely helping with childcare, women experienced resentment, loneliness, and, in some cases, severe depression. A 1961 *Observer* exposé entitled "Miserable Married Women" reported sympathetically that many working- and middle-class suburban housewives fantasized about leaving their husbands and children. The mental harm caused by life at home alone with one's children was often remarked upon, subverting the promises made in women's magazines and in modern parenting literature: one contributor noted that "the stress and strain of managing without proper facilities during children's younger years does infinite harm to the mental health of mothers *and* their families."[97]

Over the course of the 1960s, the essence of marriage was increasingly defined in terms of intimacy and mutual emotional fulfillment, rather than its legal or spiritual meanings. In a 1964 address to the NMGC, marriage counselor Peter Fletcher maintained that "its sanctity ... derives from love," and it was therefore no use preserving a marriage based only on its merits as a "social institution."[98] The legal aspects of marriage were also frequently described as merely a formal recognition of an emotional relationship that itself constituted a family as legitimate. Novelist and social critic Gillian Tindall noted that British men and women increasingly expected more from marriage as the central relationship of their adult lives. In a plea to liberalize the divorce law, she argued that a readiness to resort to divorce was reflective of higher emotional standards. A higher divorce rate signified that "we expect more from [marriage] in terms of personal companionship and individual fulfillment."[99] Some marriages, she argued, were simply "not worth maintaining" as they were "based on a situation so neurotic that it can never be rendered more stable."[100] Tindall thus strongly opposed the agenda of any public service—especially singling out the NMGC—that sought to prevent divorce. She called for a radical change in both public opinion and the work performed by Britain's marriage welfare services. In her view, emphasis needed to shift "from disapproval of divorce undertaken 'too readily and too lightly,' to disapproval of marriage undertaken too lightly."[101] Tindall was not alone in seeing divorce as an appropriate solution for many dissatisfied couples. In a 1968 *Guardian* survey of British attitudes to marriage, 71% responded that divorce was the "best way out" of an "empty" marriage.[102]

Admiring the relationship insights of Britain's psychotherapeutic marriage services, Labour MP Leo Abse mobilized a similar style of argument in Parliament. As the primary author of the transformative 1968 Divorce Reform Bill, Abse sought to replace the offense model for divorce with mutual consent following from recognition of a marriage relationship's irretrievable "breakdown." He argued that adultery and desertion were merely telling "symptoms," and the not the cause, of a failing marriage.[103] Like the Tavistock marriage therapist and the FDB caseworker, Abse pronounced the collapse of a marriage to be mutual: neither spouse was ever wholly innocent or entirely guilty. Moreover, he argued that his proposed reforms to the divorce law would nurture the democratic family, whose "basis is not legal constraint but personal affection":

> and within its comforting but not overprotective embrace, children enjoy a high status and parental concern and involvement. It is the family where ... parental authoritarianism [is] neither wanted nor enforced ... and where the greatest single need, to give a model for development of the child, is not shirked by the parent... The making of the modern family has been part of the making of the new society.[104]

Abse argued that the offense model for divorce proceedings needed to be abolished not only because it misunderstood the true basis of intimate relationships, but also because it stood as an obstacle to the creation of a fully democratic society—one that was rooted in emotional freedom. He therefore proposed that Britain's approach to divorce be replaced with a marriage "breakdown" model that was informed by a psychological view of intimate relationships. According to Abse, the law needed to support citizens' emotional needs, and "nurture not strangle" the possibility for all British marriages to be anchored in feelings of love.[105] His bill sought to create not more unmarried men and women but more stable second marriages and more secure and loving environments for children deprived of positive emotional connection.

After several years of heated debate, the Divorce Reform Bill was introduced in Parliament in February 1968. Abse had presented an earlier Matrimonial Causes and Reconciliation Bill in 1963; in it one clause—proposing that married couples be allowed to divorce following seven years of separation without any attribution of offense to either spouse—immediately erupted in controversy. The bill encountered resistance from every Christian organization in England. *The Times* declared this "remarkable display of solidarity" as a landmark event since it was the first time that all the churches of England and Wales had united on a matter of doctrine.[106] Abse dropped the controversial "seven-year clause" after deciding it would prevent the bill's central proposals from being passed—including legal changes that would allow couples to make use of marriage reconciliation services without either being seen as guilty of collusion or of having forgiven a marital offence if a divorce petition ultimately followed.[107] As he saw it, it was more important to enable couples to reconcile than to make it possible to divorce through mutual consent. In his view, "magistrates and solicitors [could] deal only with explicit surface problems" in a marriage:[108]

> To attain a real catharsis, readjustment and reconciliation, is a psychiatric task ... In my view, we shall have a right as legislators to congratulate ourselves on having an up-to-date matrimonial law only when we have built into it a conciliation service adequately manned by psychiatrists, psychiatric social workers and an adequate number of family caseworkers.[109]

Although church opposition had managed to stymie Abse's inclusion of the seven-year separation clause, the following year the Church of England's Archbishop of Canterbury appointed a group of church leaders to investigate contemporary divorce procedures and arrive at an informed decision about the matrimonial offense model. To the astonishment of many, the group's 1966 report concluded that "empty, legal marriage bonds are contrary to the public interest and ... breakdown of marriage should be substituted for the notion of matrimonial 'guilt' and 'innocence.'"[110] Explaining the meaning of breakdown, the group maintained that, "frequently, if not always, the failures in adjustment that lead to the divorce court come of failure to deal successfully with the legacy of infantile experience."[111] Embracing the contemporary, psychological interpretation of marriage as compatible with their own spiritual view, they recommended that the government concentrate on preventing breakdown and further expand existing marriage welfare services so that they reach a greater number of couples in need. The group further described Britain's marriage services as enabling spouses to "learn how to accept in the other, as well as in himself (or herself), some of the deepest elements of early infantile relationships. If both succeed in doing this, a new and more creative relationship may emerge."[112]

The archbishop's report was integrated into the 1968 Divorce Reform Bill, the purpose of which was to "recast [Britain's] divorce law by making the breakdown of marriage the sole basis of a divorce petition."[113] Rejecting the offence-based model for divorce proceedings, it emphasized spouses' mutual participation in causing a marriage to fall apart. As with Abse's earlier 1963 bill, this new bill suggested expanding and encouraging the use of marriage counseling services. William Wilson, the Labour MP and lawyer who piloted the bill through Parliament, declared himself "satisfied from talks that I have had with organisations that are skilled in reconciliation work that there is considerable scope for improvement and expansion of the work they do."[114] When the Divorce Reform Bill was passed in October 1969, *The Guardian* described it as following "a psychological approach to divorce in place of the present system of divorce by marital offence."[115]

Although the theological objections to British divorce law reform had been settled by 1966 for many of Britain's most eminent churchmen, an additional set of protests were still not fully addressed. These misgivings did not focus on reservations about the "marriage breakdown" model but instead on the financial impact of divorce on housewives and mothers. The most vocal opponent of the Divorce Reform Bill was Dr. Edith Summerskill, a respected physician, Privy Council member, and married mother who had the support of the Married Women's Association. Positioning herself as representing all married mothers, Summerskill attacked the bill as a "Casanova's Charter." She condemned it both in the press and in Parliament as "a husband's bill, drafted by a man who doubtless meant well but who failed to recognize that marriage has different values for a man and a woman."[116] According to Summerskill, since "the preservation of the home with children was more important to the wife than the husband," the dissolution of a marriage was far more devastating to women than it was to men.[117] For Summerskill and her supporters, it was considered a commonly known fact that all married men eventually developed an appetite for new lovers, leaving their more family-oriented wives saddled with the responsibility of keeping their desires in check. It was therefore the law's duty to force men to remain faithful to their marital vows. Summerskill warned that allowing greater freedom in this area would result in the destitution of vast numbers of innocent wives and children. The bleak prospect of poverty, rather than the vague promise of emotional fulfillment, was her overwhelming concern. Compared with a significant rise in unsupported mothers, Summerskill viewed appeals to emotional dissatisfaction as unimportant. She noted that, "we have not yet reached the stage of social affluence where many [husbands] can afford two wives."[118]

Advocates of divorce reform disagreed with Summerskill's grim assessment and appealed instead to the abject misery that they argued tens of thousands of men *and* women were currently experiencing in their marriages. Alex Lyon, Labour MP for York, maintained that he "did not believe life would be much altered for a woman who was divorced against her will if the marriage had already collapsed."[119] Lady Gaitskell similarly argued that, "nothing is deader than dead love," and she "refused to accept the social myth that men tire of women more easily than women tire of men."[120] In a memoir published shortly after the Divorce Act had come into effect, Abse's reply to Summerskill and other opponents of the Divorce Bill was far more cutting. He dismissed *all* of Summerskill's major campaigns—including her efforts to make boxing illegal and to prevent the birth control pill from becoming readily available to unmarried women—as stemming from a "resentment, if not envy, of male aggressiveness and sexuality."[121] Mobilizing psychoanalytic diagnosis as a tool against his opponents, Abse framed all of his campaigns for social reform—in favor of liberalizing divorce, decriminalizing homosexuality, and seemingly paradoxically, in opposition to the legalization of abortion—as working toward the wider psychopolitical end of "liberating Eros" and protecting citizens' emotional and sexual freedom.[122]

When the Divorce Reform Bill was finally passed on October 17, 1969, its implementation was postponed by more than a year to allow time to make changes to the laws surrounding the division of marital property and finances. By 1969, it had proved impossible to stem the tide of shifting public opinion when it came to beliefs about the importance of intimate relationships: emotional concerns took precedence over financial misgivings. Summerskill's campaign had, however, not been in vain. Before divorces could be made easier to obtain, new laws were drafted to ensure that divorced men's children and former wives would not be left without financial support.

While "irretrievable breakdown" became the new legal framework for understanding divorce, the old offences—adultery, cruelty, and desertion—were retained in divorce proceedings as evidence of breakdown. Although the archbishop's group had recommended an inquiry into the presence of "irretrievable breakdown" for every divorce petition brought before the court, it was decided that if either spouse claimed that their marriage had irreversibly broken down, this would be treated as sufficient evidence for the case to proceed. Contrary to Summerskill's prediction, in the years following the passage of the act, the majority of divorce proceedings were initiated by wives rather than husbands, and only 10% of divorces involved couples over age fifty.[123] The Divorce Reform Bill proved to be less a "Casanova's Charter" that left middle-aged women destitute than a means for people under forty to pursue the possibility of an emotionally fulfilling relationship.

Studies of English attitudes toward marriage at the height of Britain's "sexual revolution" showed widespread expectations of emotional satisfaction in marriage. Geoffrey Gorer's 1969 inquiry demonstrated shifting commitments across the social classes when it came to defining marital happiness in England. Gorer identified a move away from a focus on material factors toward a preoccupation with emotional concerns; he noted that the most common response to the question, "What do you think goes to wreck a marriage?" did not touch on socio-economic issues like cramped housing and financial struggles as it had twenty years earlier, but instead most often focused on relational concerns like "bad communication," "selfishness," and "conflicting personalities."[124] Gorer's study revealed pervasive expectations of emotional intimacy in love relationships among both men and women under forty-five and also showed that younger generations continued to value monogamous marriage just as strongly as their parents and grandparents did:

> In England the press, and other media of mass communication ... insisted that there was a major change in the sexual morals of the young; the "permissive society," "swinging London" and all the other clichés implied that the young were far more licentious than their elders had ever been and had an ever-diminishing regard for the importance of marriage as an institution. Such casual observations as I had been able to make made me doubt the validity of these observations; I thought the censorious commentators were confusing changes in word-style with changes in life-style.[125]

Gorer noted, however, his respondents' preference for emotional language when explaining the enduring value of monogamy. For example, when asked whether fidelity remained important even though more effective methods of birth control had become available to many, 92% of respondents gave answers that stressed the "emotional importance of fidelity" despite waning concerns about extra-marital pregnancies.[126]

The findings of a 1971 study of British attitudes toward marriage conducted by the Institute of Marital Studies (IMS) similarly revealed that marriage continued to be deeply valued across age groups and social classes. IMS researchers interpreted this as evidence that monogamy was the most natural form of human coupling. To prove this point, the study included recent population statistics demonstrating that the numbers of couples choosing to marry was on the rise despite growing tolerance for premarital sex. However much monogamous marriage was being challenged by second-wave feminists, countercultural movements, and New Left Marxists, its perceived emotional benefits continued to hold significant weight. Declining support for the virtues of self-sacrificial "adjustment" to marriage by spouses (especially wives) may, on the surface of things, appear to have set the stage for a rejection of monogamous marriage by British young people. However, in 1971, the growing number of married couples and rising proportion of married men and women who were under twenty-five demonstrated that this was far from the way things were.[127]

Widespread expectations of emotional satisfaction in intimate relationships appeared to many to dismantle, rather than bolster, marital stability by the end of the 1960s. As evidence for this, more than four hundred thousand couples divorced in the first two years following the passage of Britain's Divorce Act.[128] Divorce reformers had drawn on the vocabulary of marriage therapists and even prioritized the further expansion of reconciliation services to bring British laws surrounding divorce in line with new scientific discoveries about the eminently relational nature of human emotional development. Reformers' savvy appropriation of new knowledge about intimate relationships—however unintended by marriage therapy pioneers at the end of WWII—ended up proving to be more effective in ending marriages than therapists had been at "saving" them. Despite the surge in divorce petitions after the Divorce Act came into effect in January 1971, supporters of the benefits of stable marriage remained optimistic that the most recent (and most extreme) "divorce epidemic" might actually be a good thing for Britain. As people bravely chose to end their dysfunctional marriages, they were free to enter more emotionally fulfilling relationships and become more "self-realized" and responsible citizens and parents. Appeals to the logic of evolutionary progress were common as supporters of monogamous marriage continued to promote this specific form of relationship as the necessary path toward emotional satisfaction.

Conclusion

Britain's state-supported marriage welfare services both propelled and gave shape to changing understandings of the purpose of marriage and its function in people's lives. Not only did marriage services play an instrumental role in popularizing a new language of interpersonal psychological development and emotional fulfillment, they also provided the basis for the post-war emergence of a new kind of emotional self who expected to become "mature" and "self-realized" through marriage. By 1971—despite the relaxation of divorce laws, the state-funded accessibility of birth control to unmarried women, and the decriminalization of homosexuality—marriage counselors and therapists continued to make a persuasive case for the continued relevance of monogamous heterosexual marriage in producing mature men and women. The IMS, which was "particularly concerned with the use people make of marriage as a vehicle for developing maturity," reported its longest waiting list yet that year.[129]

For decades, scholars have noted that a transformation occurred in legal discourse and public opinion in the second half of the twentieth century—from thinking about marriage as an institution to thinking about it as a relationship.[130] Social historians Jane Lewis, Kathleen Kiernan, and Hilary Land add that the view that marriage primarily serves "public purposes" has been abandoned in favor of seeing it "as a private arrangement that maximizes individual satisfactions."[131] This reading, while not incorrect, obscures the ways that healthy emotional development was framed as deeply connected to public life in the post-WWII decades—as a basic guarantee of responsible citizenship and as a basis for resolving intractable social problems and securing a stable democratic polity. As this chapter has shown, the emotionally oriented post-war subject was brought into existence, in part, through the British government's involvement in attempting to ensure the cultivation of socially responsible citizens. Moreover, Britain's first generation of marriage therapists promoted their services as fulfilling a necessary social function: harmonious families were meant to re-invigorate public life by setting empathic social responsibility on a solid foundation—the healthy and fully developed personality. Unlike the individualizing projects that Michel Foucault's work on modern penal and psychiatric institutions has explored, Britain's marriage welfare services were anchored in experts' "discovery" that the self was fundamentally relational—interdependent rather than independent, intersubjective rather than self-sufficient.[132] Marriage therapists presented a naturalized community-centered alternative to the endlessly competitive Darwinian vision of urban industrial modernity.

Anthony Giddens has described the greater valuation of emotional life in the latter half of the twentieth century as integral to the democratization of private life.[133] In Giddens' view, love relationships have been elevated to a place of utmost importance in defining individual identities and aspirations; a model of love that is more self-expressive than self-sacrificing. This view has since been echoed in historians' explanations for reforms connected to the late-1960s sexual revolution, associating choices rooted in emotional preference with democratic freedom.[134] Giddens helps to account for the steady popularity of couples' counseling and marriage improvement literature. But he fails to consider the extent to which emotional intimacy became a value associated with a form of lifelong monogamy that many felt compelled to accept and incorporate into their lives. Giddens takes for granted that emotions are pure, in the sense of being expressive of an unmediated agentive self. However, it is important to note that the conventions surrounding emotional intimacy in the decades following WWII were centered on the production of male-breadwinning, female-homemaking nuclear families and served very specific purposes. Marriage counseling services both reflected and nurtured this. While it seems that many genuinely supported and found comfort in the increasing regard for emotional life and saw tremendous potential for freedom contained within this emerging set of values, there were also many others who were excluded from this model of mature adulthood: homosexuals, childless couples, and those who, for a variety of reasons, never married. The freedom that was associated with love relationships did not straightforwardly extend to non-childbearing individuals and couples.

By the late 1960s, emotional intimacy was seen as relying upon privacy of a kind that remained out of financial reach for most working-class families. The privacy of the marriage relationship was ideally manifested through a couple's spatial separation from the world and their commitment to monogamous exclusivity. At the same time, their unique emotional dynamic, and its impact on each spouse's personal development, involved the two of them and no one else. These various aspects of intimacy were seen as intertwined: it was through no accident of word choice that IMS marriage therapist Stanley Ruszczynski explained that it was "within the privacy of our own home" that we had "the opportunity to regress or grow, to become childlike again or adults ... Marriage asks us to be the fullness of our potential as human beings."[135] Privacy was essential for marital harmony; however, marriage therapists also emphasized the consequences of emotionally satisfying marriages for public life, since they enabled spouses and children to become the most highly developed and socially attuned selves that they could be. Integrating Britain's marriage counseling and therapy services into the welfare state gave legitimacy to their psychological reading of married life; it also provided optimal conditions for its permeation of British society at every socio-economic level, so that it might give coherent shape to the needs and expectations of a large proportion of the adult population.

Because marriage welfare services were included in Britain's publicly funded social and health services, emotions were politicized in Britain in a way that they were not in the United States, where marriage counseling services were also launched during the same decades as a service to private fee-paying clients, as well as through the sponsorship of Protestant churches.[136] In postwar Britain, as in the United States, the democratic dream of responsible citizenship was linked to an imagined ideal of psychological maturity; however, the idea that the state shared responsibility for ensuring that children and adults alike experienced healthy emotional development was peculiar to Britain. Marriage therapy services were often provided by government employees and made available as a condition of national belonging and workforce participation. This had the effect of legitimating the desire for a fuller private emotional life as a basic guarantee of citizenship. T.H. Marshall influentially argued in 1949 that Britain's social services ensured that every citizen had access to a common social heritage and in this way served to flatten class disparities and guarantee social equality. Britain's marriage welfare services contributed to this postwar ideal. Not only did they help couples develop the necessary emotional literacy to stay married, they also promoted a cross-class awareness that permanent monogamous marriages could function as a platform for psychological growth that would enable individuals to achieve their fullest social potential. This was a promise that was steeped in a quintessentially middle-class ideal of family life; however, its foundation in emotional life made it seem like a universal aspiration.

Scholarship examining the history of the British welfare state has shed light on its problematic consequences in codifying the male-breadwinning, female-homemaking nuclear family as meriting state support, not only as a social and economic arrangement but also as a personalized set of relationships.[137] Much of this work has focused on how it sanctioned adult men as active and responsible contributors and women and children as economically vulnerable dependents. This chapter contributes to the conversation by revealing how post-war perceptions of citizens' emotional needs and developmental potential were implicated in the state's decision to fund a marriage welfare service.

Ultimately, Britain's marriage welfare service made new modes of emotionally oriented existence possible and helped create new possibilities for being a fully integrated social self. These methods garnered the support of the British government and the public alike and helped a new set of values rooted in emotional health and personal development flourish. While this may have provided new freedoms for some (such as divorce seekers), it also presented a host of new barriers for others—queer men and women especially—thus creating not only new possibilities for making political demands but also a series of new obstacles and exclusions. As only certain family arrangements and sexual choices were aligned with healthy emotional maturity, all others became troubling (however curable) signs of a suspended state of development.

PART II
SEXUAL REVOLUTION AND INTIMACY REIMAGINED

PART II

5
Pursuing Connection
Queer Romance and Friendship during Britain's Sexual Revolution

> I have no wish to suggest that I regard homosexuality as a desirable way of life. It is in my view undesirable ... because it leads so often to unhappiness, to loneliness and to frustration, because it entails in many cases heavy burdens of guilt and shame on those affected by it and because it seldom provides a basis for a stable emotional relationship.
> —Kenneth Robinson, House of Commons Debate, June 29, 1960

> I fail to see why there should be one law for heterosexuals and another for homosexuals. Homosexual love can, I am sure, be just as sincere, profound and lasting as any other form of love—be it heterosexual, parental, or fraternal. The main obstacle, I feel, is not so much legal as social.
> —Anonymous, "Social Needs Survey," Albany Trust, 1968

On December 4, 1957, Colonel John Moore-Brabazon, former minister of Transport and Aircraft Production, presented a spirited celebration of sexual love in his moving—at the time, shockingly forthright—speech in support of the decriminalization of homosexual behavior:

> when we speak about the repugnance and the disgust of the act, we have to face the fact that all sexual intercourse, be it heterosexual or homosexual, if it is looked at anatomically and physiologically, is not very attractive. But along comes the glamour of love; and that is a mystical, creative, Divine force which comes over two people and makes all things seem natural and normal. And what we have to get into our heads, although it is difficult, is that that glamour of love, odd as it may sound, is just as much present between two homosexuals as it is between a man and a woman.[1]

Decades later, queer rights campaigner Antony Grey would refer to Brabazon's speech as a key insight and look back fondly on the "wisdom and compassion" of this unlikely ally, better known for being an accomplished sportsman, pioneer

The Intimate State. Teri Chettiar, Oxford University Press. © Oxford University Press 2023.
DOI: 10.1093/oso/9780190931209.003.0006

motorist, and friend to Winston Churchill.[2] Brabazon's defense of the controversial proposal to decriminalize homosexual behavior—presented two months earlier by the (Wolfenden) Committee on Homosexual Offences and Prostitution—rested on the notion that sex was a gateway to the disembodied spiritual experience of love. What many contemporaries saw as a sordid experience between "perverse" oversexed men that presented a danger to public life was refigured as "mystical, creative," even "Divine." Although he drew upon familiar tropes, Brabazon's appeal to the "mystical" when describing intimate relationships may not have resonated with many. As we saw in the previous chapter, adjectives like quiet and humdrum, or alternatively tense and conflictual, may have been more fitting descriptors, particularly for those rising numbers of men and women dissatisfied with their marriages and contemplating divorce.

Brabazon's assumption that homosexual equality was really, at its core, about access to love rather than sexual privacy was not typical of parliamentary discussion in the years leading up to homosexual decriminalization. However, a focus on intimacy rather than sex—queer people's emotions rather than their bodies—would turn out to be neither idiosyncratic nor anomalous within the homosexual law reform and gay liberation movements in 1960s and 1970s Britain. Government lobbyists and grassroots activists alike were as concerned with queer people's access to fulfilled emotional lives as they were with sexual choice, social acceptance, and an end to repressive heteronormative power imbalances both leading up to and during the years after the criminal penalties for consenting homosexual sex were removed in July 1967.

On September 16, 1967, seven weeks after the passage of the momentous Sexual Offences Act—which decriminalized private homosexual behavior between consenting male adults who were more than twenty-one years old—*The Guardian* newspaper ran an article that both celebrated and scrutinized this seemingly historic piece of legislative reform. It highlighted the lived experience of "John and Eric, who have been together for the past twenty years," who confirmed that "it hasn't made a ha'porth of difference to them."[3] Given the many restrictions that the law kept in place, the continued growth of police arrests, and the enduring stigma attached to homosexuality, the couple maintained that the "legislation they want to see now would make the man-man situation entirely comparable to the man-girl one."[4] The changes they hoped for would ensure that all expressions of sexual intimacy and love—so highly revered in the context of heterosexual marriage and the nuclear family—were viewed equally by British people regardless of gender and sexual orientation.

Many activists and organizations involved in campaigns for homosexual law reform and gay liberation similarly saw the decriminalization of homosexual behavior as insufficient on its own for introducing sexual equality. In response, they confronted social stigma and its disabling emotional effects through counseling initiatives aimed at Britain's large population of sexual minorities. The Homosexual Law Reform Society created the Albany Trust in 1958, which pursued psychosexual counseling beginning in the early 1960s. In the early 1970s every organization attached to the homophile and gay liberation movements similarly developed a counseling arm. The Campaign for Homosexual Equality (CHE) launched Friend (Fellowship for the

Relief of the Isolated and Emotionally in Need and Distress) in 1971 and the Gay Liberation Front (GLF) created the Counter-Psychiatry Group in reaction to the popular use of aversion therapies to "cure" homosexuality and, soon after, Icebreakers, a network of support groups. Gay Switchboard, an autonomous twenty-four-hour telephone referral service offering information, help, and advice to those in need, was launched in early 1974.

As this chapter will show, law reform took up only a fraction of activists' time and effort. Ensuring queer people's access to the full range of choices and experiences that heterosexuals took for granted involved far more than the elimination of legal obstacles to same-sex intimacy. The emotional weight of cultural associations of homosexuality with criminality and mental abnormality needed to be directly tackled. Following the establishment of queer counseling services in the early 1960s through the Albany Trust and the Minorities Research Group, many advocates of homosexual equality approached relationship choice as connected less to legal permission than psychological capacity.

The psychological sciences loomed large, and ominously, for sexually nonconforming people—the term "homosexual" first came into use because of path-breaking studies of sexual pathology published by German psychiatrists in the last third of the nineteenth century. In more recent decades, marriage counseling and aversion therapies alike celebrated child-producing monogamous heterosexuality as an expression of healthy psychological maturity. Developing counseling services aimed at sexual minorities required negotiating this harmful and enduring past.

This chapter explores how certain features of Britain's post-WWII constellation of sexual values were retained—particularly the end goal of stable intimacy and pathologization of promiscuous behaviors—in efforts to create well-adjusted sexual minorities who were meaningfully connected to a network of emotionally fulfilling relationships. At the same time, activists and LGBTQ+ counselors reoriented narratives of emotional maturity and expanded understandings of the social foundations of mental and emotional "health" by bringing attention to the profoundly damaging psychological impact of social exclusion and sexual stigma on sexual minorities.

In this chapter, I argue that counseling services aimed at queer people, in their pursuit of resolving the complex suffering uniquely experienced by sexual minorities, focused on making clients emotionally capable of choosing and sustaining intimate relationships. These relationships, however, far exceeded the narrow network of family relationships so highly valued in British society at the time: they were of a much broader range than that seen in the post-WWII British emotional health initiatives explored in earlier chapters. The goal of creating intimate queer relationships—which included romance, friendship, and, by the 1970s, queer activist social communities—was, I further argue, connected to broader political objectives related to both homosexual equality and 1970s socio-sexual liberation. Like the state-supported emotional health initiatives examined in previous chapters, queer counseling initiatives initially, in the 1960s, prioritized intimate emotional relationships for their central role in creating good, socially responsible, queer *citizens* who were fully included in Britain's wider national community. Early queer counseling provided at the Albany Trust promoted this. By the early 1970s, however, LGBTQ+ counselors and "befrienders" instead viewed intimate queer sexual relationships, close friendships, and supportive activist communities as foundational for creating fully liberated and self-accepting "proud" queer *individuals*.

The explosion of queer counseling services was not a practitioner-led phenomenon like many of the services explored in earlier chapters. The narrative presented in this chapter is not a top-down story demonstrating the triumph of psychological experts in an era of queer liberation. Instead, the creation and use of queer counseling involved a creative reciprocity between predominantly queer counselors and volunteer "befrienders" (often themselves former advice seekers and clients) and service users through written correspondence, telephone conversations, and in-person meetings. This was not a case of experts imposing a goal of intimate relationships onto avowedly lonely sexual minorities. Instead, counselors and those who sought their help *together* engaged in imagining what queer community and relationships could do.

This is not to say that all voices counted equally. Despite the mutual involvement of clients and service providers in identifying problems and dreaming up a more desirable future, there were clear outliers who approached these services with needs that lay decidedly beyond the capacity (or willingness) of these services to help. In the view of service providers, "good" advice seekers tended to be individuals like queer men looking to meet potential partners outside of the club scene and lesbians seeking advice on how to maintain their partner's sexual interest. They presented desires that could be channeled toward building lasting relationships. "Bad" advice seekers on the other hand, presented desires that were antithetical to this—such as, for example, having exclusively unattached sex, or a fetish for being whipped. The "good" advice seeker sought to be part of a community and showed a commitment to durable intimacy. The "bad" advice seeker sought out relationships that were transient, one-sided, and not *mutually* fulfilling. Advice seekers in general wanted help extending their sexual sociability into a world of strangers, however "bad" advice seekers did not hope to have this exploration result in either lasting romantic partnerships or ongoing participation within a queer community.

The use of queer counseling and befriending services grew dramatically in the years following the decriminalization of homosexual behavior in 1967. In 1970, the Albany Trust helped more than two thousand men and women positively accept their sexuality through in-person counseling.[5] By 1978, Gay Switchboard reported that their organization had dealt with 123,140 calls that year alone;[6] and Friend's telephone counseling services were helping more than 30,000 men and women per year.[7] Yet, historical literature on homosexual law reform and gay liberation activism scarcely mention counseling as an important concern or activity, much less assign it a place of importance alongside more familiar forms of political work, such as marches to protest homosexual discrimination and campaigns to lower the age of homosexual consent.[8] This tendency to split off the development of counseling, befriending, and support groups geared specifically toward assisting lesbians and gay men in working through "homosexual problems" like social isolation, loneliness, guilt, and shame speaks to a narrow and oversimplifying characterization of politics. I argue that, like the campaigning organizations that they were affiliated with, queer counseling and befriending worked to provide men and women who had suffered a lifetime of social exclusion access to sexual partnerships. Helping queer men and women achieve not only social acceptance, but also self-acceptance, was a necessary precursor to this. This spoke to a political movement that sought not only to enlarge the scope of freedom for sexual minorities but to help fashion the kinds of people capable of participating fully in the emotional depths of sexual liberation.

This chapter reveals connections between counseling and the politics of sexual freedom and challenges the notion that these were separate areas of activity. I argue that queer counseling initiatives were a central—although now overlooked—feature of queer liberation. Specifically, they provided a crucial space for cultivating the emotions and relationship styles that were at the heart of a projected "healthy" liberated queer subjectivity. In counseling encounters sexual minorities tested out their feelings about their sexual desires and experiences and received validation and advice as to how they should proceed in meeting someone with whom they might find love.

Additionally, I argue that counseling and befriending—its intentionally less-skilled counterpart—helped create the political scripts and goals that shaped gay liberation. Just as consciousness-raising groups provided a language and set of demands for feminists to rally around, counseling and befriending services focused on identifying the effects of the harm caused by homo- and transphobia. By 1966, on the eve of decriminalization, it was widely known that public knowledge of one's homosexuality could cost one one's job, one's family, and one's ability to find housing. The effects of loneliness and despair were, however, less commonly grappled with. It is in this register—the experience of daily suffering—that gay liberation politics would take shape in the wake of criminal law reform. It was the less precisely visible everyday aspects of discrimination—those which could not be resolved through changes in the law—that queer counseling services helped to illuminate and politicize.

Sexual Law Reform and the Persistence of Stigma in the 1960s

Although there had been a five-fold increase in the number of arrests for homosexual behavior between 1939 and 1954, there was virtually no movement to legalize homosexual sex in the decade following WWII.[9] The 1885 Labouchere Amendment, which had expanded the range of homosexual crimes to all forms of intimacy whether conducted in public or private, was occasionally raised in the press and Parliament as wrongheaded and frequently exploited for far more harmful criminal purposes, notably blackmail. In response the home secretary, Sir David Maxwell Fyfe, appointed a departmental committee in August 1954 to investigate whether the criminalization of homosexual behavior and public solicitation of prostitution interfered with citizens' right to personal freedom. The committee, headed by John Wolfenden, vice-chancellor of Reading University, equally explored questions of public solicitation and the just treatment of homosexuality. It was the latter of these questions that ended up at the forefront of public discussion.[10]

When the Wolfenden Committee's report was published in 1957, it sold five thousand copies in a mere matter of hours and ignited public conversation over the decriminalization of homosexual acts, which, since 1885, had been subject to prison sentences lasting two years. The report couched its questions within a broader philosophical defense of individual privacy and freedom of choice, rather than presenting an appeal for sexual liberation. Inspired by nineteenth-century liberal values supporting individual freedom and the small state, the report's support for decriminalization was predicated on the notion that there was a domain of "private morality" that needed to be outside the jurisdiction of the law. It was emphatic that the law's "function" was exclusively to "protect the citizen from what is offensive and injurious" and in no way meant to "intervene in the private life of citizens or to seek to enforce any particular pattern of behaviour."[11] Response to the report was highly divided. It touched upon key areas of uncertainty—tensions between Cold War anti-totalitarian values and British social democracy—that were far from being resolved, particularly at a moment when there was widespread support for state expansion and the universal public provision of schools, health services, family allowances, town planning, and basic social security.

The Wolfenden Report explicitly waged war on the endurance of Victorian moral values in British law and thus hit upon a raw nerve running through Britain's reluctantly secularizing society.[12] Sin, the committee argued, needed to be seen as entirely separate from legal matters; crime needed to be understood in terms of harm reduction rather than morality, which was a matter of private conscience. The choice of one's sexual partner—if one was an adult, of sound mind, and not harming anyone—was thus beyond the state's concern. The report's defense of privacy, however, failed to consider how, with the rise of Britain's welfare state, the most intimate areas of heterosexual private life had taken on renewed public value—from a mother's love for her child to married couples' commitment to lasting monogamy. In the movement to decriminalize sex between consenting adult men we see an attempt to establish clear limits to the state's interest in private life and a defense of privacy at a moment when it appeared to be slipping away.

It was not until the mid-1960s that Britain's MPs would show significant support for removing criminal penalties attached to homosexuality. However, the support that did exist among MPs in the late 1950s shared the Wolfenden Report's concern for citizens' right to privacy. The first discussion of homosexuality in parliament focused on the dangers presumed to be inherent to the state's participation in making moral decisions on behalf of its citizens. On December 4, 1957, Viscount (Frank) Pakenham, an Oxford don, former Labour cabinet minister, and advocate for prisoners' rights, raised the issue before the House of Lords. When Pakenham addressed the House, he enthusiastically endorsed the Wolfenden Committee's distinction between crime and sin. Approaching the document from a Christian standpoint, he argued that moral decisions needed to be made autonomously by individuals.

Pakenham was not alone in his concern that Britain's welfare state might, like a totalitarian state, compete with the church in providing moral guidance. The Archbishop of Canterbury (Geoffrey Fisher) similarly cautioned that it was "precisely the belief of the totalitarian State" that declared every sin a crime:

> That such a belief should continue is a very dangerous thing... The State and the Law are not concerned directly, as the Church is, with saving the souls of men from their own destruction. The right to decide one's own moral code and obey it, even to a man's own hurt, is a fundamental right of man, given him by God and to be strictly respected by society and the criminal code.[13]

In the eyes of many committed Christians, choice, and not coercion, was the only true basis for moral action.

Liberal arguments in support of decriminalization were immediately forced to contend with defenders of the traditional social order. The most famous of these, presented by the esteemed jurist Lord (Patrick) Devlin, criticized the Wolfenden Report on the grounds that it incorrectly presented morality as a private matter. In his widely publicized 1959 Maccabean Lecture in Jurisprudence, entitled "The Enforcement of Morals," he argued that morality was not only publicly shared by members of a given society but functioned to cement them together as a people.[14] The law, Devlin argued, needed to be used to protect against threats to social cohesion.

Devlin was not alone in defending the importance of public morality in the early 1960s, a moment when, John Wolfenden noted, many Britons were becoming aware of the existence of homosexuality for the first time.[15] A widely publicized ruling made by the House of Lords in 1961, Britain's highest court of appeal, resurrected the old charge of "conspiracy to corrupt public morals" to condemn Frederic Charles Shaw for creating the *Ladies Directory*, a guide to commercial sex in London that included contact information and, in some cases, nude photos.[16] The decision was controversial.[17] It was far from widely accepted that appeals to "public morals" were anything other than efforts to conceal an enforcement of upper-middle-class values. To many it smacked of politico-moral surveillance.

In the wake of these defenses of "public morals," public conversation began to take on greater urgency as the stakes of homosexual decriminalization were enlarged to include considerations of the law's impact on emotional health. In 1963, Oxford law professor Herbert Hart attacked appeals to "public morality," arguing that both Devlin's admonition of the Wolfenden Report and the Shaw ruling smacked of paternalism. Even worse, he argued, legal interference on behalf of a presumably cohesive imaginary "public" was psychologically damaging to those who found themselves on the wrong side of public morality. According to Hart, laws limiting an individual's sexual choices restricted the range of human experience. In explaining his disagreement, he was less concerned with defending unimpeded freedom of choice as a "value in itself with which it is *prima facie* wrong to interfere."[18] Instead, he focused on the psychological harm that he speculated was caused by the legal enforcement of sexual morality:

> interference with individual liberty may be thought an evil ... for it is itself the infliction of a special form of suffering—often very acute—on those whose desires are frustrated by the fear of punishment. This is of peculiar importance in the case of laws enforcing a sexual morality. They may create misery of a quite special degree. For both the difficulties involved in the repression of sexual impulses and the consequences of repression are quite different from those involved in the abstention from "ordinary" crime. Unlike sexual impulses, the impulse to steal or to wound or even kill is not, except in a minority of mentally abnormal cases, a recurrent and insistent part of daily life. Resistance to the temptation to commit these crimes is not often, as *the suppression of sexual impulses* generally is, something which *affects the development of balance of the individual's emotional life, happiness, and personality*.[19]

Hart's psychological reasoning moved into territory that was less commonly explored by traditional utilitarian thinkers, extending beyond preoccupations with the human inevitability of pleasure-seeking and pain-avoidance—Bentham's "empire of pleasure and of pain"—and into the arena of desire and the consequences of its forced suppression.[20] According to Hart's logic, "the repression of sexual impulses" had psychological consequences that the law urgently needed to consider.

When parliament overwhelmingly voted in favor of support for the passage of a Sexual Offences Bill that would decriminalize homosexual acts in July 1967, it was to support citizens' right to privacy rather than a call for sexual liberation. In his final speech to the House of Lords, Lord Arran, the bill's sponsor, noted that a change in the law did not—and perhaps could never—indicate social acceptance:

> Homosexuals must continue to remember that while there may be nothing bad in being a homosexual, there is certainly nothing good. Lest the opponents of the Bill think that a new freedom, a new privileged class, has been created, let me remind them that no amount of legislation will prevent homosexuals from being the subject of dislike and derision or at best of pity.[21]

As is clear in Lord Arran's final address, the passage of the act was not intended to usher in a new era of full homosexual equality. Indeed, the most prominent reasons for favoring homosexual law reform in the mid-1960s stemmed from concerns about blackmail and police witch hunts.[22] Indiscriminate prosecutions—not infrequently leading to suicide—were given increasing public exposure by the Homosexual Law Reform Society. Emphasis in parliament, however, was given to how fear of arrest prevented homosexuals from openly pursuing medical treatment that might "convert" them to heterosexuality.[23]

The act itself also had severe limitations. Historian Jeffrey Weeks describes it as "hardly a trumpet-call to freedom."[24] Not only did it exclude Scotland and Northern Ireland and not apply to the army and navy, but it introduced harsher penalties for sex with underage men ("minors" were identified as under twenty-one) and public solicitation. This resulted in more policing and a rise in prosecutions for homosexual offences. In addition, the Sexual Offences Act did not alter the public view of homosexuals as promiscuous, often predatory, and a threat to the family.

The act's defense of privacy was also woefully ineffective in overturning social stigma. First, the meaning of "in private" presented in the act was highly restrictive. It was meant to indicate not only spaces that were shielded from public view—such as the private residence of a property owner—but one where a third party was unlikely to be present. "Public" sex referred not only to sex that took place in a public lavatory, but any sex act that could *potentially* be seen by another person. The legal protections that the act afforded to sex "in private" excluded a wide range of intimate encounters: not only sex in a secluded place outdoors but also sex in shared rented accommodations as well as sex in a separate room of a private residence where a social gathering was taking place.

More importantly, emphasizing the "private" status of sex did not shield it from postwar heteronormative values, especially at a moment when heterosexual intimacy had become increasingly connected to aspirations for the public good. Birth control, marriage, child rearing, and divorce were all publicly regulated: the government was deeply invested in heterosexual relations. Since queer sex did not belong to the reproductive field that created child-producing families, it could be written off as unproductive and unimportant. Archbishop Fisher had proclaimed at a 1957 Church Assembly debate that homosexuality did not pose a threat to the family in the way that adultery and other extramarital heterosexual relations did since it did not lead to unwanted "illegitimate" children. Gesturing toward a more fitting criminalization of adultery and premarital heterosexual sex, Fisher proclaimed that, "If homosexual sin is criminal, then heterosexual sin is doubly criminal."[25] Lord Brabazon similarly presented homosexuality as inconsequential in his passionate defense of decriminalization in the House of Lords in 1957: "These people are self-eliminating. They do not breed. They do very little harm if left to themselves."[26] Since homosexual sex was non-reproductive, it was presented as having no real consequence (negative *or* positive) in relation to broader society.

In 1960s Britain, the defense of private sexual choice revealed tensions in the welfare state's commitment to protecting intimate family life in the decades after the war. Sarah Igo points out that discussions about privacy in the United States in the postwar decades were "really arguments over what it meant to be a modern citizen," making claims as they did about "the latitude for action and anonymity a decent, democratic society ought to afford its members."[27] In the postwar British context, these were also discussions about the consequences of individual actions for "society" as it was then being reinvented. As Igo notes, claims to the right to privacy invoked assumptions about the kind of person (white, male, adult) that could be relied upon to behave responsibly. They also, I argue, involved decisions about how society was produced and might potentially be transformed. While Devlin saw the "public" as bound together by a common morality, the lawmakers who decriminalized homosexual behavior "in private" were more concerned about protecting a public that they believed was produced and reproduced in families.

Not only were the potentially reproductive aspects of heterosexual sex key to determining government interest, but family love—both marital and parental love—had become increasingly valued as the bedrock of civic life. Imagined as an ideally stable and lasting bulwark against the instabilities of the twentieth century, heterosexual relationships—geared toward the production of children—were seen as the most reliable foundation for a thriving society. To render homosexual sex "private" as the basis for removing it from criminal law statutes was to potentially banish it from the public interest that heterosexuality was becoming increasingly enmeshed within. When it came to sexual and emotional life, the liberal value of privacy conflicted with Britain's intimate state. One form of intimacy—hetero, stable, loving, child-producing—was being accorded far-reaching public value whereas as another—queer, fleeting, pleasure- rather than love-oriented—was presented as having no relationship to the state and public life.

Following the decriminalization of homosexual acts in 1967, homophile activists and organizations shifted focus to homosexual stigma and its effects. They launched psychosexual counseling services to help queer men and women "adjust" to their sexual orientation and form meaningful relationships. Although they would continue to defend citizens' right to sexual privacy, they saw greater urgency in ensuring that queer people's private sexual choices were as publicly valued as those made by married monogamous child-producing heterosexuals.

Expanding the Scope of Sexual Reform: Counseling Sexual Minorities

Although it was the support of Parliament that ultimately produced a change in the law impacting homosexual behavior in 1967, government lobbyists were central to making this happen. Discussions of homosexuality in Parliament following release of the Wolfenden Report failed to inspire much support for reform among most MPs until 1964. Unwavering opposition was even expressed by members, such as Lord Denning, who backed the liberalization of the divorce law during the same years. In response to government intransigency, supporters of homosexual law reform had published letters in Britain's major newspapers championing the Wolfenden Committee's proposals and quickly generated a movement for reform. University of Wales lecturer Tony Dyson published the most seminal of these in *The Times* on March 7, 1958, having managed to secure the signatures of thirty-three influential public figures, including Isaiah Berlin, Julian Huxley, Jacquetta Hawkes, Bertrand Russell, and J.B. Priestley.[28] The letter led to the formation of the Homosexual Law

Reform Society (HLRS) just two months later on May 12, 1958, under the chairmanship of sexologist Kenneth Walker.[29]

Despite the clear need for an organized lobby with a respectable public face to urge on the government's consideration of the Wolfenden proposals, legal reform was only ever one—and, to many of the actors involved, narrow—objective of the sexual reform movement. The HLRS immediately created a registered charity in May 1958 that was devoted to the longer-term goals of reform: overturning the social stigma attached to homosexuality and promoting the psychological health of criminalized homosexual men. It was named the Albany Trust after the Piccadilly residence of J.B. Priestley and Jacquetta Hawkes (The Albany), which had been the location of its early meetings.

Homosexual men's mental health struggles were highlighted as a priority because, as early HLRS member Antony Grey explained, "the present British laws against male homosexual behaviour" were "responsible for a great deal of neurosis and some severe mental illness."[30] Like Herbert Hart, who also brought attention to the damaging psychological consequences of legal repression that same year, Grey noted that psychological "difficulties" resulted "primarily from fear and a degree of repression which makes sex a problem that is impossible for the homosexual individual to solve with peace of mind."[31] For this reason, members of the HLRS and Albany Trust believed that a movement to bring about homosexual equality needed to address not only the legal features of homosexual repression but the psychological outcomes of that repression as well.

Members of the trust did not, however, originally set out to create a counseling service. The way that this happened was, in many ways, a tribute to the need that many queer men and women felt for a venue where they could openly talk through their emotional pain, uncertainties, and desires for different kind of life. Inspired by the Kinsey reports' transformative impact on understandings of sexuality, the Albany Trust had initially set out to gather extensive data on the lives of British homosexuals with the intention of changing public opinion. It soon also became a referral service for physicians, lawyers, and psychiatrists sympathetic to the needs of people with same-sex sexual desire. Yet their office quickly became,

> the constant destination of a stream of requests for help. Many of these were for professional help or for advice on treatment. Some were from poor, wretched people who felt they had come to the bitter end, and were contemplating suicide. Others simply wanted someone to talk to, who would listen unreprovingly to their tale of woe.[32]

By 1963, in response to steady demand for psychiatric help, the trust had begun to offer non-directive counseling in-house on an ad hoc basis to help sexual minorities to "adjust" to their sexual orientation.

The trust's approach to counseling consciously departed from the aversion therapies that had become popular in the decades following the war.[33] Rather than viewing conversion to heterosexuality as a solution for symptoms of depression and despair, the trust offered clients "constructive adjustment in the face of social and legal problems rather than 'cure.'"[34] Demand for counseling stayed at between 100 and 150 clients per year until 1967, when—following the addition of an experienced full-time social worker to the staff alongside the partial decriminalization of homosexual behavior—client numbers shot up to over 500.[35] Most new clients were described as requiring "help in accepting their own sexuality, help fitting in to a predominantly heterosexually orientated society, help in meeting other homosexuals under normal circumstances, help to fight loneliness."[36]

The historical relationship between psychiatry and same-sex desire is fraught and complex, extending far beyond the growing use of aversion therapies in the post-WWII decades. The term "homosexual" first emerged in the latter decades of the nineteenth century as a psychiatric diagnosis, and its associations with mental disease—despite the challenge this presented to contemporary associations between homosexuality and sin—opened up new possibilities for medical surveillance, classification, and forcible "cure." Despite this, historians of queer sexuality have also revealed the liberatory potential of sexual diagnoses, revealing how they were embraced and revised by predominantly middle-class, white, male homosexuals who sought greater public visibility and social acceptance.[37] The Albany Trust's support for psychological treatments that deviated from a disease framework for understanding homosexuality was not new. The Wolfenden Report, which had argued against straightforwardly accepting the mainstream medical view of homosexuality as a disease, nonetheless included extensive discussion of "therapeutic measures." Doubtful of the efficacy of "converting" homosexuals to heterosexuality, the report instead addressed the benefits of treatment focused on encouraging greater sexual discretion and geared toward "better adaptation to life in general."[38]

Taking its lead from the Wolfenden Committee, and despite its complete refusal of homosexual pathology, the trust approached "treatment" as playing an essential role in bringing about sexual equality. Focusing less on encouraging discretion and instead on helping homosexuals "come to terms with" their sexuality, Albany Trust leadership saw counseling as a promising support toward creating emotionally well-adjusted sexual subjects. The therapeutic encounter was meant to help clients develop language for the invalidating pain caused by social injustice and, in the process, create a more positive view of homosexuality with a view to successful integration in a more sexually evolved society. Trust leadership did not envision a positive future in queer sub-cultural communities. Grey saw this as working against large-scale change in cultural attitudes to sexual diversity.

Given the trust's commitment to social integration, its vision of sexual "adjustment" was not only not critical of heteronormative sexual values—such as monogamy, lifelong marriage, and shared emotional intimacy—but actively celebrated them. Promiscuity was associated with psychological ill-health, in addition to what Grey described as "disagreeable" (gender-crossing) personal features, such as "affectation of manner and dress."[39] Grey argued that none of these ostensibly "deviant" behaviors were inherent to homosexuality itself but were derived from homosexuals' "non-acceptance, and often positive rejection, by society," which caused them to "rebel."[40] Grey did not challenge common male homosexual stereotypes but instead explained them as socially induced and, therefore, capable of being changed.

For Grey and others at the Albany Trust, the enormous task of sexual "adjustment" relied upon collaboration with trained experts. The style of counseling that they advocated and eventually practiced, particularly following the inclusion of an experienced caseworker on staff from 1967 onward, was non-directive, non-hierarchical, and client centered. Given that treatment of homosexuality had long been cornered by psychiatric professionals, it made sense that counseling aimed at sexual minorities in the 1960s was more explicitly expert-oriented than the sexual and marriage counseling services offered by volunteer lay counselors through the NMGC. According to David Mace's 1948 handbook on marriage counseling, the ability to counsel young married couples on sexual matters derived more from personal experience with successful marriage than specialized training and skills.[41] At the trust, however, any appeal to shared experience was far more complicated. Fear of criminal associations and a desire to maintain sexual respectability meant that the trust's public face was almost exclusively heterosexual and married. Aside from Grey, counselors working with sexual minorities both with and alongside the trust tended not to share their clients' experiences as a sexual minority.

Despite the Albany Trust's and NMGC's differing commitments to expertise in counseling, the trust's counseling goals quickly came to resemble those of marriage counselors. Counselors wanted to help their clients become capable of sustaining a monogamous intimate relationship. Antony Grey—who was himself happily partnered from 1958 until his death in 2010—saw relationship stability as not only "desirable in itself" because it led to happiness but as also playing a key role in overturning damaging homosexual stereotypes of "promiscuity, importuning and public indecency."[42] In a 1964 funding proposal, trust leadership emphasized the longer-term political goals of counseling: "By converting the individual into a complete and intact personality, we shall be going the right way about it to educate the public."[43] In counseling sessions, clients were informed of the social causes behind their inability to establish a lasting relationship. They were alerted to the important contribution that they could make by living a respectable life in overturning negative public perceptions of homosexuality.

In addition to 1960s conventions attached to sexual respectability, Grey's own rather conventional sexual biography certainly played a role in the value that trust leadership attached to stable intimacy. Grey understood his own homosexual inclinations as primarily "emotional" and love-oriented rather than "physical" and overwhelmingly sex-focused:

> Like many who are homosexual, my first awareness of my attraction was emotional, not physical... from kindergarten school until university, I fell in love with a succession of my fellow-students. And I do not say "fell in love" lightly; these loves

were as tender, as longingly passionate and as agonizingly frustrated as any that I have experienced in my adult life ... A good deal of physical sex went on between boys at school, of course ... but emotion hardly entered in. I found these boyishly randy pastimes enlightening and enjoyable, but they did not satisfy my yearning for an ideal companion.[44]

He recorded in his memoir that he had been "mostly celibate" until he was thirty-two, when he met his life partner. Throughout his long career as a psychosexual counselor, Grey sought to make the kind of lifelong partnership that he himself had experienced become as common in the queer world as it was among heterosexuals. Although success in counseling was not measured in terms of statistics relating to desertion and divorce, its purpose, as it was for many marriage counselors, was to inculcate clients with the capacity to sustain lasting relationships that were anchored in emotional connection.

Grey was not alone in prioritizing solutions to deviant homosexual behaviors, rather than either rebutting homosexual stereotypes or challenging the value of British heteronormative sexual ideals. Michael Schofield, path-breaking British sociologist of homosexuality, similarly spotlighted promiscuity as an unfortunately common relationship mode pursued by most homosexual men in the 1960s. As historian Chris Waters points out, Schofield was crucial in shifting the focus among human and social scientists from viewing homosexuals as suffering from pathology to belonging to a social minority.[45] Yet, in all of his studies of homosexual men in the 1950s and 1960s, he affirmed the denigration of undesirable homosexual traits and behaviors—including feminine affect, lack of stable employment, and fleeting sexual encounters—and confirmed their prevalence among large sections of the queer population. He was careful, however, to disproportionately attribute promiscuous lifestyles to men who had either received psychiatric treatment or been incarcerated for homosexual behavior.[46] In a comparative 1965 study of three "homosexual types"—convicts, psychiatric patients, and "others" who had never been either—he pointed out that those in the "other" category (around 30% of his respondents) were far more likely to be able "to accept and carry on a satisfactory and lengthy relationship with another man" since they experienced their homoerotic feelings "as much emotional as sexual."[47] Not only were they far more likely to carry on romantic relationships lasting more than a year, they also tended to be affluent, have large networks of friends, and be "less likely to appear feminine."[48] Schofield's comparison between homosexual "types" demonstrated that the less socially desirable features that were typically associated with homosexuals actually resulted from encounters with repressive institutions—white middle-class gay men tended to avoid these and thus maintain (healthy) sexual respectability.

The trust's goal of making monogamous relationships possible was also shared by many clients. Many of the men and women who contacted the trust emphasized their despair as connected to the absence of a stable long-term partnership. For example, a young man in Menorca, Spain, wrote to the trust in June 1966, requesting help in meeting someone with whom he might become romantically involved:

> As for myself I am feeling *extremely* frustrated and becoming more so ... I feel empty, lonely, and long for a deep emotional attachment to someone like myself (my age) with whom to share my life and home. I want to feel needed and to need in return.[49]

Similar expressions of sad longing were present in letters from queer men and women in relationships who were concerned about their relationship's fragility given the enormous pressure of being a sexual outsider. In 1968, Grey became an ongoing counselor to Jonathan, who worried that his partner Michael, who wanted to date other men, was going to leave him.[50] Other clients told of suffering connected to their spouse's bisexuality, infidelity, and indecision about which partner they ultimately wanted to be with. A young woman, who had been married to a bisexual man for eleven years—having always known of his "homosexual tendencies" but earlier thinking "it would work itself out"—underwent several counseling sessions with Grey hoping to "preserve homelife both for the sake of her husband and her children."[51] Her husband—who was also seen by Grey several times—similarly confessed he "still had loving feelings" despite his "deep emotional involvement homosexually."[52] Although Grey noted that cases of bisexuality and multiple partners were more difficult to help resolve, it was clients, not trust counselors, who often led the process of identifying the romantic relationship that worked best for everyone (husband, wife, children, and new partner).

In 1967, the trust experienced a post-reform jump in the demand for counseling. Upon his return from a 1968 trip to the United States to meet with gay rights organizations, Grey found the Albany Trust's office

> just as fraught as it had been when the parliamentary campaign was reaching its climax. It became even more so; now homosexual people felt there was a freer climate in which to seek help for their social and emotional difficulties, their first chosen port of call was the Albany Trust.[53]

The demand for help, he noted, "was nationwide and in the first twelve months after law reform the annual number of people approaching the Trust more than doubled and continued to climb."[54] The number of clients receiving counseling at the trust rose to over two thousand in 1970, a twenty-fold increase in comparison to the early 1960s.[55] Not only were more people requesting emotional assistance in the wake of reform, but clients' sexual problems had become more diverse. In addition to gays, lesbians, and bisexuals, self-identified transvestites and transsexuals were key recipients of the trust's work after 1965. In this broader range of clients, we see the beginnings of an incipient LGBTQ+ identity. What tied the trust's diverse client body together as a group was their shared emotional experience of social alienation.

Herbert Hart's discussion of the psychologically harmful effects of the law may not have been a major feature of Parliamentary discussion, which focused more on emotions related to the fear of prosecution rather than the pain of repression. However, at the Albany Trust—located as it was on the front line of help-related referrals and counseling for sexual minorities—confusion, alienation, shame, and despair quickly became the basis for understanding the serious need for legal reform. The goal of making "deep, mature" relationships possible was not only important for individual happiness, it also had an important political purpose in the pursuit of equality, working against public perceptions of promiscuity and prostitution, and preparing queer people for participation in the post-reform world of monogamous sexuality. Much more was at stake than the despair experienced by large numbers of queer men and women. In counseling, Grey saw the possibility of full social inclusion: homosexuals and heterosexuals alike would share equally in the promises of stable intimacy.

This commitment to queer respectability and mental health in the form of monogamous relationality would change in the early 1970s with the post-Stonewall emergence of a gay liberation movement in Britain. As the next section will show, queer counseling (and allied befriending services) became less committed to a goal of romantic monogamy and more interested in fostering queer relationality writ large.

Queer Counseling and the Pursuit of Intimacy in 1970s Britain

The Albany Trust's psychological health initiatives had, from their earliest days, been focused on ending queer men and women's social alienation and feelings of despair. According to surveys investigating the "social needs" and relationship experiences of queer men and women conducted over months spanning 1969–1970—more than two years after the passage of the 1967 Sexual Offences Act—the vast majority of the 2,700 respondents continued to suffer deeply from social isolation.[56] The legality of homosexual relations in private between adults had not amounted to full social equality or anything close to "liberation." Not only did police arrests continue to rise, a dramatic indication of a lack of inclusion at the local level, but social attitudes remained largely unchanged.

Despite significant increases in the number of people approaching the Albany Trust in the years following the 1967 Act, sharing their ongoing and "unmanageable feelings of guilt" and experiences of "fear, ostracism, and bigotry," the trust leadership decided in 1970 that they would no longer take on more counseling cases themselves.[57] Counseling individuals in order to cultivate queer respectability was seen as less immediately effective in tackling homosexual and trans stigma than large-scale research into the needs of Britain's queer population. Research, ideally organized through a well-funded British Sex Research Institute, was seen as more promising in directing policy change and supporting improvements in social services for queer people.[58] The trust thus directed would-be clients toward those services that had been providing experienced counseling for decades, partnering with suicide-prevention, marriage counseling, and sexual health organizations like the Samaritans, the Family Planning Association, and the NMGC.[59] This outsourcing of counseling referrals remained in place until October 1974, when a yearly grant of £10,000 began to be received from the Voluntary Services Unit, enabling the trust to hire additional staff and become more directly involved in providing front-line help.[60]

Despite the trust's decreased involvement in counseling in the early 1970s, the number of queer people receiving counseling rose dramatically. This coincided with the high point of queer liberation in Britain. Following the Stonewall riots in New York City in the summer of 1969 and launching of the GLF in the United States in July 1969 and in the UK in October 1970, the CHE created Friend in May 1971 as a gay counseling and befriending service.[61] Given the record number of queer adults and young people empowered to "come out"—encouraged by positive political associations with openness and self-acceptance—and lack of services to help sexual minorities cope with their internalized homophobia, Friend saw itself as "well placed to help with these problems."[62] It placed high value on befrienders being open about their sexuality since they could demonstrate "from personal experience it's possible to lead a full, happy and productive life":

> We can help people not only with our counselling skills, but also by example. By being openly gay, we're proof that gays don't have to conform to the unhappy, neurotic stereotypes invented for us by others.[63]

Appealing to the importance of real examples of positive queer experience as central to the counseling and befriending experience, Friend rejected the strict need for training in specialized counseling techniques (increasingly promoted by the Albany Trust in the 1970s). In training volunteer befrienders, Friend focused on close listening and providing friendship when appropriate. Friend began its work in May 1971 with only a couple of dozen befrienders, all of whom were openly homosexual. It soon became clear that the demand for befriending services provided for queer people by queer people was much greater than anticipated. By November 1972, the London office had brought in an experienced counsellor to assess client needs and London Friend was open five nights a week for callers to telephone in.[64] By early 1973, Friend had become an independent national organization—relaunched as separate from CHE—with seven local groups and approximately fifty consultants and befrienders.

Friend was not the only service purporting to meet the needs of the self-confessedly lonely queer person. The counseling scene both expanded and transformed during the first half of the 1970s as each organization within the "homophile" and gay liberation movements developed a counseling arm. Queer counseling services launched during these years were linked to the goal of queer liberation. The clearest example of this was Icebreakers, whose mission was to provide help by using only proudly queer-identified activists: healing was understood to take place within the context of shared experience. When Icebreakers was first launched by the GLF in 1973, homosexuality had yet to be removed as a psychiatric condition from the *Diagnostic and Statistical Manual of Mental Disorders*.[65] Icebreakers' roots lay in the GLF's counter-psychiatry group, and its objective was to not only provide emotional support to those who suffered from queer discrimination but also counter the long history of queer oppression that psychiatrists had both directly and indirectly supported and enacted. Merging their Marxist-inspired call for large-scale structural change with an antipsychiatric imperative to purge capitalist structures of psychiatrically legitimated power imbalances, Icebreakers' agenda was political to its core. Taking their lead from the feminist cry "the personal is political," they organized support groups as consciousness-raising cells.

Although not nearly as outspoken against the psychiatric and allied professions as Icebreakers, Friend (whose origins lay in the more politically moderate CHE) was also deliberately operated by openly queer befrienders who answered telephone calls, responded to letters, and met with advice-seekers in person. As at Icebreakers, the reasons for this were both psychological and political: befrienders were meant to serve as positive examples of queer self-acceptance, offering evidence of eventual psychological relief, at the same time as befrienders encouraged clients to become active participants in queer organizations and sub-cultural communities. Even after Friend was relaunched as an independent counseling organization in 1972, it continued to receive most of its requests for help through CHE referrals and, in turn, frequently encouraged clients to join CHE social groups as a means for resolving their emotional problems.

The massive growth in counseling, befriending, and self-help support services at the height of gay liberation was thus not separate from gay liberation politics but reflected the view that the resolution of sexual minorities' emotional problems was deeply connected to the advancement of emancipatory sexual politics in the 1970s. This story has, however, been largely relegated to the margins of histories of 1970s queer political radicalism. Jeffrey Weeks refers to the existence of early support groups as "conservative and tiny," yet "an important first step":

> This fear of public opinion, and the deep internalization of guilt and secrecy, had a corrosive effect on people's lives. *The existence of support groups, however conservative and tiny*, had therefore had an important impact. As a result of these many found their sense of identity and self-esteem had been immeasurably strengthened. *This was an important first step*.[66]

Weeks is far from idiosyncratic in bracketing off confessional pro-queer speech within political spaces—like pride marches, demonstrations against anti-gay factions like the Christian Festival of Light, and government lobbying—from confession in the intimate space of the counseling or befriending encounter. In the case of the former, the purpose of pro-queer speech was to challenge and transform public opinion. Counseling services were, instead, ostensibly meant to help individuals accept and adjust to the life that they—privately—wanted to live.

An alternative view to this—and one that acknowledges the political objectives of queer counseling and befriending services—disrupts assumptions of hard and fast distinctions between public and private. Intimate relationality was, for these queer befrienders, counselors, and many clients, itself a political act and foundation for political community. Queer scholars such as Lauren Berlant, Michael Warner, Lee Edelman, and Deborah Nelson have shown that constructions of private life have been deeply informed by needs that might more typically be understood as quintessentially public: state actors, participation in market activities, and cultural values have played key roles in producing its boundaries. They have also shown that the conventions of intimacy—its associations with emotional depth, sharing, and the transcendence of individual boundaries in the twentieth-century West—are themselves the outcome of collective processes of imagination and are embedded in power relationships. What has been less explored, however, is how the very experience of intimate relationality has itself functioned as a mode of publicness. Against the Habermasian reading of the public sphere as governed by rationality, Berlant points out that intimate attachments "make people public, producing transpersonal identities and subjectivities."[67]

Intimacy is thus not merely "public" because public entities like the state and market invest it with meaning and value. It became public within the context of queer counseling and befriending services because it provided a means for creating what were seen as liberating, humane, and wholly egalitarian social alternatives. As Berlant puts it, "intimacy builds worlds"—worlds that exclude some populations to cement others (wherein intimacy is seen as only possible in a heteronormative space like the nuclear family) and worlds that foreground inclusion (wherein intimacy becomes the means for producing sub-cultural communities as well as more inclusive national and transnational communities, a bridge that connects all worlds). The version of intimate relationality that was being cultivated at queer counseling and befriending sites did not hinge upon an ideal of married child-producing monogamy. The production of children was not the intended outcome of queer intimacy; yet durable relationships—romantic, friendship, community—were.

Counseling and befriending services were important sites of initiation into an alternative, emotionally oriented queer public. The written responses of counselors and befrienders to advice seekers typically began by attempting to create a sense of shared emotional experience. Phrases like "many people in your situation feel this way" and "I used to feel as you do now" preceded befrienders' advice, addressing letter writers' feelings of isolation.[68] Correspondence very often continued back and forth for several weeks, months, even years, before the advice seeker became either willing or able (such as when the person was writing from prison) to meet face-to-face and even participate in one of Friend's weekly social gatherings.

A sense of common hardship set the initial tone of communications and provided the befriender with the opportunity to model the longer-term emotional purpose of the advice seeker's current suffering: after overcoming their own alienation, they now felt optimistic and open to the many opportunities that queer social life had made possible. Befrienders—often themselves having once been on the other end of Friend correspondence—demonstrated a self-accepting, friendly, and open disposition as a positive outcome of establishing contact with a queer self-help organization like Friend. Some would immediately share their own experiences of coming out and the months that followed—many now had queer flatmates, a network of close friends, and had formed one or more fulfilling romantic relationships.

Requests for advice were most often framed within a larger narrative of loneliness and shame. Although letter writers were typically very open about their emotional hardships—resulting not only from their stigmatized sexual desires but often also from age, socio-economic factors, and differing cultural backgrounds that led them to feel cut off from the queer social scene—the act of putting these into words was fraught with uncertainty. Correspondents described their struggle in finding the words that best described their current situation, the events that were most relevant to mention, and the emotions that felt most suitable to convey. The act of writing was not infrequently mentioned in letters as a safe first step toward forming connections with other queer people and less challenging for many than either calling to speak to another queer person over the phone or meeting in person. Letters were typically read by befrienders as communicating deep sadness, which was often intended, but this was commented upon even when the advice seeker was contacting Friend about practical issues, with questions about housing or employment opportunities. Even in these cases, befrienders would invite deeper confession; their responses would open with sentences that reflected difficult emotions back to the letter writer, such as, "You sound very lonely and I know that it can be difficult to reach out for help."[69]

Advice seekers who wrote to Friend saw the possibility of friendship as very seductive. Replies to their first round of correspondence most often expressed relief at having finally, at long last, encountered the mutual understanding that might only be found in communication with someone with similarly painful experiences. The goal of communication with queer counseling and befriending services was, in many ways, mutually negotiated and agreed upon. Letters written to Friend shared many similarities, and yet whatever the problem and ideal outcome imagined, there was seldom a clear road map to its resolution. These included requests for advice on how to go about meeting people with whom one might form an authentic romantic connection outside of the club scene, questions about how to find housing when openly homosexual, as well as inquiries relating to intimacy challenges, such as how one might go about negotiating a significant age difference, divergences in class backgrounds, and varying levels of sexual experience. Many exchanges showed both advice seeker and befriender working together to arrive at an ideal solution.

Although Friend's correspondence showed a strong commitment to helping self-confessedly lonely correspondents establish intimate connections with others, unlike at the Albany Trust the focus was not always on developing monogamous relationships. For example, when a young couple, David and Gordon, approached Friend asking for advice about moving in together (from finding a landlord willing to rent to a homosexual couple to managing changing relationship dynamics), Friend counselor John Peterson advised the men to exercise caution in their decision as the intensity of cohabitation often destroyed rather than stabilized intimacy. He instructed them not to "ape heterosexuality" and invest all their emotional needs in their relationship:

> lots of people assume that all their needs (to give and take) can be fulfilled by one person and this is very rarely true and more particularly with same sex partners. Most of us need a network of relationships (I don't necessarily mean sexual of course) to be fulfilled. Living together of course can be a joyful experience, so long as it isn't an effort to "ape" heterosexuality, but many people find it too heavy and often say that it has shortened their relationship, because it was too demanding.[70]

Advice like this was not exclusively given to men. Lesbian befrienders similarly affirmed the importance of "a network of relationships" for personal fulfillment. When, for example, an anonymous woman approached Friend expressing shame at carrying on sexual relationships with multiple female friends, her befriender advised her to abandon the notion that non-monogamous sex was somehow wrong. If anything, "making love certainly enriche[d] a friendship":

> there is nothing to be ashamed of ... if you can go further than the majority of women and include physical love-making in your relationships with other women, then the better for you (and the sizeable minority of women sharing this gift with you) ... the more intimate and exciting are the possibilities of such relationship.[71]

It was a commitment to intimate relationality—a capacity to form close relationships and friendships—rather than an appeal to a specific kind of relationship (monogamous, child-producing) that was actively promoted and cultivated at Friend.

Although Friend correspondence typically functioned as a consciously friendly and upbeat introduction to a welcoming queer community, with invitations to meet in person or attend social groups usually extended, there were notable exceptions. For example, Mark, who wrote to Friend complaining of his inability to form emotional connections with his sexual partners, was counseled to abandon his focus on physical appearance. In response to confessing to being sexually drawn exclusively to men of a specific physical type—handsome, hairy, and well-endowed—his befriender pointed out that he seemed to be "getting tired of pursuing such men and want something more—perhaps someone you can like and love as a person and not just as a body."[72] He then advised Mark to focus on building emotional connections with his sexual partners and to "try for a while to not consider only handsome, hairy men and try to find a situation where you can meet different sorts of people, not only those who instantly appeal to you sexually."[73]

Not only were advice seekers dissuaded from pursuing fleeting physical encounters, but correspondents with certain fetishes were offered little help in satisfying their desires. For example, in the autumn of 1979, Friend counselor Philip Conn advised a middle-aged advice seeker against indulging in his fantasy of being "thrashed" by an older man. His correspondent, George, described as around fifty, divorced for ten years, and "possibly homosexual," had stated that he had a "deep-seated longing" to show himself "freely to an old man wearing my long pants" and "to receive a thrashing from him."[74] He believed that this would "cure" him of "this ridiculous desire which has been with me for some time."[75] George sent several letters to Friend asking for help finding a man who might discreetly help him live out his fantasy. He explained that his uncle had assumed this role on several occasions, however, he had recently become unwilling and threatened to expose George to his mother (who was then very ill) if he did not stop asking.

In response to George's initial letter requesting help with introductions, befriender Richard McCance had advised that he put a personal advertisement in *Gay Times* describing the person that he hoped to meet—over seventy, gray-haired or bald, and "highly trustworthy." When no one responded to his ad, George wrote back to again ask for help. At this point, Philip Conn let George know that there was nothing that Friend could do for him:

> I cannot see that I can help you very much, if you really want to realise your ambition to be thrashed by an old man while you are wearing long pants. You seem to feel that this will "cure" you. But I cannot see why this should be the case... There are lots of people around who have strong wishes to engage in unusual activities associated with sexual feelings. While it is the case that the feelings can diminish over time, and the activity even be socialized, as with the organisations for transvestites and rubber lovers, this probably happens because such people have ample opportunities to satisfy their needs. You, however, crave one and only one experience.[76]

Conn was bothered not by the fact that George's request was "unusual" in and of itself, but that its rarity likely precluded him from forming connections with similarly oriented individuals. Unlike people with latex fetishes, who existed in growing numbers, George's fetish was seen as isolating him from others. Conn thus responded negatively to George's insinuation that he himself might be willing to accommodate his needs:

> I am not old enough to perform the rite. And even if I were I would be unlikely to acquiesce—at least if you expected to be freed from your wish thereafter. What I would have done, had we met, would have been to discuss with you quite what your desire was, how you felt about it, and whether you wanted to be free of it. And my "cure" would not have entailed encouraging you to enact it.[77]

In communications between George and Conn, unlike most Friend correspondence, there was a clear lack of support for the advice seeker realizing their desires.

Even in exchanges with self-identified pedophiles—however controversial their sexual interest—befrienders showed compassion in response to descriptions of deep loneliness and repeated failed attempts at establishing lasting love relationships.[78] In response to longing for romantic relationships—a distinctive marker of a "good" queer—befrienders communicated understanding and empathy.

The emotional tone of correspondence was an important feature of queer initiation. Recent work by David Halperin on gay (male) initiation brings attention to the social practices and cultural identifications at work in producing gay male subjectivity. Halperin describes homosexual subjectivity as involving far more than desire for homosexual sex. It emerges out of a range of social and emotional practices cordoning off mainstream gay male culture, practices that produce "not only identification but disidentification."[79] On this account, being gay or "queer" "refers not just to something you are, but also to something you do."[80] And, like many other social practices, one can do this well or badly: performing with a high level of fluency, missing the mark, or failing to even try. Gay initiation teaches self-identified gay men how to properly perform gayness. While the subject of Halperin's book focuses on the music, theater, and cinema that has been appropriated and reinterpreted as quintessentially "gay"—and is perhaps seemingly far from the work of counseling—his approach, namely bringing our attention to gay male initiation and the social practices of gayness, is deeply relevant. The psychosexual initiatives that this chapter examines played an important role in fashioning a queer subjectivity that was embedded in lasting relationships. Becoming a well-adjusted sexual minority far exceeded issues of desire and sexual practice. It involved social practices meant to end alienation. Making peace with one's sexuality and becoming a "good" queer meant becoming part of a queer community and embedded in a network of meaningful queer relationships.

At Friend, "good" queer correspondents communicated loneliness but without self-indulgence or self-pity. They communicated awareness that their isolation was connected to an experienced absence of meaningful connections. For example, the tone of Michael's letters, a young man in prison for sexual offences, was discussed among Friend workers as problematically "self-indulgent and demanding." In response, intimate one-on-one (as opposed to official business), correspondence was discontinued. As one befriender, who had been "careful to strike a balance between a friendly, yet reserved tone," put it:

> He obviously feels very lonely, but I have become increasingly concerned about the tone of his replies; I've found them increasingly self-indulgent and demanding. I have explained that "Friend" is made up of part-time volunteers, but it seems that he <u>expects</u> to be visited periodically and sent up-to-date copies of *Gay News* etc. whilst in Broadmoor and a full-time rehabilitation service upon his forthcoming release. He seems to think that we can take all the effort and difficulty out of his life... In the circumstances I feel that it would not be wise to continue correspondence with [Michael] on a one-to-one basis.[81]

Other correspondents expressed concern that they might be seen as self-pitying and self-centered by befrienders.[82] Toby, an agoraphobic man who identified as homosexual, complained of the lack of sincere relationships to be found in "facilities for gays in London" (a category in which he included Icebreakers, the CHE, and Gay Switchboard). He wondered why he had been unable to experience anything more than casual sexual encounters, and if there was something especially off-putting about him: "I hope that this letter doesn't make me sound to be full of self-pity... I've been let down and been in contact with those who seem to care only for their own personal pleasure."[83] Others worried about the damage that homosexual discrimination had done to their capacity for authentic human connection: "I really don't know how much damage emotional repression does to a person but judging by the periodic explosions I have it surely can't be too beneficial!"[84] This expression of self-doubt elicited a sympathetic response from a befriender: "let me first of all express my total sympathy with your troubled state of mind... one's sexuality is tied up with so many other facets of individuality that a repression of one's sexuality must also affect much of what makes up our relationship with the world."[85] The solution to correspondents' complaints was to join queer social organizations:

> I am sorry to read that you have been finding yourself increasingly isolated and unhappy of late. Your letter makes it clear that you see the difficulties and strains of your life and emotional needs very clearly... But our social groups do offer you still the only alternative to the dispiriting round of soulless discos of which you speak, and a very real forum for friendly, long term links with other gays, of all ages.[86]

This was suggested so often that some correspondents explicitly asked not to be given the advice that they should join a club or other queer organization:

> I have tried all the usual "remedies" such as joining clubs, societies, evening classes and the like in an endeavor to force some interest into my life, but with no avail... I have no idea what else I can do; perhaps you could suggest some course of action or perhaps put me in touch with someone with similar problems whom I might contact, but please, no "gay" societies or organisations.[87]

In their communications, counselors and befrienders modeled the candid intimacy that they hoped to foster. The private details of personal pain were met with warm sympathy and expressions of hope that suffering would be temporary. Their proposed solutions—participation in gay social organizations and events, meet-ups through Friend, face-to-face meetings with counselors, a more optimistic attitude—were centered on initiating their correspondents into a particular version of the queer social world: one dominated not by discos and casual sexual encounters but by club meetings, friendship, and sincere emotional exchange. Not only were these services meant to help heal emotional pain, they were also presenting—and helping cultivate—a relational life for queer men and women.

Conclusion: Counseling for Intimacy

During the same late-1970s moment that conversations about the disabling effects of queer isolation were happening at Friend, Antony Grey and Edward Shackleton, former diplomat and key participant in the rise of Britain's evangelical right, were engaged in a heated debate. The key issue circulated around whether Shackleton and his colleagues at the Gables, a recently launched experiment in Christian sexual counseling, should represent their ministry to confused and struggling queer men and women as "counseling." Questions surrounding the ethics and effectiveness of guidance in counseling were at the forefront of their impassioned exchange. Grey was adamant that counseling should be non-directive and ultimately help clients make their own autonomous decisions. He appealed to standards set out by the Standing Conference for the Advancement of Counselling to defend his view. Shackleton disagreed and, appealing to the dictionary definition of the term, argued that "giving counsel" was akin to giving advice. He believed that counseling needed to provide queer clients with direction on how to overcome same-sex sexual desire. Only this, he argued, would end their psychological pain.

Far more was at stake in Grey and Shackleton's disagreement than deciding on the correct meaning of the term counseling. Grey consistently brought discussion—which unfolded over more than a dozen letters in 1978[88]—back to the question of freedom in its many dimensions, moral, legal, and political. He repeatedly emphasized that counselors needed to allow their clients a "full measure of freedom," and was adamant that there should be no interference with the individual's right to choose how they lived their lives. This was congruent with the Cold War origins of marriage counseling—David Mace had similarly emphasized client freedom as the cornerstone of marriage guidance work. Grey went so far as to liken Shackleton's assumption about the sinful nature of homosexuality that pervaded his work to the moral presumptions that animated authoritarian regimes. Good liberal that he was, Grey defended the individual's right to choose as the core expression of a person's individuality. It was this commitment to radical non-judgment and respect for sexual freedom that had caused the Albany Trust to lose public funding in the wake of Margaret Thatcher's 1979 election, following a scandal—initiated by Mary Whitehouse—over the trust's provision of counseling and advice to known pedophiles.

Grey's claim that non-directive counseling was value-free was perhaps not entirely accurate. As Grey himself discovered in the decades following the Albany Trust's founding, there was much more to queer counseling than simply making clients capable of making choices about their sexual lives. Much more was required to undo the negative effects of homo- and transphobia than simply helping the client achieve greater self-awareness. Counseling aimed at sexual minorities in the 1960s and 1970s paid close attention to only some of the specificities surrounding the emotional pain described—that which related to the client's sexual experiences, interests, and desires. Race, class, gender, ability, and age were far less often addressed, and when they were, they were seen as factors accentuating the original problem, that is British society's intolerance of queer sexualities.

Was there anything "queer" about the counseling and befriending that was aimed at queer people in the 1960s and 1970s? Did their focus on healing the psychological effects of discrimination against sexual minorities cause them to operate differently from other counseling services? Definitions of counseling ranged in the mid-1970s, but, according to the Standing Conference for the Advancement of Counselling in 1975, tended to coalesce around the following three themes: counseling was understood to be a "person-to-person form of communication marked by ... subtle emotional understanding," it was "centred upon one or more problems of the client," and it was "free from authoritarian judgements and coercive pressure by the counsellor."[89] As a mode of intimate communication between strangers aimed at resolving personal problems, counseling was meant to unmask painful parts of the client's life and invest these with new meaning. Bill Logan from Gay Switchboard has emphasized the peculiarly transformative intent of queer counseling as it was directed toward shifting the client's life story from a heterosexual narrative framing to a queer one. To achieve this, the counselor engages in "queer listening," which Logan describes as marked by "a special kind of curiosity":

> We are especially interested in those elements of the story that do not fit within a compulsory heterosexuality. We listen to the heartache, we empathise with the sense of confusion our callers may be experiencing, we reflect back the grief they feel, but we also maintain a curiosity which seeks to make possible an expanded exploration of the gay element of the story.[90]

Although Logan was trained in a conventional Rogerian non-directive client-centered approach, counselor Christopher Behan points out that there was something distinctly new and different about the counseling style developed at Gay Switchboard: "the description of the work on Switchboard as 'Rogerian' does not sufficiently describe what I think is happening there. I think Bill's description of the work on the Switchboard as 'queer listening' is more rich and experience-near." Behan sums up the counseling that happens at Gay Switchboard as drawing upon conventions in counseling, but as itself producing something new—a "copying that originates."[91]

What precisely was being originated? Unlike many counseling agencies—whether the Samaritans or the NMGC—the services provided at the Albany Trust in the 1960s and organizations like Gay Switchboard and Friend in the 1970s actively sought to make counseling, and those who participated in it, agents for social change.[92] Through the meaning-giving agency of counseling services, the emotional suffering caused by internalized homophobia could become one possible foundation for a uniquely queer relational subjectivity. The proposed solutions to emotional pain centered on promoting new forms of relationality—LBGTQ community, unmarried coupling, romantic friendships. These rivaled monogamous marriage as the central, and most important, relationship of adult life. Queer relationality would emerge out of internalized homophobia as the positive resolution to isolation and despair.

This chapter has considered the important role that counseling at sexual law reform and gay liberation organizations played in cultivating models of queer relationality that were at once emotionally "healthy" and politically useful. By the late 1960s at the Albany Trust, this was more closely focused on the cultivation of sexual minorities who were able to create and sustain committed monogamous relationships; by the mid-1970s at Friend, queer emotional "health" was more broadly connected to a vision of harmonious relationality that went far beyond monogamous intimacy. The possibility of engaging in intimate relationships (including close friendships with people with similar emotional experiences) was long in the making. Clients first needed to overcome the major struggles that many lesbians, gay men, and bisexual people experienced—loneliness, social isolation, and the potentially debilitating impact of stigma.

The queer subjectivities described in this chapter were very much in process. The narratives developed reciprocally in written counseling and befriending exchanges revolved around the need for human connection, whether in the form of sex, romance, friendship, family, or community. Epistolary encounters were directed toward making socially isolated queer men and women relational subjects. This was very different from simply helping people meet potential partners. This was a project of self-making. Counsellors and befrienders modeled a relational style that would help clients themselves make ostensibly better choices about their sexual conduct and their lives.

The immense value attributed to intimate relationships in the homosexual law reform and gay liberation movements was not a foregone conclusion. This chapter has explored how conventions and expectations surrounding private life were actively remade as fundamentally emotional and relational at a moment when privacy seemed to be slipping away. There was a reassertion among supporters of the Wolfenden proposals of the value of private individual choices at a moment when much that was quintessentially private (notably, heterosexual love, sex, and family) had come to hold public value. In queer counseling initiatives we see the rise of visible efforts to make same-sex intimacy equally seen as embodying the public value attached to heterosexual love.

In the 1970s, with the rise of an active gay liberation movement, queer counseling services worked to create a queer political community that was geared toward transforming Britain's exclusionary heteronormative social world into one humanely rooted in intimate friendships and romantic relationships. At these services, relational incapacity was reconceived as a pathological outcome of social stigma. A restored ability for intimacy was seen as central to both positive queer identity and liberating social change.

6
Inherently Unstable
Adolescent Sexuality at the Boundary of Private Life

> To pass from childhood to adulthood takes a long time and whilst the majority make the physical changes, all too few manage to make the psychological ones.
> —Edward Griffith, "Adolescence," 1969

> An immature choice is not a free one.
> —The Policy Advisory Committee on Sexual Offences, June 1979

On March 10, 1976, *The Times* ran an editorial vehemently opposing a recent proposal by the National Council for Civil Liberties (NCCL) that the government lower the legal age of sexual consent to fourteen. Entitled "For the Protection of Adolescents," William Rees-Mogg, *The Times* editor and father of four children under fourteen, urged that the age of consent remain as it was—sixteen for heterosexual intercourse and twenty-one for homosexual relations—on the basis that "social values and standards should so far as possible protect adolescents from the emotional damage" resulting from early sexual exploration.[1] Although he was both conservative and a committed Catholic, Rees-Mogg did not appeal to moral arguments to make his case. Instead, he mobilized recent psychiatric discoveries that showed a gaping disparity between the rate of adolescents' physical development following puberty and the slower pace of their emotional development. While young people were physically maturing earlier than their parents had, he noted that there was "no shortage of evidence that their emotional development does not keep pace with this earlier physical advance."[2] He urged that evidence revealing the fragility of adolescent emotional development underscored the law's important role in ensuring young people's growth to healthy maturity.[3]

Rees-Mogg was not the only concerned parent to interpret a lowering of the age of sexual consent as a threat to young people's healthy emotional development. In the weeks that followed, *The Times* received dozens of letters affirming that there was "a world of difference between emotional and physical maturity,"[4] and opposing "any change in the law which would lower the age of consent."[5] Although correspondents expressed concern about teenage pregnancy, abortion, and the spread of venereal disease among young people, they stressed that the psychological dangers were still more severe, and more frightening because they were less clearly understood.[6] Foremost among these was the perceived risk that prematurely sexually active girls would become psychologically stunted and incapable of taking on the emotional responsibilities of marriage and motherhood. *Times* readers equally worried that young men involved in same-sex sexual relationships were at risk of having their sexual orientation fixed as homosexual, thus denying them the possibility of marriage and children. Although correspondents conceded that many adolescents resembled adults by age sixteen, they argued that they were still children in the ways that mattered most—the emotional purpose of sex was still beyond their grasp, and they were incapable of forming lasting intimate relationships.

The stakes of this public discussion of teenage sexuality felt especially urgent to participants. A few months earlier Britain's home secretary, Roy Jenkins—an open defender of sexual liberty as the cornerstone of a civilized society—had appointed a special Policy Advisory Committee on Sexual Offences (PAC) to direct the government in deciding whether the age of consent should be lowered. The decision to pursue the issue was prompted by several public appeals, of which the NCCL's had only been the most recent. Campaigns launched by the CHE in 1971, the Quaker Society of Friends in 1972, and the Sexual Law Reform Society (SLRS) in 1974 had similarly urged that the age of sexual consent be equalized for homosexuals and heterosexuals and lowered to fourteen to coincide with adolescents' earlier pubescence.[7]

At first glance the controversy over the legal age of consent seemed to result from a straightforward clash of values between conservatives and liberals, with outraged parents and emerging defenders of "family values" on one side and civil rights organizations and proponents of sexual freedom on the other. A closer look, however, reveals that this conflict over the purpose of the law largely centered on heated disagreement over young people's developmental needs. Both pro–family values pressure groups and medical and psychiatric organizations submitted memos to the PAC opposing any changes to the age of consent, and did so on the grounds that sexual exploration "would place greater responsibility and anxieties upon young people when they are not sufficiently mature to accept them."[8] At the same time, the PAC collected material from homosexual youth and sexual law reform organizations indicating that contemporary legal restrictions were psychologically harmful to young people— including evidence from gay teenagers and teenage mothers indicating that the law in its present form variously caused emotional damage and interfered with healthy sexual and emotional development. Similar to the views of 1970s LGBTQ+ counselors and befrienders discussed in chapter 5, the social reformers and young people discussed in this chapter prioritized access to intimate sexual relationships as foundational to every person becoming fully relational and emotionally whole. Intimate sexuality was once again seen as having crucial far-reaching *personal* outcomes, but here such relationships were more specifically presented as ensuring young citizens' right to healthy emotional maturity.

Despite the lack of resolution surrounding adolescents' emotional needs, in 1981 the Criminal Law Revision Committee announced that the ages of consent for heterosexual and homosexual sex would remain as they were. This chapter examines why appeals for change to the age of sexual consent were ultimately unsuccessful despite the central participation of teenagers in the campaign for reform, the outcome of which ostensibly affected them alone. Petitions to extend the right to sexual privacy to consenting teenagers were part of a wider set of conversations seeking to clarify—and, for some, re-define—both the scope of the criminal law relating to sexual offences *and* the state's responsibility toward children's developmental needs. These were discussions that had been ongoing since the end of WWII but had become especially urgent in the late 1960s. When homosexual sex was decriminalized in Britain in 1967, the decision was based on the conviction that the state should not intervene in adults' private lives. It was decided that the law needed to respect individuals' "private responsibility" for their "own actions" as that "which a mature agent can properly be expected to carry for himself without the threat of punishment from the law."[9]

Claims that adults had a right to sexual privacy required immediate qualification: what was the proper range of adulthood? Who belonged within its boundaries? In the decades following WWII, British young people had become increasingly visible social actors—they worked, spent money, married, and had children. In recognition of this, the legal age of majority was lowered from twenty-one to eighteen in 1967, allowing eighteen-year-olds to vote, buy property, draw up wills, and marry without parental consent.[10] It thus seemed to follow that even younger adolescents might be capable of responsibly engaging in sexual exploration with their peers. The greater availability of state-provided contraceptives following the passage of the 1967 Family Planning Act further bolstered the view that teenage sexual activity no longer needed to be condemned since teenage pregnancy and venereal disease could be avoided. Why, sexual law reformers asked, should pubescent adolescents not be left to responsibly act upon their sexual impulses with their peers if no one was harmed? Teenagers themselves became involved in the campaign for legal change. Young mothers shared the difficulties they experienced in not being able to publicly acknowledge their children's fathers—most of whom were between sixteen and nineteen—for fear of bringing about their criminal conviction. Gay teenagers also spoke openly about their harrowing experiences; descriptions of police abuse—including forced confessions of sex with suspected homosexuals—mental illness, alcoholism, drug abuse, and suicide attempts ended up at the heart of the campaign to lower the age of consent.

To understand how the legal lines distinguishing adolescent from adult sexuality were drawn in the wake of Britain's "sexual revolution," this chapter focuses on how the psychiatric targeting of adolescence as a period of emotional instability became a defining point of political debate. I argue that attention to adolescence as a medico-psychological problem after WWII ended up setting the terms for the exclusion of many teenagers from the sexual rights that were then being granted to adults. Psychiatric efforts to raise empathic awareness about "normal" adolescent emotional instability through teen parenting guides as well as through adolescent mental health services ended up providing a seemingly sound scientific basis for establishing limits to teenagers' claims to maturity and denying appeals for greater freedom from parental and state protection. The idea that adolescents were psychologically fragile framed discussions of what should be variously managed or encouraged when it came to young people's sexual desire.

This chapter reveals that the post-1945 preoccupation with the dangers of adolescent sexuality—which reached its crescendo in the 1970s—was focused on rising concerns about the precariousness of childhood emotional development. It examines the deliberate exclusion of adolescents from state protections surrounding the private life of adults in Britain when public support for a less paternalistic society was at its height. In doing so, it sheds new light on how private life was imagined during Britain's "sexual revolution" as primarily devoted to enabling adults access to both profoundly relational and personally enriching emotional experiences.

This chapter reveals that by the mid-1970s the expectation that private life should be centered on a lifelong monogamous relationship was linked to an idealized view of adulthood. Beliefs about the emotional instability of young people presented a crucial barrier to claims that they should have the same right to privacy as adults. Speaking on their own behalf with the authority of experience, gay teenagers and teenage mothers needed to overcome a compelling range of psychological claims that prevented them from being taken seriously. At the heart of these discussions loomed troubling uncertainties about what constituted emotional maturity, when it began, and how it was best secured.

Examining the controversy surrounding adolescent sexuality offers insight into how young people fell perilously in between the emotional categories of childhood and adulthood created in the decades following WWII. By the 1970s, emotional maturity—however psychologically unclear—underwrote the acceptability of social reforms predicated on citizens' right to freedom from state intervention. Since adolescents lacked the emotional maturity that made them capable of being responsible for their sexual choices, they were considered too immature to be granted freedom to make such weighty decisions. In debates over adolescent sexual consent, we see a liberal model of freedom conflict with a new emotional view of the capacity for autonomy: adults' freedom was dependent on their completed psychological development. As the foundation for monogamous marriage and responsible parenthood, emotional maturity endowed individuals with the right to a state-protected private life. Adolescents were denied this because it was widely believed that their emotional development could be easily "perverted," thus permanently rendering them incapable of marriage and responsible parenthood.

Psychiatry and the Management of Adolescent Emotional Turbulence

When adolescence was first identified as a distinct stage of human development in the early twentieth century, its hallmark features—including turbulent mood changes, hyper-sexuality, and heightened suggestibility—were emphasized as developmentally necessary despite the threat they posed to modern civilized societies. Both American psychologist G. Stanley Hall and Sigmund Freud stressed the inevitability of youthful "stress and storm" as well as the need for its careful management in making psychologically healthy adulthood possible.[11] Hall's path-breaking 1904 study of adolescence equally emphasized the functional necessity of youthful emotional struggles as well as the importance of parents, doctors, and schools in preventing young people from succumbing to inner crisis. Freud similarly explained adolescents' "hysterical disposition" in his 1905 *Three Essays on the Theory of Sexuality* as a necessary challenge to overcome toward the goal of healthy sexual maturity. How young people redirected their erratic emotions played a crucial role in determining whether they would develop sexual neuroses as adults.[12]

Although Hall and Freud were both recognized pioneers of developmental psychology by the early twentieth century, it was only after WWI that the figure of the inherently unstable adolescent became a focus of social concern.[13] In response to a wartime surge in juvenile crime, many psychologists, social workers, and educators proposed new approaches to pedagogy, styles of parenting, and penal reforms that would help young people successfully manage the restlessness, volatilities, and anti-social behaviors common to adolescence. The young person's environment—particularly their family life—became a more prominent concern in the 1920s and 1930s as adolescents, like children, were seen as still highly malleable and thus vulnerable to pathological social influences. Psychologists and social workers connected to Britain's child guidance movement and psychoanalysts at the newly launched Institute for the Scientific Treatment of Delinquency focused on adolescent clients' relationships with family members and often included parents (and sometimes also siblings) in their treatment plans.[14]

Although these interwar mental health initiatives continued to stress adolescents' inherent emotional instability, they helped introduce more leniency toward young offenders and made crime prevention initiatives seem credible. This can be seen in the reduction in custodial sentences for young offenders beginning in the 1920s and preference for supervised probation:[15] by 1938, only 10% of young people found guilty of indictable offences were sent to reform schools.[16] It can also be seen in the growing enthusiasm for youth clubs as a way of re-focusing the "primitive instincts" that drew young people to petty crime.[17] Juvenile court officer Basil Henriques advocated youth clubs as a form of crime prevention—echoing Boy Scouts' founder Robert Baden-Powell—as he stressed that adolescent boys, in particular, needed constructive outlets to sublimate their "natural effervescences and high spirits."[18]

The perception that adolescent acting-out was a medico-psychological problem rather than a moral failing intensified in the decades after WWII as a range of pressing mental health problems were identified as first (and sometimes solely) expressing themselves during the teenage years. Schizophrenia and manic depression—diagnoses given to the vast majority of patients in Britain's overpopulated psychiatric hospitals—were found most frequently in individuals between thirteen and eighteen.[19] By the early 1960s, depression, suicide, and drug and alcohol abuse, were flagged as mental health crises that particularly affected the adolescent population.[20] Not only were young people increasingly burdened with psychiatric diagnoses, but psychologists also frequently lamented adolescents' resistance to conventional forms of therapy. Psychoanalysts Moses (Moe) Laufer and Anna Freud—both pioneers in developing specialized psychological services for adolescents—explained that the treatment of adolescent patients was a "hazardous venture" requiring new strategies for care since these clients were emotionally erratic.[21] A decade later, Tavistock psychotherapist John Evans noted adolescents' ongoing unsuitability to psychotherapy since they were no longer candidates for play therapy and also not yet able to verbalize their internal conflicts as adults could.[22]

With the post-war ascendance of environmental explanations for mental illness, many psychiatrists interpreted the rise in mental health problems among adolescents as a sign of their inherent difference and an indication that they were more affected by the rapid transformations of the age.[23] This focus on environment fueled innovations in specialized psychiatric services for adolescents. Moe Laufer launched the Young People's Consultation Centre in north London in 1962; adolescent units were established at the Tavistock Clinic in 1960 and the Cassel Hospital in 1964; and adolescent counseling was introduced to a handful of schools in 1965.[24] Practitioners at these services approached adolescents' social world as riven with interpersonal conflict, exacerbated by the massive social dislocations of the post-WWII decades. School counselors were trained to concentrate on their clients' unstable relationships—with parents, siblings, peers, and teachers—as a dominant focus of their work.[25] A propensity for conflict and relationship instability was assumed to equally characterize boys *and* girls. Although boys were seen as more aggressive and girls were more likely to be described as showing heightened sexuality, gender differences were downplayed as having any important bearing on the treatment of adolescent emotional problems.[26]

At the same time as Britain's adolescent mental health care services grew at a rapid pace, psychiatrists helped fuel a growing industry of parent and teen advice literature. Stressing the "normal abnormality" of adolescence, mental health professionals emphasized their strengths in helping parents shepherd their children through these psychologically complex years. In "Teenagers Today," a 1968 booklet produced by the NAMH, psychiatrist Gordon Stewart Prince stressed that since adolescence was "naturally and normally a time of emotional turmoil, or violent surges of mood, of conflicting longings and fears" all teenagers were in urgent need of psychologically attuned parental guidance.[27] Doris Odlum, NAMH vice-president and key popularizer of child and adolescent psychology, went even further to warn that parents' lack of psychological understanding often caused their adolescent children "a great deal of damage instead of helping them through this difficult stage of development."[28]

Advice authors stressed that psychological damage could be avoided with the right parenting approach: emphasis was placed on empathy, communication, and emotional connection between parent and teenage child.[29] Postwar reforms in educational policy meant that young people stayed in school at least a year longer than they had before the war and since many deferred the post-war requirement of National Service and remained in higher education, this lengthened the time that they lived with their parents. Teenage parenting advice treated this extended cohabitation of parents and their adolescent children as a further opportunity for guiding teenagers.[30]

Parenting advice authors' emphasis on openness was set in opposition to the authoritarian and emotionally distant Victorian model of the parent-child relationship. The latter was presented as breeding insecurity, stunting individuality, and preventing healthy maturity. More importantly, however, parents' openness with their children was encouraged for avoiding social harm: close relationships enabled parents to maintain stricter supervision over their increasingly independent children. Postwar studies of adolescent psychology stressed the many dangers that young people's increasing separation from their families needed to be guarded against. For example, Anna Freud and Michael Rutter both warned that adolescents' emotional fluctuations made them more likely to frivolously transfer loyalty from one potentially dangerous political cause to another.[31] Odlum highlighted the dangers of adolescents' mental suggestibility. She worried about young people being an easy target for consumer fads, warning that advertisers particularly preyed on them:

> they utiliz[e] every weak point in the adolescents' psychological development, above all his immature sexual emotions, his insecurity, his fear of rejection, his desire to be accepted by his fellows as sophisticated and attractive, and his need to impress the adults with his independence and maturity.[32]

She was also concerned about young people's "herd" tendencies, noting that the 1954 novel *Lord of the Flies* had correctly demonstrated that when in groups, teenagers could "do terrible things ... that they would eventually regard with horror, and be quite incapable of carrying out on their own or in cold blood."[33] With the science of parenting broadening from an earlier prewar focus on babies to a new postwar focus on teenagers, advice authors fittingly compared adolescence to early infancy, describing it as a "second period of instability," but with potentially more troubling consequences since adolescents had established independent links to the world beyond their family home, and their lives were far more difficult to monitor and control. Emotional closeness was meant to healthily nurture adolescent children's ongoing development at the same time as it prevented young people from undermining the already tenuous foundations of postwar society.

Confronting Adolescent Sexuality

Of the many dangers that young people were seen as presenting in the decades after WWII, their burgeoning sexuality was at the forefront of concern. Rising rates of teenage pregnancy and venereal disease among teenagers inspired alarm, and recent medical discoveries pointing to adolescents' earlier pubescence contributed to panic that adolescent sexual desire seriously threatened public welfare.[34] Parent advice literature included guidance on sex education, with advice authors stressing that parents needed to play a central role not only in teaching their teenage children about the facts of reproduction and its associated risks, but also—more crucially—in imparting the correct attitude toward exploring relationships with peers of the opposite sex. As an NMGC pamphlet on teen parenting explained, while it was important that daughters "understand what sexual intercourse is and the risks involved ... It is even more important that she should understand what love and marriage really mean, and that she may be spoiling her future happiness if she has sexual intercourse beforehand."[35] Gynecologist Margaret White invoked the psychological consequences of sex in her parent advice manual, emphasizing that "A woman's deep involvement in sexual intercourse can change her whole personality." If she engaged in sex during adolescence, according to White, there was a strong likelihood that she would become not only "promiscuous," but also possibly "disillusioned, sexually frigid, and incapable of spontaneous affection."[36]

Parent advice authors often insisted that their opposition to premarital sex was not for moral reasons, and they urged parents to adopt their own informed understanding.[37] Marion Hilliard was clear that she was "not a person whose morals are shaped by convention," yet she "sternly advise[d]" that young people not engage in sex: "They are too young to cope with it" even if their interest in it "fills their minds and bodies."[38] NMGC counselor Alan Ingleby invoked the Christian entreaty against premarital sex not for moralizing purposes, he argued, but because it was a familiar way of presenting his own updated view of chastity's positive impact on personality development:

> Jesus was less concerned that people should conform ... than that they should become "whole" persons. Are we perhaps too greatly preoccupied with morality which measures chastity in terms of whether or not full sexual intercourse takes place, and too little in terms of those qualities of care and consideration, unselfishness and kindness, loyalty and integrity, without which no true chastity exists?[39]

Ingleby urged that premarital chastity "enhance[d] and enrich[ed]" relationships "in the long run."[40] Although she was not a churchgoer, Odlum also defended the Christian valuing of premarital abstinence since it emphasized, "the vital importance of the relations that we have with one another."[41] She stressed that every society, whether "good or ill," was built upon "the way in which each individual deals with his or her own sexual demands."[42] Acknowledging that chastity was challenging for many teenagers, Odlum warned parents against discouraging masturbation.

Adolescents' sexual ignorance became a major public concern in the mid-1960s in the wake of revelations in US sex surveys concerning teenagers' active sex lives.[43] Newer British studies highlighted the large number of sexually active girls who revealed that they thought they could not get pregnant without having an orgasm and boys who thought a girl could avoid pregnancy if she held her breath during sex or if they had sex standing up. Sex researcher Michael Schofield revealed that, of the more than 1,800 adolescents he had interviewed in 1964, 56% of boys and 13% of girls claimed to have received no sex education at school and over half could not answer basic questions about common sexually transmitted infections. Ignorance prevailed across the social classes. When she was eighteen in 1961, Sheila Rowbotham knew little about sex despite her middle-class education. Even after she had entered her first sexual relationship, she reported that "I remained as ignorant as ever about sex. Mel [her boyfriend] was not forthcoming either; it was sheer luck that I didn't get pregnant."[44] Rowbotham's commitment to monogamy might, however, have afforded some relief to many in the face of medical reports declaring widespread teenage promiscuity.[45] Britain's most respected medical journals published reports showing that the incidence of venereal disease was growing fastest among young people and that teenage pregnancies were rapidly on the rise by the late 1960s and interpreted these trends as signs that teenagers were not only sexually uninformed, but also incapable of monogamy.[46]

By the end of the 1960s, many educators and physicians supported introducing a comprehensive sex education program in British secondary schools for pragmatic reasons: they wanted the number of teenage pregnancies and sexually transmitted infections in young people to be radically reduced. Surveys of parents also showed that there was widespread support for sex education in schools (particularly since they often felt the gaps in their own sexual knowledge to be too large to offer their children adequate education).[47] Despite this, as with most subjects in British schools, no national curriculum was introduced, and the actual provision of sex education classes in British schools remained widely inconsistent.[48] Information about sex was typically provided in one lecture by a health visitor, and only if the school's director arranged it. A 1976 study of sex education in British schools summed up the situation as "chaotic" and "haphazard" despite the frequent "goodwill" of headmasters and education authorities.[49] Young people participating in education surveys consistently indicated that they wanted to know more, not only about the facts of sexual reproduction but also about child rearing, family life, and relationship problems.[50] Thank you letters sent to one visiting sex education lecturer in 1972—midwife Nancy Zinkin—consistently expressed gratitude for telling them "quite a lot of things that [they] did not know about," including information about venereal diseases and contraceptives.[51] Students frequently emphasized their enjoyment of the lesson and their hope that she would "come again soon." One girl noted that she had told her parents about it, "and they said they were glad I was told in school because it would be a difficult job for them to tell me."[52]

Although there was much support for sex education in schools, a notable—and increasingly vocal—segment of the British population believed that young people were becoming more sexually active because of their increased exposure to sex. While film and television were of greatest concern, critics also denounced sex education in schools outside of biology lessons (and even then regarded only the communication of "basic scientific facts of sexual anatomy and physiology" as necessary).[53] Sex education critics were especially worried about discussions of sex being included in health education courses. As a result, in 1971, the same year that teenage pregnancies had surpassed one hundred thousand—including more than twenty thousand abortions—an unflinchingly realistic sex education film, twenty-three-minutes in length and innocuously titled *Growing Up*, incited a major backlash against young people's exposure to depictions of sex. The film's creator, Martin Cole, co-director of the recently established Institute of Sex Education and Research, had wanted to highlight the pleasures of sex for young people. Cole rejected the pedagogical convention of using diagrams to demonstrate the stages of human development and convey information surrounding sexual reproduction. *Growing Up* instead showed viewers the naked bodies of young boys and girls who participated in the film's making, including close-up shots of their genitals, while Cole narrated details pertinent to the developmental stage on display. Most controversially, the film included scenes of a young man and woman masturbating and ended by showing a young couple having sex. Although the film educated viewers about how they might experience pleasure in sexual exploration, its final message emphasized young people's unsuitability to parenthood and cautioned teenagers to "never make love without taking the proper precautions."[54] Cole hoped that the film would be shown in schools as part of a comprehensive sex education program that communicated that sex was an entirely natural part of young people's physical and emotional development.

In the weeks following the preliminary screening of *Growing Up* in London's west end, controversy erupted over the question of how British youth should properly be exposed to information about sex. Two sixteen-year-old girls who had attended the screening were receptive to the film's approach and emphasized to a *Guardian* reporter that, "this is the sort of film that is needed."[55] Mary Whitehouse of the Clean Up TV Campaign was also present and decisively denounced it as a "rotten film" that depicted young people as "animals."[56] Shortly after this, the Archbishop of Canterbury declared that *Growing Up* (and any similar material) would not be shown in Church of England schools; he especially disparaged the film's separation of sexual pleasure from procreation within marriage.[57] Margaret Thatcher, then Minister of Education, similarly announced being "very perturbed" at the prospect of the film being used for sex education. She urged school administrators to take "utmost caution" in considering whether it would be shown.[58] Jennifer Muscutt, a young teacher who appeared in the film's segment on masturbation, was placed on indefinite suspension from her job at a Birmingham technical college.[59] Critics also demanded that Cole be forced to resign as genetics lecturer at Aston University in Birmingham on the grounds that he was "perverted."[60]

In the months that followed, campaigns to keep sex education out of British schools intensified; most critics held that parents were most appropriately suited to teach young people about proper regard for sexual life.[61] Leading the movement was a non-partisan pressure group calling itself The Responsible Society that had recently been formed to promote "family values" and protect Britain's youth from the current cultural "obsession" with "sexual gratification."[62] Among the group's founders were Brian Windeyer, vice chancellor of London University, Martin Wight, eminent international relations scholar, and Pamela Hansford Johnson, novelist and wife of C.P. Snow. The Responsible Society was created to help cultivate "responsible attitudes towards marriage and family life" and transform Britain's "permissive society" into a "responsible" one.[63] The group's founders formulated an agenda that prioritized the production and promotion of medical and sociological research into the beneficial impact of stable family life. Appeals to facts rather than moral arguments, they maintained, would go much further toward cultivating the "principles of responsibility which are essential to social and mental health."[64]

Sex education was only one of The Responsible Society's targets. Britain's emerging movement to protect "family values" also sought to quash attempts at providing contraception to young people. The recently launched Birth Control Campaign (BCC)—a pressure group formed to counter the growing threat of global overpopulation—had attracted The Responsible Society's attention since efforts to provide contraception to young people was one of its major aims, alongside promoting vasectomies for men uninterested in having children and abortions for unwanted pregnancies.[65] Although the BCC attracted the support of MPs from all party backgrounds and had an impressive list of doctors and politicians on its advisory council, the group sparked significant opposition when it began demanding that the Department of Health empower physicians to provide birth control pills to girls under sixteen without the requirement of parental consent.[66]

Despite public reaction against the BCC's focus on teenage sex in preventing overpopulation, in May 1974 the Department of Health changed its parental consent policy and removed all barriers to adolescent girls receiving prescriptions for the birth control pill.[67] For many, including members of the Medical Defense Union, this decision was long overdue. Caroline Woodruff of the Brook Advisory Centres—which until the implementation of the 1967 Family Planning Act were the only family planning clinics that made the birth control pill available to unmarried women—described the move as an appropriate response to young people's changing sexual habits. Even though the birth control pill had been introduced in 1961, it was still only being prescribed to a minority of British women, most of whom were married.

Not only was the sexual behavior of teenage girls acknowledged as a problem by the Department of Health in 1974, but the same issue re-emerged later that year in discussions of Britain's ongoing economic decline. In a highly publicized speech by Sir Keith Joseph, the Conservative former secretary of state for social services, at Birmingham's

Grand Hotel on October 19, 1974, the poor sexual choices of teenage girls were identified as the underlying reason for Britain's economic crisis.[68] Joseph stressed the need for more state-funded birth control services directed at poor teenage girls, emphasizing that teenage pregnancy was a "tragedy for the mother, the child and for us":

> a high and rising proportion of children are being born to mothers least fitted to bring children into the world and bring them up. They are born to mothers who were first pregnant in adolescence in social classes 4 and 5. Many of these girls are unmarried, many are deserted or divorced or soon will be ... They are unlikely to be able to give children the stable emotional background, the consistent combination of love and firmness which are more important than riches. They are producing problem children, the future unmarried mothers, delinquents, denizens of our borstals, sub-normal educational establishments, prisons, hostels for drifters. Yet these mothers ... are now producing a third of all births.[69]

Although Joseph conceded that he may be "condon[ing] immorality," he urged that it was the "lesser evil, until we are able to remoralise whole groups and classes of people."[70]

The issue of whether teenagers should be encouraged to use birth control became front-page news in the days after Joseph's address. Several prominent members of the Conservative Party openly supported his position.[71] However, not only did many parents express concern for Joseph's "encouragement of immorality," but anti-poverty activists joined in the conversation, criticizing the former secretary of state for social services for promoting behavioral reasons for poverty and for scapegoating the poor as the primary cause of economic problems that were structural in nature. Sexual law reformers also made their criticisms known, taking issue not with Joseph's call for a national re-moralization (which queer rights activist Antony Grey welcomed as "brave") but with his declaration of war on Britain's "permissive society."[72] Joseph placed not only teenage pregnancy, drug and alcohol abuse, and "vandalism" under the capacious umbrella of "permissiveness" but also state intervention in the economy as well as political commitments that did not prioritize "private enterprise."[73] As Antony Grey pointed out, Joseph's promotion of birth control services for teenage girls was rooted in the false assumption that Britain's economic problems were rooted in young women's emotional immaturity and corresponding inability to fully love their children.

Several participants in the debate argued that teenage sex was inevitable and that family planning services therefore needed to expand their reach to include teenage girls. Most, however, continued to present any encouragement of sexual activity among adolescents as a threat not only to Britain's future but to sexually active teenagers themselves. Sex education literature aimed at adolescents and their parents embedded information about sexual reproduction within a larger message about young people's emotional unpreparedness for sexual relationships.[74] The participants in the sex that was described were often identified as a "man and a wife in the privacy of their own house," and sex education manuals warned young people of the many risks associated with sexual activity. Contraceptives were described as unreliable in protecting against both unwanted pregnancy and venereal disease. And medical treatment for the latter was described as uncertain, especially if an infection was diagnosed too late. Furthermore, an overriding focus on reproductive sex often meant that little space was devoted to homosexuality. It was typically given only a brief explanation and a trivializing nod to its preponderance during the "immature phase" of adolescent sexual development.[75]

That teenage sexuality held such a complicated place in public opinion helps explain the Ministry of Education's ongoing reluctance to establish a comprehensive nationwide sex education program for British schools.[76] Moreover, that attempts to expand the reach of British birth control services sparked so much opposition had much to do with their targeting of teenagers by the early 1970s. Public opinion polls showed that the majority of Britons supported providing free birth control to any adult who sought it out. Ecological arguments concerning the catastrophic dangers of overpopulation were generally accepted even if the connection between poverty and family size—and population density more broadly—was most often linked to "third world" nations. However when connections were drawn between population size and teenage motherhood in Britain, defenders of "family values" were adamant that adolescents were still children and therefore emotionally unprepared for sex.[77] They argued that teen pregnancies resulted from too much information rather than a lack of information: the media's oversaturation with sex was infecting the suggestible minds of the young and emotionally immature who, they maintained, felt social pressure to experiment with sex.

This was a moment of intense polarization in British responses to adolescent sexuality. On the one hand, Whitehouse's Clean Up TV Campaign called on the BBC to stop media "filth" from infecting the minds of good Christian girls and the Responsible Society vowed to protect children from Britain's increasingly sex-obsessed culture.[78] At the same time, activists connected to the Birth Control Campaign and Zero Population Growth and medical staff at the Brook Advisory Centres saw adolescent sexual desire as a major threat to the future of humanity (particularly Western middle-class humanity). The search for answers as to why young people were more likely to engage in sexual exploration in 1974 than they had been fifteen years earlier led politicians, physicians, and activists to scrutinize both the nation's moral climate as well as changes in adolescents' lifestyles. For many, the flourishing of "permissive" values and the expansion of sexual freedom meant that the law more than ever played a critical role in protecting children's right to a healthy childhood.

The Controversy over the Age of Sexual Consent and the Politics of Emotional Maturity

In the summer of 1974, during the same moment that volunteers for the Birth Control Campaign were visiting cafes and night clubs in London's trendy Camden area to educate young people about the use of contraceptives, public debate was exploding over whether the age of sexual consent should be lowered. The Young Liberals had recently launched a campaign to persuade the Liberal Party to make homosexual inequality an electoral issue. The age of consent provided a foothold into the fight against homosexual discrimination in Britain since the age for homosexual consent was twenty-one while the age of consent for heterosexual intercourse was sixteen for girls and eighteen for boys. Jeremy Thorpe, leader of the Liberal Party—whose rumored homosexuality would become a public conversation in 1976—refused to take a stance on the issue.[79] Following Thorpe's lead, most Liberal candidates were reluctant to make homosexual equality an electoral issue for fear of alienating voters. The Young Liberals responded by openly criticizing the Liberals, describing the party's leadership as out of touch with rising popular support for protecting civil liberties.[80]

Although the Young Liberals were not the first to demand a change to the age of consent, their campaign was especially timely. The British Medical Association had recently published a report identifying the legal age of consent as contributing to rising rates of teen pregnancy and venereal disease. The report suggested that young people's fear of punishment for engaging in unlawful sexual acts made them afraid to seek medical help.[81] The Young Liberals' campaign also coincided with the publication of the SLRS report proposing comprehensive reforms to the laws surrounding sexual offences. An appeal that the legal age of sexual consent be lowered to fourteen for both heterosexual intercourse and homosexual relations appeared alongside proposals that brothels be legalized and rape treated as a form of physical assault rather than as its own special category of offense.[82] The report's authors argued that lawmakers and the public alike treated "sexual cases" more emotionally than "nonsexual cases," and punished these offenses with unreasonable severity.

More than simply an issue of providing a fair basis for punishing criminal acts, members of the SLRS saw the intrusion of the law into private sexual life as morally problematic. According to their chairman, Bishop John Robinson, it interfered with individuals developing their own autonomous moral compass. As he put it, the laws seeking to protect "public morality" prevented Britain from becoming a "more mature society":

> I don't think it is the function of the law to legislate on moral issues in the sense that it is there as a sort of moral policeman ... What I think the law is there to do is to protect people's liberties against exploitation ... so that people are free to be mature human beings as much as possible.[83]

According to Robinson, the state should not interfere with citizens'—even young citizens'—sexual lives as it prevented them from becoming fully mature adults.[84]

The Responsible Society promptly attacked the SLRS report, describing it as "totally evil."[85] Whitehouse also immediately criticized the report's "total unconcern for the pressures under which the young grow to maturity":

If the age of consent were to be lowered there is no doubt that the contraceptive merchants and the so-called "liberal thinkers" would put enormous pressure on the 14-year-olds, and it would inevitably appear that society had given promiscuity its blessing.[86]

Whitehouse argued that the law needed to be used to dissuade adolescents from engaging in sexual relations because they were "*not* prepared for sexual experience."[87] This was a developmental reality that, she argued, the law needed to protect.

There was nothing new about placing adolescents' development at the forefront of discussion, as Robinson and Whitehouse had. Both proponents and opponents of changes to the legal age of sexual consent had mobilized competing claims about adolescents' degree of maturity for several years. According to Marjorie Jones, a supporter of reform, the minimum age for sex should coincide with puberty which, physicians confirmed, began on average at age thirteen.[88] On the other hand, Ambrose King of The Responsible Society described the campaign to lower the age of consent as a "direct psychological assault on children."[89] It was in response to confusion surrounding the law's relationship to young people's developmental needs that Home Secretary Roy Jenkins set up the PAC, in December 1975, to investigate whether any legal change was necessary. Specifically, the PAC was charged with sifting through all relevant medical and sociological findings and with collecting data on public opinion.[90]

In 1976, when it became clear that the PAC was not only considering the matter but had accepted evidence from the NCCL in favor of lowering the age of consent to fourteen, many expressed serious concern. Political commentator Ronald Butt published a provocative piece in *The Times* on January 22, 1976, arguing that British people did not truly desire a change in the legal age of consent but had been "hypnotized into silence ... by any self-appointed 'expert' who stands up to testify as though to a revealed and absolute truth, that even the most unspeakable beastliness is therapeutically 'good' for somebody."[91] Butt criticized Jenkins for yielding to pressure groups like the SLRS and the NCCL at the expense of citizens' wellbeing. In contrast, those in favor of lowering the age of consent focused on adolescents' maturity (physical *and* emotional) as the basis for their right to sexual privacy. SLRS member Tim Beaumont responded to Butt by stressing that the adolescent was "as, if not more, capable of making [decisions] as adults are."[92] Beaumont, a former Anglican priest who had found church values to be at odds with his liberal commitments, focused on the ethics of the state's involvement in private life:

> The main objective of the report of the working party of the Sexual Law Reform Society, of which I was an enthusiastic signatory, was not to encourage various sexual practices of which Mr. Butt does not approve but to limit the power of the State to interfere in people's private lives ... For instance, the proposals on lowering the age of consent are less to do with moving an absurd and arbitrary age limit to an equally arbitrary but slightly less absurd [age limit] than in restoring the

power to make decisions to the adolescent (who is often as, if not more, capable of making them as adults are).[93]

Not only did Beaumont view adolescents as mature enough to make sexual decisions, he also encouraged adolescent sexual experimentation as both normal and healthy:

> The sexual side of life (if there is any side that is not sexual) is an important part and ... we must wish everyone a happy and fulfilled sex life. To achieve this their sexuality must be allowed to develop naturally, and knowledge and advice should be readily available as they grow up."[94]

The SLRS membership more broadly argued that the only laws children required for their healthy development were those that ensured they would be reared in a loving family. Their 1974 report thus suggested that care and protection orders be extended to age eighteen so that young people from "bad or broken homes" were guaranteed stable adult guidance as they themselves grew to mature adulthood.[95]

Butt and Beaumont presented two very different approaches to youth protection. While Butt believed that adolescents needed protection against their developing sexual desires, Beaumont maintained that the criminalization of adolescent sexuality interfered with important opportunities for sexual, as well as emotional and social, development. The SLRS, in common with the NCCL and the CHE, was emphatic that sexual exploration was a necessary part of healthy adolescent development. The problem of fixing an appropriate minimum age of sexual consent had been a recurring issue in Britain for almost a century, however in the mid-1970s the protection of children's emotional development had become a priority. In the late nineteenth century, when prostitution involving girls as young as thirteen had come to public attention, controversy over consent had centered on child prostitution and the need to protect prepubescent working-class girls from predatory middle-aged men. According to the narrative popularized by Josephine Butler, Lord Shaftesbury, and W.T. Stead, pre-pubescent girls had high sexual value for men but were themselves entirely asexual.[96] Increasing the legal age of consent from thirteen to sixteen had been intended to accurately reflect the fact that girls under sixteen were still physically non-sexual. The law was meant to protect them from the unwanted advances and exploitation of older men.

Despite Freud's "discovery" of children's sexuality and widespread dissemination of his theories of sexual development over the course of the twentieth century, young adolescents continued to be viewed by many as asexual and requiring protection from adult male sexual urges. Between the end of WWI and the mid-1950s, there were several attempts to further raise the age of female sexual consent to seventeen (and even eighteen), however none were nearly as well-organized as Butler's efforts in the late nineteenth century.[97] In the years following WWII, British newspapers were filled with alarming reports that sexual crimes against young girls were "increasing every day."[98] In response, a group of physicians and judges headed by

Doris Odlum campaigned to introduce harsher legal penalties for sex with underage girls. They argued that the psychological damage resulting from sexual assault was so life-altering that convicted offenders needed to undergo psychiatric treatment while in prison to prevent them from reoffending.[99] None of the proposed changes to the sexual offences law were introduced until 1956, and the press continued to fixate on the ongoing rise in sexual assaults committed against underage girls alongside panicked discussion of the growing visibility of prostitution and homosexuality. In winter 1953, the *Daily Herald* declared Britain had entered an "age of indecency" with sexual crimes "seeping into" daily life "like filth from a broken sewer."[100]

The middle-aged male sexual predator was not only an important feature of discussions of the age of consent for girls, it also dominated considerations of legal reform surrounding underage homosexual activity. The Wolfenden Committee's 1957 recommendations in favor of decriminalizing homosexuality included that it remain a criminal offense for young men under twenty-one to engage in homosexual acts and further, that the penalties for sex with underage men be increased from two years imprisonment to five. The reason given was that young men were extraordinarily suggestible—especially in their relationships with older male authority figures, in particular teachers and university professors—and their sexual orientation was still unstable. The concern was that their sexual preferences would be shifted off their "natural" heterosexual course. Committee members argued that it was highly likely that sexual experimentation with an older man rendered a young man incapable of ever sustaining a monogamous heterosexual relationship.

When the Sexual Offenses Act was passed in 1967, its inclusion of the Wolfenden Committee's suggested age of sexual consent for homosexual relations was immediately controversial. As indicated in the Wolfenden Committee's report, it signaled that men under twenty-one were not "sufficiently adult to take decisions about [their] private conduct and to carry the responsibility for their consequences."[101] It thus effectively extended the sexual and emotional boundaries of childhood for homosexual men to twenty-one. The Sexual Offenses Act did not present an uncontroversial view of adulthood; later that same year, the Latey Committee on the Age of Majority recommended that the age of majority, which was then twenty-one, be lowered to eighteen.[102] While the Latey Committee granted that eighteen-year-olds were more mature than they had been in previous generations, it was decided that the age of consent for homosexual intercourse should be twenty-one, with some in the House of Lords arguing that it should actually be as high as thirty. The reasons given consistently revealed anxiety surrounding Britain's many intimate homosocial communities made up of young men and their vulnerability to the influence of respected middle-aged men. Despite medical consensus that sexual orientation was fixed by early adolescence—sixteen at the latest—the public continued to hold that youthful male sexuality was in flux and easily "corrupted."[103] The danger here was not rape or prostitution—as it had been in discussions of young girls' consent—but the spread of homosexuality. In continuing to criminalize homosexual sex that involved men under twenty-one, the Sexual Offences Act 1967 effectively sought to prevent homosexuality from continuing to take root in the male psyche.

While fears surrounding the threat of middle-aged male sexual predators remained an important feature of discussions of adolescent sexual consent in the 1970s, much more pressing were concerns about emotional harm and disrupted psychological development resulting from underage sexual activity. In a letter to *The Guardian*, religion lecturer Reverend John Meeres described sex between underage teenagers as "mutual exploitation for immediate satisfaction" that inevitably resulted in "a lower level of self esteem."[104] National newspapers were not the only venue for opinions on the harm caused by teenage sex. In a letter to her local newspaper in Welwyn Garden City, an anonymous mother stressed that underage girls who behaved as though "ready for sexual intercourse" were especially in need of being "saved from their own sexuality."[105] She warned that, "Just because they like doing it is not to say that responsible adults should stand by and watch them go headlong into danger."[106] In decriminalizing homosexual sex only for consenting adults over twenty-one, the Wolfenden Report similarly affirmed the need to protect young people from the harmful effects of sex. To this end, the report invoked two different sets of legal rights: one for adults and one for children. While adult citizens had a right to privacy, children had a right to state protection. Although homosexual acts were no longer necessarily deemed "perversion" in the case of adults, they remained in all cases "perverse" acts for children (which, here, meant any man or boy under twenty-one).

For sexual law reformers, scientific evidence showing that adolescents routinely experienced sexual desire presented an important rebuttal to arguments that sex was emotionally harmful to young people, particularly young girls. Medical evidence demonstrating that girls and boys matured earlier than they had in the previous century was at the heart of the defense of adolescent sexual activity.[107] Whereas young girls in the early twentieth century were not beginning to menstruate until age seventeen, by 1971 girls were beginning to menstruate at thirteen on average, with some reaching maturity by age ten. The argument thus followed that a legal age of sexual consent set at sixteen no longer reflected the biological reality of teenage girls who now had better access to nutrition and hygiene.

In addition to physicians noting the earlier onset of puberty, the frequent lack of enforcement of the law prohibiting Under Sixteen Intercourse (USI) reflected British police officers' growing perception of adolescent female sexual agency. Criminologist Robert Mawby's examination of Sheffield police records from 1971 to 1972 showed that in practice not every girl under sixteen was treated as a victim of unwanted sexual attention. In several cases, Sheffield police officers saw the real victim as the man entrapped by a knowing younger woman:

> The police frequently adopted a position whereby they directly assessed the extent to which the girl had lost the right to victim status. In seven cases, for example, it was asserted that the girl had enticed or encouraged the man to have intercourse, i.e. he was more of a victim than she was. Two quotes from the files illustrate this

point neatly: "... a morally loose person, and in view of her age, a danger to men." [and in another file] "she frequents low class Arab cafes where girls of low morals and persons with criminal records congregate. She would appear to be of low morals herself and is undoubtedly the instigator in those offences committed against her. This is not a case where an innocent young girl has been seduced by older, more experienced men."[108]

Police saw the real perpetrators in such cases as the morally suspect girls who seduced older men into sexual encounters. These perceived "Lolitas"—who were embedded within a fantasy of sexual danger surrounding the precocious maturity of young working-class girls—had Sheffield police treating the sexual consent laws with profound skepticism.[109]

Just as some police questioned the sexual innocence of underage (especially working-class) girls, some physicians noted that "emotionally deprived" girls developed an abnormal predilection for seducing older men. One physician from a family planning clinic who submitted evidence to the PAC noted that, "The individual case histories of these younger girls show a high incidence of broken homes, parental neglect or rejection ... I find that the majority of the under-16s who attend are using their sexual relationship to gain 'love' or attention or for revenge on their parents."[110] Some physicians also openly questioned the view that adolescents—and even children—experienced psychological harm from sex with considerably older adults. In a letter to *The Times*, Professor Ivor H. Mills of Cambridge University's Department of Investigative Medicine argued that children who have had sexual contact with an adult still tend to "develop normally."[111] Mills noted that the worst case he had seen—a twelve-year-old girl who had attempted suicide following the persistent sexual advances of a lodger who was then living in her house—had soon resolved itself. He noted that, "a few years later" the girl in question was "happily married" and had a family.[112]

Although some physicians and psychologists linked the earlier age of menstruation to an earlier desire for sexual activity, such views were not uncontroversial. In their evidence to the PAC, the British Medical Association focused on adolescents' emotional unreadiness for sex, maintaining that "Emotional maturity does not accompany the physical process and adolescence is frequently a time of great emotional instability."[113] The Royal College of Psychiatrists echoed this view, stating in their evidence that adolescents were not sufficiently emotionally mature to assume the responsibilities of parenthood. They lamented the difficulty of measuring emotional development, emphasizing that "intellectual understanding, or even the actual experience of sexual intercourse are not good indicators of maturity."[114]

The argument of emotional immaturity was equally mobilized by those opposed to lowering the age of consent for homosexual relations in the late 1970s. During discussion in the House of Lords in 1977, Lord Baden-Powell was adamantly against any change to the age of homosexual consent, maintaining that lowering the legal age would only make boys between the ages of fifteen and twenty more vulnerable to emotional trauma resulting from homosexual advances:

> the effect on these young people when an approach has been made to them by an older person—a not uncommon experience—is traumatic. They are not mature enough to know how to cope with and rebuff the advance ... These young people, after such an encounter, affect much bravado in front of their peers but it does have a deep and lasting impression on them beyond reasonable bounds, as they are haunted by the fear of further approaches which they will not be able to contain.[115]

Mental and emotional health were central to Baden-Powell's understanding of what the consent laws were instituted to protect. He speculated that if a boy were to "succumb" to an advance, "the awful effects on that young person's mind [would be] beyond comprehension."[116]

Young people were also key participants in the campaign to lower the age of consent. Since there was enormous uncertainty surrounding adolescents' desires—the genuine existence of homosexual adolescents was even frequently brought into question—gay and bisexual teens were motivated to participate in the sexual consent debate so that the law might be changed to reflect their actual needs. In 1978, the Joint Council for Gay Teenagers (JCGT) was formed with the help of the CHE to create public awareness of queer teens and their social isolation. The JCGT consisted of representatives from gay youth groups and support services, all of which had only recently been established. Their first initiative—a survey of gay support services—was inspired by the "firm impression among gay help services that the number of telephone calls from teenagers has risen markedly over the last two years or so."[117] The group found that more than 6,500 young people between fifteen and twenty-one had contacted gay support services in 1977.[118] The sizeable number of young queer people in need gave the JCGT's political cause the quantifiable urgency that it needed, prompting members to follow up with an in-depth report arguing that the legal age of consent needed to be abolished. They presented their findings and recommendations for change to the PAC in July 1979.

Entitled *I Know What I Am*, the JCGT's report drew upon excerpts from ninety-eight intimate personal accounts by young queer men and women aged between fifteen and twenty-one.[119] This collection of firsthand perspectives offered the public a new view into the everyday experiences of gay, lesbian, and bisexual teenagers, providing information that "originate[d] not from the traditional clinical or penal setting, but from ordinary life."[120] The report emphasized that homosexual teens were aware of their homosexuality at a young age, often long before becoming sexually active. Zoe, a nineteen-year-old from Islington, stated that she had experienced "gay feelings all my life," and eighteen-year-old Alan, from Lewisham, wrote that while he knew he was gay when he was thirteen, he thought that he "was the only gay in the world."[121] Several contributors recounted confessing homosexual feelings to friends and family members and being told that they were "going through a phase."[122] The report also stressed that gay, lesbian, and bisexual youth experienced social alienation and a shameful sense that they were abnormal and revealed that this often led to violent confrontations and suicide attempts. Contributors shared these private details to convey the disastrous consequences of feeling sexually abnormal. Paul, a nineteen-year-old from Birmingham, confessed that he often "became so depressed" that he "felt like killing" himself.[123] Another boy, eighteen-year-old Derek from Streatham, a largely working-class neighborhood in South London, described forcing a younger boy into a sexual encounter because he felt angry all the time.[124] All of the contributors commented on the importance of gay support networks—primarily the phone-in centers Lesbian Line and Gay Switchboard—in ending their isolation.

I Know What I Am concluded with an appeal to abolish the legal age of sexual consent, pleading that:

> Until this happens, young gay people will continue to suffer, partly because anyone who wants to offer them constructive advice will be constantly at risk of the law. But even if a minimum age of 16 for homosexual men were adopted (the same as the present age for lesbians), there would still be a growing number of requests for help from gay people below that age, while agencies offering help remain at risk.[125]

Contributors described the hopeless feeling that came with being turned away by gay help services because they were too young. James from Northampton swore that, if he did not "meet someone soon," he was certain to "do something" he would "regret."[126] Others described the stress and humiliation of a lengthy trial following police discovery of a homosexual relationship with a partner over twenty-one. Nineteen-year-old Glyn described how his "life was wrecked" by the experience: "I didn't go to school for three months. I was recovering from a nervous breakdown."[127] The case had spanned nearly a year, and his twenty-two-year-old partner was ultimately sentenced to eighteen months in prison.

The key misperceptions that JCGT members felt they needed to overturn were first, that middle-aged homosexual men sought to "convert" young men and boys to homosexuality, and second, that sexual orientation remained unfixed throughout adolescence. They argued that the age of sexual consent served less to protect adolescent boys from emotional injury than to protect "the boy from his own actual or potential homosexuality."[128] This was a law that was meant, above all, to preserve heterosexuality as the socio-sexual norm. Linking the JCGT's mission to the gay rights movement more broadly, members argued that they wanted to help create a world where young homosexuals could experience their sexual development as a process that moved them toward greater emotional and sexual connection:

> A vital part of helping gay people to lead happy and fulfilling lives (just as it is for heterosexual people) is to provide them from an early age with positive advice, with others whose lives can act as models for their own, and the opportunity to

experience relationships and emotions ... At present it is only that fortunate minority of gay teenagers aged under 18 who have contacted gay help services who are able to grow up without first going through a long period of isolation, private torture and rejection.[129]

Gay men and women, they argued, not only had a right to sexual freedom as adults, they also had a right to a normal adolescence. The denial of this through measures like the age of sexual consent was pointed to as harmfully "prevent[ing] teenage homosexuals from legitimately exploring personal relationships and thus from coming to terms with their true identity."[130] Moreover, noting the psychological importance of monogamous love relationships, JCGT members maintained that the age of consent law could "make it difficult for them to eventually find a close personal relationship which can be sustaining and healing, and which can provide the possibility of individual growth and development."[131]

Many supporters of sexual law reform saw these teens' proposal to abolish the age of consent as too extreme. The only other group to make a similar appeal was the Working Party on Pregnant Schoolgirls and Schoolgirl Mothers who had published a study of teenage mothers' experiences earlier that year (entitled *Pregnant at School*). Like *I Know What I Am*, *Pregnant at School* offered insight into the social rejection and shame that adolescent mothers commonly experienced and laws surrounding the age of consent intensified. The study's subjects described how it felt to be labeled "promiscuous" when they refused to name their child's father (out of genuine fear that he might be prosecuted).[132] Equally troubling was the reported frequency of guilty feelings that young mothers experienced in response to having participated in a criminal act. Arriving at conclusions that paralleled those in *I Know What I Am*, *Pregnant at School* argued that the legal age of sexual consent should be abolished so that young girls could, without shame, seek out the medical and social services they desperately needed when they became pregnant:

> In order to reduce pregnancies amongst schoolgirls we argue ... for legal changes and ... for improvement in sex education within schools. These recommendations, if adopted, would also go some way to helping a girl who becomes pregnant by encouraging her to come forward for advice and care at an early stage in her pregnancy.[133]

Both *Pregnant at School* and *I Know What I Am* demonstrated through firsthand accounts that the criminalization of adolescent sexual activity placed great emotional strain on young people. Sociologist Ken Plummer echoed this in evidence submitted to the PAC, emphasizing that the young homosexual "neophyte comes to perceive his initial experience with increasing anxiety and possible guilt."[134] Basing this observation on his research conducted on homosexual communities in London, Plummer emphasized that having one's sexual desires stigmatized often hardened into psychological pathology over time.

Although advocates of sexual law reform were sympathetic to the experiences conveyed in *I Know What I Am* and *Pregnant at School*—and drew extensively on these reports to formulate their own arguments for change—appeals to abolish the age of consent were consistently sidestepped. After receiving evidence from dozens of medical, educational, and political organizations, in 1981 the PAC settled on keeping the age of consent for heterosexual intercourse at sixteen for girls and eighteen for boys and proposed lowering the age of consent for homosexual relations to eighteen. The PAC's recommendations to the Criminal Law Revision Committee agreed with evidence provided by the Royal College of Psychiatrists, the British Medical Association, the Medical Women's Federation, as well as six teaching organizations. All of these groups agreed that adolescent emotional instability was "best counteracted by a legal framework that makes all relationships more secure rather than more vulnerable to disruption."[135] Appealing to adolescents' healthy emotional development as a primary consideration in their decision, the PAC report stated that when young people engaged in sexual experimentation, their "gradual development to sexual maturity can be affected."[136] They concluded that because "immature choice[s]" were not "free," the law needed to protect young people from endangering their fragile emotional development.[137]

Despite the PAC's recommendation in 1981 to lower the homosexual age of consent to eighteen, the Criminal Law Revision Committee decided that, in the interest of public opinion, the legal ages of consent for both heterosexual intercourse and homosexual relations would be kept as they were.[138] Whereas change may have seemed promising to many sexual law reformers in the early 1970s—in the wake of late-1960s legal reforms surrounding homosexuality, divorce, and access to birth control—by 1981 it had become clear that any alteration in the sexual laws affecting young people was not possible. After seven years of intense effort, the campaign to lower the legal age of sexual consent had largely come to an end.

Teenage Sex in the Age of "Family Values"

Whether or not a "sexual revolution" took place in Britain after 1963 has been the subject of lively debate. Proponents of this view have argued that a "revolution" in sexual mores did in fact occur and was propelled by the public provision of contraceptives to women and accompanying emphasis on sex as primarily for pleasure rather than reproduction.[139] Opponents, in large measure influenced by Michel Foucault, have argued that the "incitement to discourse" surrounding sex was actually an indication that sexuality was becoming more heavily policed.[140] What is certain—and argued even by the fiercest supporters of the sexual revolution thesis—is that adolescents under the age of consent were not fully included in this transformative shift in sexual mores. In 1981, just as in 1963, adolescent sexuality was seen as a danger from which young people needed protection. Ultimately considered much closer emotionally to children than adults, adolescents were denied the right to a private sexual life that had recently been afforded adults with the passage of the Sexual Offences Act in 1967. Reactions against the dangers of Britain's "sexual revolution" were made on behalf of children for whom sex was seen as a damaging threat to healthy emotional development.

The 1981 decision against lowering the legal age of sexual consent did not, however, dissuade teenagers from engaging in premarital sex. In March 1982, the teen magazine *19* published the results of a survey showing that more than a quarter of girls under sixteen had had sex: "27% of the 6000 women who answered an intimate questionnaire had lost their virginity before reaching the age of consent. One in 10 of these were 13 years old when they first made love, three in 10 were 14, and six in 10 were over 14."[141] The article pointed out that "the sexual consent laws are being widely flouted," but offered "a crumb of comfort" in the fact that "87% of women found sex without affection unsatisfactory."[142] By the end of the 1980s, there were clear signs that a greater proportion of British teens were having sex. Although the numbers of babies born to teenage mothers had decreased over the previous two decades—after rising in the late 1960s and peaking at just over 82,000 in 1971—young girls were having far more abortions and were more commonly being prescribed birth control; more teens were also being treated for sexually transmitted infections.[143] Teenage girls' interest in sex and love relationships fueled the market for teenage magazines. Hundreds of young girls wrote to advice columnists seeking guidance on how to approach their first sexual encounter and on choosing the best forms of birth control; many also asked about abortion versus adoption as the best solution to an unwanted pregnancy.[144]

Homosexual teenagers also became increasingly open and unashamed about their interest in sex and relationships as the 1980s progressed. This could be seen in the growing numbers of gay youth venues, gay social groups at universities, and gay festivals and summer camps that became central to the gay youth movement after 1981. In the wake of political defeat, gay youth groups shifted their attention onto queer teenagers' social alienation and directed energy toward creating opportunities for young people to develop friendships and networks of community support. Toward this end, Gay Youth Movement (GYM), founded in 1981, organized a yearly festival called Gayfest, where gay teens could come together and enjoy a wide selection of films, theater, cabaret, and discos. Their 1982 flier boasted "everything from religious celebrations to S&M workshops!"[145] GYM also began holding yearly summer camps for queer men and women under twenty-six in 1981. The summer camps provided young people—although it was mostly young men who attended—with the opportunity to come together for a week and enjoy swimming, sports, and campfires as well as relaxation sessions, gay self-defense classes, workshops on a variety of subjects ranging from drama and dance to intimacy sessions, and groups discussions on the experience of coming out.[146] GYM also produced a regular magazine, *Gay Youth*, in which they publicized social events for queer youth taking place across the country. All of GYM's many activities were directed toward normalizing gay teens' intimate relationship experiences.

While the early 1980s saw the development of a more cohesive and publicly visible gay youth movement, young people were also increasingly marginalized from the gay rights movement. This could be seen as early as 1982, when, during the annual Gay Pride parade, GYM were forcefully prevented from setting up an information stall and not permitted to sell issues of their magazine or march together as a group.[147] The unwillingness of Gay Pride organizers to support a movement celebrating the sexuality of gay men under twenty-one only intensified over the course of the 1980s, particularly as the AIDS crisis provoked additional discrimination against homosexuals. The plight of the under-twenty-ones was left to queer youth to manage on their own, contributing to a widening generation gap within the queer community.

In the early 1980s the growing visibility of adolescent sexuality coincided with the development of a cohesive movement opposing the distribution of birth control to underage teenagers. While the Department of Health's 1974 circular supporting the prescription of birth control pills to underage girls without parental consent had been controversial at the time, a re-issuing of a slightly amended version in 1980 prompted a 1984 court decision to make parental consent a legal requirement for girls under sixteen. The campaign's organizer, Victoria Gillick, a Catholic mother of ten (including five daughters), argued that birth control prescriptions given without parental consent "aided and abetted" illicit sexual intercourse. "Everyone," she urged, "must surely know that all under-age girls are 'vulnerable.'"[148]

The early success of Gillick's campaign was helped enormously when it attracted the support of the Conservative government. Prime Minister Thatcher was an enthusiastic advocate and named Gillick an important figure in promoting the Conservative "family values" agenda. Although the 1984 decision in favor of Gillick was overturned in 1985, following an appeal by the Department of Health and Social Services, in 1987 the "Gillick competence" ruling offered a compromise.[149] It was decided that girls under sixteen would only be prescribed birth control without parental consent if they showed that they understood the consequences of sex. Gillick thus had a lasting impact by casting doubt on whether adolescents could be seen as capable of fully comprehending what sex was and what it entailed. Surveys conducted in the 1990s of teachers, doctors, and young people showed that enormous uncertainty remained concerning what was legal when it came to adolescent sex. Historian Jane Pilcher notes there remained tremendous ambiguity "in current perceptions of the proper scope of children's autonomy interests ... especially evident around the issue of children and sex."[150]

This chapter brings the stakes of private life in the post-1960s era into perspective. As privacy came be widely articulated as a fundamental right of adult citizens by the end of the 1960s, it became necessary for the precise limits and meaning of adulthood to be established. If it could be argued that adolescents were adults in many important respects—as the Latey Committee successfully argued in their 1967 proposal to lower the age of majority to eighteen—then it became especially important to clarify how teenagers remained closer to childhood than adulthood in assessments of their emotional and sexual development. In 1979, gay rights activist Micky Burbidge observed that, "The ability to give mature consent is not merely a function of individual 'emotional maturity,' as the PAC implies. It is, on the contrary, a socially determined feature of a particular relationship."[151] The Royal College of Psychiatrists had also been clear about this in their evidence to the PAC in 1976 when they had sought to clarify the full meaning of sex:

> Sex is of course not just a matter of sexual potency and fertility, but a complex commitment of two partners who are together capable of preparing for, and building, a family, so that "going steady," mutual respect and helpfulness, maintaining work, finding lodgings, buying a cot and a pram, handling the two sets of grandparents amicably, may be better criteria of maturity than physical or intellectual attainment.[152]

Over the course of the five years that the PAC collected evidence, it became clear that however much young people's actual desires and experiences might differ from an ideal of adolescent asexuality, their political demands would not be taken seriously because adolescents were considered incapable of creating stable middle-class families.

In the decision against lowering the age of consent, political and economic concerns were elided with claims about adolescents' emotional immaturity. Although it may have been clear that most young people could not hope to economically sustain a male-breadwinning, female-homemaking nuclear family, the explanation for their unreadiness to become parents was always focused on their emotional capacities. As Keith Joseph argued in 1974, the poor—or the socio-economic classes 4 and 5 whom he associated with "unmarried or single-parent teenage households"—should not be denied children because they lacked money, but because they were incapable of giving their children enough love.[153]

Middle-class assumptions about what adolescence should look like were crucial to teenagers' exclusion from sex life. Marion Hilliard described this time of life as one ideally devoted to education and learning more broadly. Sex and relationships should come after this. However, the reality for many thousands of working-class teens was a life of work and financial responsibility from as early as age sixteen (and even younger for some). Lorna Sage remembers envying those middle-class young people who could relate to the experiences described in songs by Elvis Presley as having "a second chance at childhood" that she and her fifteen-year-old peers in the working-class Welsh village of Hanmer were denied. Instead, they were expected to leave school, earn a living, and get on with the responsibilities of adulthood: "In Hanmer ... you couldn't afford to be a teenager, you were supposed to go out to work at fifteen, or if you were still at school you had your sights fixed on the future."[154]

That teenagers were considered incapable of creating stable, middle-class families was one crucial hurdle that they faced in making a successful case for sharing in the right to privacy. Compounded with this was the danger that sex posed to their emotional development. The Criminal Law Revision Committee's decision against lowering the legal age of sexual consent marked out adolescents as children. Similarly, when Lord Brandon ruled in favor of Victoria Gillick in 1984, he claimed to do so on the grounds that girls under sixteen did not yet entirely qualify as "persons."[155] Because they were still in the process of becoming adults—and still sexually undeveloped—Lord Brandon decided that it should be illegal to provide underage girls with birth control without parental consent.

Much as the controversy over sexual consent was underwritten by a need to codify the relationship of citizenship to sexual freedom, equally at the heart of the debate was the concern that sex was itself developmentally harmful to children. The focus on sexual predators and child prostitution at the heart of the late-nineteenth-century campaigns of W.T. Stead and Josephine Butler animated this set of late twentieth-century discussions and debates far less than the perceived prospect of the lifelong emotional damage that may ensue from children acting on their sexual desires. In the controversy over the age of consent, there was not only a reaction against teenage parenthood but also a rejection of teenage sexuality. In concluding that teenagers were still emotionally children, by the early 1980s their sexuality had become so controversial that it seemed safest to keep discussion of it out of Parliament.[156]

The 1970s were a crucial moment of possibility in the development of sexual rights. The equation of sexual freedom with stable monogamous love excluded young people—who were seen as inherently emotionally unstable—from making supportable claims to sharing equally in this new area of human rights. Those opposed to young people's share in late-1960s sexual "liberation" appealed to the requirements of healthy development. They did not view young people's *expressed* needs as having an authentic relationship to their *real* needs. While sexual reform advocates argued that the criminalization of adolescent sexuality interfered with much-needed access to sex education and family planning services, arguments in favor of protecting children from the pathological consequences of their emotional immaturity won the day. This chapter has shown that the closing down of the age of consent debate by 1981—due in part to the Conservative government's support for "family values"—was underwritten by an infantilization of adolescents that had been ongoing for decades. British teenagers in the 1960s were the first generation to grow up in a welfare state; every political initiative that they attached themselves to and every consumer fad that they experimented with were viewed as pathologically connected to having been set adrift from traditional family networks of dependence and obligation. By 1981, support for adolescents' right to a private life had largely dissipated because they were widely believed incapable of creating stable relationships. Adulthood came to be understood in opposition to the emotional instability of adolescence as a developmental category that pertained primarily to emotional life. Emotional maturity guaranteed that one could choose freely and responsibly. It thus came to mark the natural limits of the state's power to intervene in private life.

7
"Home Is for Many a Very Violent Place"
Healing from Family Violence in 1970s Britain

> Because we, as a society, have buried our heads in the sand, we do not wish to recognize that the injuries sustained behind the front door, at the hands of a partner who is supposed to love and cherish you, can be so much worse. The bruises and bones can heal, but the internal personal damage will take years to mend. A woman or man who has been mentally tortured by his partner will show far worse damage than that of the occasional furious fistfight. The slow corroding of a personality that occurs with unkind treatment takes a lot of healing.
> —Erin Pizzey, *Infernal Child*, 1978

> Home is for many a very violent place.
> —House of Commons Select Committee on Violence in Marriage, 1975

On June 12, 1974, Keith Parkin, co-founder with child psychiatrist Alick Elithorn, of the emerging fathers' rights organization Families Need Fathers (FNF), passionately defended divorced men in *The Guardian*. He wanted to see an end to women receiving preferential treatment in custody decisions, and a change in court and social service partiality toward mothers as the parent optimally suited to childcare. He called attention to the crucial role that fathers played in child rearing, gesturing beyond the financial contributions that men were expected to make to children's upbringing. Fathers, he argued, were as important as mothers in nurturing their children's healthy emotional development. He was adamant that "the ability to give love, warmth, and stimulation is not the prerogative of females alone."[1]

To bring social recognition to fathers' emotional value, FNF set out to expose the "myth of a mothering instinct" and challenge the pervasive assumption that "real love and empathy for the child comes [only] from its mother."[2] Unlike most contemporary movements concerned about children's emotional wellbeing, FNF was critical of the state's involvement in family life. Noting that presumptions about mothers' emotional value had become enshrined in Britain's legal, health, and social services, FNF argued that the government promoted a vision of the family that excluded men from activities relating to childcare. In their view, the state dangerously romanticized the mother-child bond, and, because of this, failed to protect the true psychological interests of the child.

FNF immediately met with criticism from across the political spectrum. Jill Tweedie—whose former husband had abducted their two children following the breakup of their marriage—was the first of several feminists to challenge the group's agenda in the wake of Parkin's impassioned plea. She argued that FNF was acting in bad faith when members claimed that men could equally perform the emotional work that women had labored for centuries to develop: "on the whole fathers are, at best, absentmindedly fond of their children and, at worst, extremely irritated by them."[3] In Tweedie's view, men could not have it both ways. They could not expect their wives to spend every waking hour caring for their children when married and claim the right to a central place in their children's upbringing when divorced. If they were sincere, they would support revisions to expectations surrounding married men's childcare responsibilities. She insisted that their demands were nothing more than a vengeful assertion of child ownership:

> when it comes to custody, the ugly side of paternity too often emerges. The man, furious with a wife whose one sin may have been her cessation of love for him, threatens a fearful battle for the children he has until now virtually ignored ... Punishment, vengeance, possessiveness—these are, sad to say, the main motivations behind too many men's wish for custody of their children today.[4]

Tweedie—along with many FNF critics—argued that women had for centuries developed an emotional competency for childcare. Their greater aptitude for childrearing might not be rooted in biology, she noted, but it had been cultivated for too long to suddenly be dismissed as fiction. Judges in family law courts were equally unsympathetic to fathers' petitions for custody. Men's stories about their failed efforts to obtain custody often included judges' proclamations that "a man's brain ... should be used for working and not for turning himself into a mother."[5] Courts and feminists alike were skeptical about men being given responsibility for their children's upbringing, especially their emotional care.

FNF's challenge to the British idealization of the mother-child relationship was far from exceptional in the mid-1970s. For example, Lee Comer wrote in her 1972 Marxist feminist manifesto "The Motherhood Myth" that it was chiefly mothers who propped up the post-WWII Bowlbian myth of maternal deprivation as truth. She argued that it allowed them to rationalize "gross possessiveness" toward their children, but that it was "destroying" mothers and children alike:

> When we have learnt to disengage ourselves from the children we care for, liberating them from the pressure to conform to our image of them, we will be loving them without violence. In the process we will be going some way toward liberating ourselves.[6]

And, for very different reasons than Comer, Erin Pizzey, the founder of the first organization to provide refuge to women fleeing violent marriages—Chiswick Women's Aid (CWA)—also publicly questioned presumptions of women's inherent capacity to provide stable non-violent love. By the end of the 1970s, Pizzey insisted upon women's complicity in family violence. She maintained that many abused women were not passive victims. Rather she argued that "violence-prone" women were drawn to such relationships because of their childhood experiences, and many also "beat their own children."[7] Following the publication of Pizzey's psychological assessment—most fully laid out in her 1982 book *Prone to Violence*—Women's Aid organizations cut off all association with her, seeing her as "victim blaming." In a 1983 piece in *Spare Rib*, "Who Needs Enemies with Friends Like Erin Pizzey?," feminist Liz Kelly described Pizzey's book as poorly researched and "voyeuristic" and its overall message "dangerous."[8]

The spotlighting of less-than-ideal, even "bad," mothers who had failed their children was nothing new. But what was striking about the range of criticisms that were levelled in this transformative post-1960s moment was the persistent unwillingness—even on behalf of ardent critics of the maternalist emotional ideal—to abandon the view that children's early relationships were crucial for their healthy development. Priority was consistently placed on children's emotional life. As one *Guardian* reader, John Hills, put it in 1978: "Sadly, you see, women have not done an especially good job of mothering, in providing the kind of 'maternalism' children are believed to require at the outset of their lives."[9] Something needed to be done. Whether the solution lay with fathers assuming a more central role in childcare or with "violence-prone" women and their children being housed in peaceful community-run refuges, the assumption was that all children *needed* to experience unselfish nurturing care to grow up to become emotionally healthy adults. Mothers might have failed in many cases, but the priority given to emotional intimacy in childhood did not waver. If anything, as this chapter will show, its perceived value only deepened.

In the 1960s and 1970s, the white middle-class nuclear family was implicated in maintaining a range of oppressive social forms, including late-industrial capitalism, patriarchy, and societies with high rates of violent crime, by antipsychiatrists, feminists, and advocates of battered women's refuges. However, solutions to these complex social problems were not seen as requiring an abandonment of the emotional values linked to the nuclear family in the post-WWII decades. Instead, critics continued to emphasize the importance of stable interpersonal intimacy in righting the violence, power imbalances, and hypocrisies that plagued post-WWII British society. Proposals for family reform focused on emotional life as central to solving the serious social problems that they illuminated. Few wanted to jettison the belief that children's relationships with their caregivers played a pivotal role in producing future inclinations and behaviors, including the capacity for authentic agency, the ability to experience empathy, and the propensity for violence.

Despite their apparent failures, women continued to occupy a central place in British commitments to children's access to emotional intimacy in the 1970s. The belief that women were especially well suited to making intimacy possible in their families was, if anything, reinforced following exposés spotlighting violence perpetrated within middle-class families. Critics highlighted the emotional effects of family violence as particularly damaging because psyches, they noted, healed far more slowly and unevenly than bodies. Antipsychiatrists, feminists, and defenders of abused women argued that violence produced more of itself, leading to a never-ending cycle of violence if no intervention was introduced. The outcome was a range of damaged individuals, including abusive husbands, depressed housewives, and schizophrenic teenagers. The worst forms of violence were presented as *emotional* in nature, and women featured prominently in both their enactment and resolution.

In many ways 1970s repudiations of the white middle-class male-breadwinning, female-homemaking nuclear family were new. However, the psychologically informed interventions leveled by feminists, antipsychiatrists, and advocates for abused women were grounded in ongoing concerns about children's healthy emotional development that had been pervasive in Britain since WWII. Although British second-wave feminists developed Marxist critiques of the patriarchal nuclear family, as Sheila Rowbotham points out, many were reluctant to reject the experience of motherhood and the idea that it was socially important: "Instead we wanted new relationships and conditions in which we could have children and lead fuller lives."[10] For some feminists, Rowbotham noted, the mother-child relationship was upheld as politically important, since the emotional skills involved in childcare helped maintain women's propensity toward peaceful non-aggression.[11] Antipsychiatrists declared the family to be psychiatry's co-conspirator in labeling inconvenient people "mad." At the same time, however, they positioned themselves in "anti-hospital" therapy as caring surrogate mothers to help heal their clients' emotional injuries.[12] In the many different, intersecting debates surrounding British families' contributions to social oppression and psychological harm, mothers maintained a central, yet deeply fraught, place in therapeutic discourse and the popular imagination. Although some Britons may have challenged presumptions of women's *natural* suitability to childcare, the 1970s backlash against the nuclear family held fast to the possibilities that women's capacity for intimacy had promised, despite its demonstrated failures, to fulfil.

This chapter examines several intersecting areas of psychologically informed political action that sought to expose the white middle-class family as perpetrating forms of violence that resulted in severe psychological damage. Critics of the family presented emotional violence as interfering with healthy psychological development and, in turn, full personal liberation. Unlike the post-WWII priority placed on preventing political violence (such as international warfare and authoritarian governance) through the protection of children's emotions, here we see a targeting of emotional violence as itself the violation that was the most urgent problem. It was this less visible yet insidious mode of violence, they argued, that produced gender-based oppression, schizophrenia, and abuse within families. This chapter reveals the enduring preoccupation with the lasting impact of early emotional life in this era of privacy and permissiveness, spotlighting the intensified importance of mothers' emotional labor even though family intimacy was increasingly shown to have a violent dark side.

Emotional Violence and Schizophrenia

In 1971, South African psychiatrist and Marxist David Cooper pronounced the "death of the family" a needed solution to widespread social oppression and mental distress. He declared a two-fronted war on mainstream psychiatry and the white middle-class nuclear family, arguing that the two colluded in undermining authentic agency and upholding an oppressive status quo. He maintained that psychiatrists extended family repression when they took charge of difficult family members and labeled them "schizophrenic." Their interventions rendered their patients even more impotent.

Cooper indicted the white middle-class nuclear family for producing the symptoms associated with schizophrenia, which caused an immediate sensation: the timing was right for his message to be widely received. It was written soon after Edmund Leach had decried the family as "the source of all of our discontents" in his highly publicized Reith Lecture.[13] And it was published less than a year before Philip Larkin's attack on the family as a major perpetrator of psychological damage, warning readers to "Get out as early as you can, and don't have any kids yourself."[14] Cooper's psychopolitical critique found a responsive audience and he quickly became a major voice in Britain's rising backlash against the family.

Anthropologist Gregory Bateson had presented a similar hypothesis for the family's causal role in producing schizophrenia in 1956, which he termed the "double bind." Radical psychiatrists like Cooper, however, propelled this idea further into public consciousness by framing it as an exaggerated version of the typical experience growing up in a Western middle-class family. As Cooper's colleague and friend Ronald D. Laing had explained it in his bestselling 1960 study *The Divided Self: A Study of Sanity and Madness*, schizophrenics were the grown-up children of exacting parents who had fed them conflicting messages their entire lives. These were the children of parents who promised love but consistently withheld it. The experience felt familiar to many young "baby boomers" who had grown up in 1950s Britain.

Cooper presented mental illness as resulting from dysfunctions in the "microsocial" world of personal relationships. He coined the term "antipsychiatry" in 1967 to not only denounce psychiatry's harmful impact on patients but also to describe his anti-institutional approach to healing traumas rooted in interpersonal emotional life. Antipsychiatric therapy was grounded in community-based practices that Cooper and Laing had experimented with at various "anti-hospitals" across London. Cooper's anti-hospital Villa 21 was launched in January 1962 in a former insulin coma ward at Shenley Hospital, a sprawling psychiatric hospital located on a rural estate north of London. Villa 21 adhered to therapeutic community conventions, and staff did not reject the notion that patients suffered from a mental affliction. Cooper was adamant, however, that the idea of the expert—and the power abuses that had long marked institutional psychiatry—had no place in therapy. Healing was instead supported by the collective involvement of men and women who had themselves previously experienced emotional breakdown and "sufficiently explored their own interiority and their own despair."[15] Therapy mainly consisted of patients' engaged participation in community life and regular group discussions that allowed patients to explore their family experiences. One patient, "Mr. G.," related that, "often, as we discovered in our discussions, the cause of someone's breakdown could be traced to his relationship with his family, particularly his parents."[16]

Not only did residents receive an education in the emotional dangers of family life, but the many visitors that passed through the ward were familiarized with Cooper's understanding of mental affliction. Playwright David Mercer—who made several visits to Villa 21 while collecting material for his controversial play *In Two Minds*—presented Cooper's critical perspective on the family to a wider national audience when his play was shown on BBC television on March 1, 1967. The play's inspiration was born out of Mercer's own hospitalization for nervous breakdown in 1957. However, his focus on the development of schizophrenic symptoms in an adolescent girl who had been emotionally abused by her mother and sister more closely resembled Laing's best-selling case studies. Kate, the play's protagonist, suffered repeated verbal attacks from the women in her family, while her father failed to intervene. Over time, Kate's self-esteem was so severely eroded that she became incapable of living independently. She was taken to a psychiatrist who diagnosed her as schizophrenic and advised that she be placed under constant medical care.

Mercer's play was later remade by British social realist filmmaker Ken Loach into the critically acclaimed film *Family Life*.[17] Both the play and film versions were produced in a documentary style, giving viewers the unsettling feeling that they were observing real events. Villa 21's "Mr. G." later described Mercer's play as a perfect rendering:

> accurately reflect[ing] the story of more than a few of my fellow patients while I was there but with the difference that, after the usual treatment, they found their way to a place where more understanding of their situation was available.[18]

Despite this creative revision, "Mr. G." expressed "hope that it is possible to show this film in mental hospitals throughout the country" as he believed that many were trapped in similarly destructive family relationships.[19]

Psychiatrists' response to *In Two Minds* was—unsurprisingly—overwhelmingly critical. Some were primarily troubled by Mercer's misrepresentation of Kate as schizophrenic, when they believed that she was depressed.[20] However, most were disturbed at the close similarities between Kate's family experiences and Laing's case studies detailed in *The Divided Self* and his follow-up 1964 study of eleven schizophrenic young women, *Sanity, Madness and the Family*. Mercer had drawn on Laing's work in his research, and Laing had been a consultant for the play. Psychiatrist William Sargant, who championed physical treatments like electro-shock therapy and psychosurgery for schizophrenia, accused Mercer of creating propaganda. The two faced off on the BBC television program *Late Night Line Up* soon after *In Two Minds* was televised. Mercer denied Sargant's accusations that the play functioned solely to promote antipsychiatry, arguing that his aim had been to reveal the true relationship between mental illness and the family through an artistic medium.

Although Mercer shared the antipsychiatric view of the nuclear family as oppressive, radical psychiatrists and those sympathetic to their criticisms were deeply ambivalent about the mother-child relationship. Like US psychiatric descriptions of the cold and controlling "schizophrenogenic mother," Mercer depicted Kate's mother as an uncaring woman and her father as weak-willed.[21] Kate's story, like all of Laing's case studies, revolved around a troubled relationship between an apparently schizophrenic young woman and her mother. Her father's contribution to her condition lay mainly in his refusal to protect Kate from her cruel mother. In Laing's case studies, mothers similarly sought to control their daughters' lives. In every case, mother and daughter butted heads because of stark generational differences in their ideas about a woman's destiny. Julia, described in *The Divided Self*, "had a great deal to say about her mother. She was smothering her, she would not let her live."[22] In *Sanity, Madness and the Family*, Laing described eighteen-year-old Maya Abbott as showing the normal signs of growing up, but her parents (especially her mother) refused to accept that she was no longer an obedient little girl. Claire Church complained that "mother never wanted me to grow up" and that "she didn't like me to have my own ideas about things."[23] Lucie Blair similarly struggled to be her own person, and always relied on her mother for advice. Laing pointed out the obvious problems with this:

> her mother could only give her advice based on what she herself knew. Her daughter was struggling for autonomy, self-confidence, trying to be a person, but Mrs. Blair, if she had ever glimpsed what this meant, had given up years ago.[24]

In every case that Laing documented, it was clear that the patients' mothers lacked the maturity and absence of possessiveness that were the hallmarks of truly loving parents.

Laing especially emphasized patients' mothers' misunderstanding of normal adolescent development: they reacted to appropriate assertions of independence as symptoms of mental illness. In the encounter between Maya Abbott and her mother that led to Maya's psychiatric hospitalization, Laing noted that in her mother's recollection, "Maya attacked her for no reason. It was the result of her illness coming on again."[25] Maya's memory of the event, however, differed remarkably:

> She was dicing some meat. Her mother was standing behind her, telling her how to do things right, and that she was doing things wrong as usual. She felt she was going to snap inside unless she acted. She turned round and brandished the knife at her mother, and then threw it on the floor. She did not know why she felt like

that. She was not sorry for what had happened, but she wanted to understand it. She said she had felt quite well at the time: she did not feel that it had to do with her "illness." She was responsible for it.[26]

Laing summed up Maya's behavior as not particularly noteworthy—it "might have passed unnoticed in many households as an expression of ordinary exasperation between daughter and mother."[27] He consistently pointed to examples of youthful rebellion that he believed were entirely normal signs of maturity progressing, but that the patient's mother had misinterpreted as signs of pathology.

The focus of Laing's research showed his prevailing interest in the mother-child relationship. Of the twenty-four hours of interviews conducted with Claire Church and her various family members, fifteen were with mother and daughter together, whereas three hours were spent with Claire alone, and only one hour involved both mother and father present.[28] Of the nineteen hour-long interviews investigating Lucie Blair's condition, thirteen were with mother and daughter, five with Lucie alone, and only one with mother, father, and daughter present together.[29] Of the forty-five hours of interviews with the Abbotts, twenty-nine were with mother and daughter, and only eight with mother, daughter, and father.[30] In each case, the focus of the investigation into the afflicted individual's family relationships was on their relationship with their mother.

Laing's preoccupation with mothers' special role in producing schizophrenic symptoms was also evident in the "anti-hospital" therapy that he helped develop. Between 1965 and 1970, at Kingsley Hall in East London, where Laing launched his most famous "anti-hospital" initiative, dozens of diagnosed schizophrenics embarked on unmedicated healing "journeys." Residents were encouraged to regress to early infancy and return in time to a renewed, and more authentic, state of adulthood. The therapists at Kingsley Hall were distinguished as such not because they possessed special insight into schizophrenia, but because they were compassionately curious about difficult emotional experiences. They nursed, supported, and communicated their love for residents as they regressed. They held, bottle-fed, and even silently took abuse from them in the process. In short, they acted like the loving, unconditionally supportive, and self-sacrificing mothers that residents had lacked as children.

The "journey" of one resident, nurse and budding artist Mary Barnes, was described in detail by Barnes and her primary caregiver, American psychiatrist Joseph Berke, in a 1971 book that the two co-authored, *Two Accounts of a Journey through Madness*. Much of Barnes's retelling of the affliction that brought her to Kingsley Hall centered on her relationship with her mother, whom she described as unsupportive and dominating: "Mother always said she liked us best as little babies. It seemed we were then as dolls more easily to her."[31] At Kingsley Hall, Barnes allowed herself to fully regress to a state of infantile nakedness and incontinence. This period of her stay was narrated in childlike monosyllables, and the therapy that she described receiving showed close similarities to the maternal care an infant might receive:

Suck, suck … Suck the bottle. Not long to wait. Get me a car. Home. Naked. Bed … The car comes, Wait, Suck, Play ball. Lay with my Teddy. Therapy. The car. Home. Clothes off. Wet the bed. Cuddle Teddy … I told Ronnie [Laing], "I could put my shit all over you, you would still love me."[32]

Barnes repeatedly tested her therapists' unconditional acceptance. Berke's unwavering devotion was especially significant in this regard. Even when covered in her own feces, it was important to Barnes that "Joe was not afraid. He bathed me."[33] When she refused to eat solid food, he fed her from a bottle. And, when she bit, punched, or kicked him during an angry tantrum, he allowed her to exhaust her anger and always immediately forgave her: "Bite, punch, punch, in the end, when I was exhausted with screaming and growling and hitting, Joe took me into the kitchen. He gave me a drink of milk, then put me to bed."[34] When Berke's friends visited Kingsley Hall with their baby, Barnes became jealous: "I was Joe's baby still wanting to be held. Too much, the idea of seeing Joe with another baby."[35]

Berke referred to Barnes during this phase of her recovery as "Baby Mary." Like the good Bowlbyan mother, he offered her his full devoted attention as her therapist:

> During the early stages of our relationship I was tempted to exclaim, "Mary, you want the breast, you want my breast, you want me to take care of you just like a baby at the breast, you want me to love you, let me take care of you, let me feed you, let me give you nice warm loving milk." But it became obvious that it wasn't words that mattered so much as deeds, and even when deeds and words coincided and were seemingly accepted by her, the ensuing state of relaxation could revert to one of agony for the barest of reasons. All I had to do was turn my head, or look inattentive, or blink an eye while feeding her, and Mary began to pinch her skin, twist her hair, contort her face, and moan and groan. Worse shrieks following if I had to leave the room and get involved in another matter at about the time she was due for a feed.[36]

He explained his participation in Barnes' healing process as enabling her to replace " a 'bad' internalized relationship (her identification with her original mother), with a 'good' one (her identification with 'Joe') … it laid the basis for her uncovering her 'real self' … the ultimate lesson was that the source of herself is herself, not 'Joe' or anyone else."[37]

It was through her relationship with "Joe," her surrogate mother, that Barnes ultimately arrived at what she believed was a truer and more complete version of herself. Honest expression of authentic selfhood was the foundation for Laing and Cooper's existential solution to the psychopolitical ills of the postwar age. Full engagement in community life was not prioritized as it was at the Cassel Hospital in the 1950s and 1960s; instead, the way toward true healing lay with the afflicted individual's retreat into mother-child oneness with their therapist.

Despite their psychopolitical critique of the family for its involvement in creating both symptoms of mental illness as well as pervasive exploitation under capitalism, radical psychiatrists were deeply ambivalent about the mother-child bond. As much as Barnes needed to liberate herself from her internalized childhood relationship with her controlling mother, her recovery centered on Berke dutifully mothering her—feeding her, bathing her, and loving her during her temporary return to infancy.[38] The loving mother figure was embraced in therapy for its emotional benefits. Although Laing and Cooper challenged the prevailing biological view of mental illness, they did not cease to offer treatment to those saddled with psychiatric diagnostic labels. As a complicated figure in the schizophrenic's "journey" toward wholeness, mothers took on a pathogenic as well as a liberatory role. Although the nuclear family had taken on a host of negative associations, mother love continued to hold a transcendent emancipatory place. In its highest form, it offered redemption for the emotionally violent and love-destroying late-capitalist Western world.

The Political Is Also Personal: Emotional Violence and Women's Oppression

Radical psychiatrists' revised schizophrenia diagnosis and their experiments with "antihospitals" generated significant public sympathy, particularly among the educated middle-classes. *The Divided Self*, for example, was discussed far more frequently in popular publications like *The Guardian* and *New Statesman* than in medical journals.[39] Feminist activist Sheila Rowbotham emphasized the life-changing impact of Laing's work in shaping her radical consciousness in the 1960s: "When I read the anti-psychiatrist R.D. Laing's *The Divided Self* I, along with many others, decided that here was a metaphor for my discontent. Split in two, it was as if one part of me had begun to observe the other."[40] Through Laing's work, Rowbotham was provided with new meaningful concepts for understanding her "inward rustlings of resistance."[41] By the early 1970s, there were hundreds of news pieces and magazine articles describing most forms of mental illness—from mild to severe—as the outcome of damaging middle-class values and expectations.[42] For many, like Rowbotham, personal suffering became a spur to political action.

Antipsychiatrists' psychopolitical analyses were fertile ground for a new generation of feminists eager to untangle the complex relationship between women's social oppression and everyday family experiences.[43] In her landmark 1971 socialist feminist work *Woman's Estate*, Juliet Mitchell, a major voice of British second-wave feminism, ranked antipsychiatry's importance alongside anti-Vietnam war protests and the strike for equal pay at the Ford factory in Dagenham in the emergence of Britain's Women's Liberation Movement. The 1967 Congress of the Dialectics of Liberation and Cooper's Antiuniversity were mentioned as particularly inspiring to the women's liberation agenda in the late 1960s.[44]

Mitchell, who was David Cooper's partner, saw her feminist political understanding as fundamentally indebted to psychoanalysis and radical psychiatry. Here Mitchell departed from the more usual American feminist tendency to dismiss Freud because of his misogyny. In 1974, she explained in an interview in the feminist magazine *Spare Rib* that before turning to psychoanalysis she "just didn't have the concepts, the terminology, to think about women."[45] Psychoanalysis had helped her to grasp the family's role in producing male and female psyches and, ultimately, to understand why women so often enabled their social oppression.

Mitchell was equally inspired by radical psychiatry, despite its lack of attention to gender-based mental oppression. Her widely-read books—*Woman's Estate* (1971) and *Psychoanalysis and Feminism: Freud, Reich, Laing and Women* (1974)—addressed this by pushing antipsychiatry in a feminist direction. While Laing was concerned about the psychological harm produced by seemingly normal families, Mitchell was more specifically interested in how *women* were psychologically damaged in families. She pointed out that Laing's second book, *Sanity, Madness and the Family*, had focused entirely on young female schizophrenics living in East London, yet had failed to consider their experiences as bearing any relationship to their gender. The only thing that he saw them as having in common was their schizophrenia diagnosis.

This absence of attention to women as a special category of the oppressed had also been on display at the 1967 Congress for the Dialectics of Liberation. Not only was the list of speakers overwhelmingly male, but no one addressed women's situation in late-capitalist society. The event's maleness has since been criticized as a blind spot. When six working-class women invaded the stage to denounce the organization of the event near the end of the two-week gathering, they were met with "little audible reaction from a stunned crowd."[46] One of Cooper's patients, David Gale, later reflected that for the women present, "The Dialectics of Liberation Congress was just one more kick in the teeth, delivered by superstars in the blissfully unreflective male firmament of hot new radicalism."[47]

Despite so many antipsychiatrists' insensitivity to gender, Mitchell drew upon Laing's "politics of experience" to understand how the personal and the political were intertwined in women's lives.[48] She went a step further than feminist contemporaries like Hannah Gavron—whose sociological examination had shed light on working-class housewives' "captivity" and social isolation within their families—by stressing the family's psychological production of women. As she explained, "the family does more than occupy the woman: it produces her. It is in the family that the psychology of men and women is founded."[49] Reminiscent of arguments made more than a decade earlier by French existentialist feminist Simone de Beauvoir, Mitchell contended that growing up in male-breadwinning, female-homemaking families (especially white middle-class families) often prematurely halted women's psychological development.

Mitchell's illumination of the psychological effects of family life flew in the face of attachment theorist John Bowlby's presentation. Bowlby had described girls as developing into empathetic, supportive, and socially cooperative women within stable loving families. Mitchell, on the other hand, presented women as often dependent, jealous, conservative, irrational, excessively emotional, and even violent because of their oppressive upbringing. She stressed that no person could "inhabit a small and backward world without it doing something to you."[50] In Mitchell's view, feminist politics needed to move beyond problems like unequal wages, unfair employment hierarchies, and the devaluation of housework, and confront the psychological underpinnings of women's oppression:

> However inegalitarian her situation at work (and it is invariably so) it is within the development of her feminine psyche and her ideological and socio-economic role as mother and housekeeper that woman finds the oppression that is hers alone. As this defines her, so any movement for her liberation must analyse and change this position.[51]

Mitchell would take her commitment to psychoanalysis as a basis for transforming gender oppression a step further in 1975 and undergo training at the British Psychoanalytical Society to become a practicing psychoanalyst. This was one year after the publication of *Psycho-Analysis and Feminism: Freud, Reich, Laing and Women* and her rise to prominence as an intellectual leader of British second-wave feminism.

In merging feminism and psychoanalysis, Mitchell saw herself as instead resuscitating inquiries that had been pursued in progressive psychoanalytic circles in the 1930s. She noted that this promising line of study had been abandoned during the war and further displaced after WWII by Britain's state-sanctioned idealization of the mother-child relationship. Even Laing had not rejected the developmental priority that Bowlby had given to this all-important "primary" human connection. Mitchell, however, was more concerned with mining Laing and Esterson's predominantly female case studies for their uses in better understanding feminine psychology.

Since Laing and Esterson's studies of female psychiatric patients focused on their relationships with their mothers, Mitchell was attentive to what they revealed about the impact of the mother-daughter relationship on the female psyche. Further, Laing's case studies highlighted the emotional turmoil resulting from the ever-widening post-WWII generation gap, which had a greater impact on young women than on their male contemporaries. The world was changing more rapidly for women, and it was becoming increasingly difficult for mothers and daughters to establish common experiences and shared concerns. Escalation of conflict between young women and their parents (especially their mothers) showed the urgent need to better understand the psychological roots of female oppression.

The antipsychiatric inspiration behind Mitchell's feminist critique of the family was neither idiosyncratic nor exceptional. Sheila Rowbotham, for example, reported a similar experience. Rowbotham's reading of *The Divided Self* in 1966 not only caused her to identify herself as "divided"—inwardly uneasy despite giving the appearance of being happy in her self-consciously egalitarian romantic partnership—it also prompted her to examine her relationships with men. Like several of her Marxist feminist contemporaries, Rowbotham had attended the 1967 Congress. On hearing Laing speak on "institutional violence," Rowbotham had concluded that "Social control was ... embedded within the texture of daily life."[52] She noted that this was "an idea which the women's movement," of which she was an early participant, "was later to adapt."[53]

Laing's *The Politics of Experience* also provided feminist activist Lee Comer with the tools for critically unpacking the British idealization of mother love and the Bowlbian theoretical framework that helped support it. In her 1972 manifesto "The Motherhood Myth," Comer condemned women's appeal to "Bowlbyism" as a seemingly laudable rationale for possessive child-rearing. Directly citing Laing, Comer argued that what passed for mother love was in fact "emotional violence" that erased the child's unique individuality:

> Is it loving a child to make yourself the centre of its universe?... Most of what goes under the guise of good parental care is an elaborate rationalization of gross possessiveness... Laing, in his book, *The Politics of Experience*, expressed this point very forcefully: "From the moment of birth... the baby is subjected to these forces of violence, called love, as its mother and father have been and their parents and their parents before them."[54]

Comer targeted women as "constantly reinforc[ing]" Bowlby's "mythology" for their own gain:

> women have embraced the mythology so wholeheartedly that it is they themselves who constantly reinforce it. If really pushed, they would admit that their children could do without their fathers, grandmothers, school, peer group, etc., but, deprived of their mothers, the children would fall apart.[55]

Love, for Comer, meant supporting the child in forming many social relationships.

In Comer's view, the inclusion of more people in the child-rearing process—fathers, grandparents, daycare providers, friends—would not only liberate women from the shackles of motherhood, it would also promote children's emotional well-being. In Comer's feminist work, we see a critique of the family that also re-affirmed child-rearing as crucial in shaping psychological development—in this case, childcare kept not solely in the hands of one person. It was "emotional incestuousness" (as Comer described it), and not the hard work of child-rearing itself, that introduced *both* the death of women's freedom and the emotional problems that so many children and adolescents struggled with.

Since emotional pain was interpreted as demonstrating the need for socio-political change, the feminist practice of consciousness raising—and its creation of a common language for seemingly idiosyncratic private struggles—became key for overturning women's oppression. Many second-wave feminists disagreed with similarities dismissively proposed between consciousness raising and the psychotherapy session, however its agenda of creating change by bringing to light previously unspoken pain was strikingly similar. For Mitchell, it was no wonder that consciousness raising was often compared to psychoanalysis, even if the intent behind such claims was derisive. When psychotherapy was mobilized for political ends, its aims were similar. For example, Karen Horney's interwar feminist psychoanalysis refused to view female clients' psychological troubles solely as outcomes of their unique experiences and family history. She instead explored their connection to a social history that was shared by all women, using therapy to spotlight painful common experiences.[56]

In providing language for women's unspoken common experiences, the most daring thing one could do was to publicize women's honest accounts of motherhood. The feminist magazine *Spare Rib* repeatedly broke new ground by including confessions of maternal dissatisfaction. In the early months of its existence, Michelene Wandor, *Time Out* poetry editor, contributed a scathing condemnation of motherhood as a source of emotional harm that psychiatry could not cure:

> What began as a dream of love and security, a challenge, the building of a home and family, becomes a nightmare. The sounds the children make become torture, you feel guilty because it isn't their fault; housework is meaningless, the day doesn't seem worth getting through. No-one can understand that you've simply been driven mad and that it isn't a condition that pills or therapy can cure (though both may relieve you). I use the term "mad" to describe a state of dislocation in which you don't know where or who you are ... No woman can emerge from it undamaged, and most women are damaged severely. It's just that the signs are dismissed; they're "neurotic," or "hysterical" or "unnatural." On the surface women cope, children are pretty healthy, the family façade is maintained. But the price we pay is too great.[57]

As the mother of two young sons, Wandor spoke from experience. The solution, as she saw it, was the wholesale replacement of the isolated and "emotionally incestuous" family with "more communal forms of living."[58] She found her own family situation so dissatisfying that, after twelve years of marriage, she divorced her husband, literary agent Ed Victor, the year after this article was published.

Interviews with Lee Comer and Ann Oakley published in *Spare Rib* presented similar confessions giving critical insight into the conditions of motherhood. Both drew from their experiences to make broader observations about the dehumanizing impact of women's social roles:

> It was no longer the things I'd done, said or been which identified me to myself and equipped me to confront the world but, instead, my role. I had a womb and since it had been pressed into service, it now marked me out as, occasionally subhuman, but mostly ignorant and inferior.[59]

Spare Rib's inclusion of such criticisms of motherhood did not sit well with many readers. Letters to the editor showed disappointment at the magazine's frequent presentation of motherhood as a mere social role. Many readers reported that the satisfaction they received from their full- or part-time employment—even in fields requiring a university education—was incomparable to the "joy of creating and rearing a child."[60] As Sheila Rowbotham has since pointed out, the "dilemmas of mothering" impacted most British feminists in the 1960s and 1970s, but few pursued childlessness as a desired solution. As many saw it, "To dismiss the delights of mothering denies intense and passionate aspects of women's lives."[61] Although Women's Liberation feminists wanted more freedom for women to choose how to live their lives, many, including Rowbotham, insisted that being a mother was not only deeply personally fulfilling, but also socially important.

Although feminists like Lee Comer and Michelene Wandor were critical of "emotionally incestuous" ideals surrounding responsible childcare, they nevertheless insisted that children's early relationships were developmentally important. This was not meant to put additional pressure upon mothers, but to provide alternative approaches to child-rearing that would produce positive political change. As Lee Comer pointed out, "yes, we are shaped by our families, but families are shaped by the system."[62] Such attention to the impact of family structures and dynamics on the female psyche was similar to Laing's "politics of experience" in its focus on interconnections between the personal and political. It was, however, presented in a far more gender-conscious register.

At a fundamental level, the politics of women's liberation feminists and antipsychiatry both connected private family experiences to inequalities in the public world of work and social power. Antipsychiatrists and British second-wave feminists alike brought attention to the emotional violence that families routinely enacted against their socially vulnerable members. This was a mode of violence that had a lasting psychological impact, producing people who were incapable of assuming positions of power, competing in the public domain of work, and pursuing their own self-directed goals in the world. The victims of such emotional violence were silenced, psychically erased, and rendered unimportant (even inconvenient) as they were shunted off to the psychiatric hospital, the prison, and the seemingly "normal" middle-class family home.

The "Cycle of Violence" and British Efforts to End Domestic Abuse

Emotional violence was not only a major concern of antipsychiatrists and second-wave feminists in the 1970s. An emerging battered women's refuge movement that brought public awareness to the routine physical violence perpetrated in white middle-class families also emphasized the especially damaging impact of emotional violence. Erin Pizzey, who founded CWA in 1971, would consistently point out that while "bruises can fade... Even the most balanced of women needed time to recover from the emotional damage that had been meted out to them by callous and vicious partners."[63]

When the pervasiveness of family violence came to public attention in the 1970s, efforts to end the violence, at both grassroots and governmental levels, focused on its lasting impact through the warping of not only abused women's psyches but also and even more alarmingly their children's. Following many conversations with women housed at CWA and extensive correspondence with abused women across the country, Pizzey concluded that a "cycle of violence" operated in violent families. When giving evidence before the government-appointed Select Committee on Violence in Marriage in February 1975, she was adamant that boys from violent homes grew up to be violent toward their spouses (and, often, their children as well) and girls became the recipients of violence as adults. Like Pizzey, expert investigators appearing before the committee during its five-month-long examination of domestic abuse in 1975 insisted that family violence was not only more widespread than previously believed but that its psychological impact was especially profound.[64] Not only did it beget violence in future generations, it was also the foundation for modern "violent societies," marked by rising rates of violent crime and widespread desensitization to violence in the media.

The identification of men as perpetrators and women as passive victims had, by 1975, become a central feature of most discussions of family violence. It was a view that was largely shared by the experts, activists, and staff at women's refuges who submitted testimony to the Select Committee on Violence in Marriage. It was also prominently featured in the committee's 580-page final report. The report—which included transcripts of interviews with experts as well as individuals affected by family violence—presented family violence as primarily a male problem and most often the outcome of experiencing violence at home as a child.[65] As a solution to the potentially unending "cycle of violence," it recommended ejecting violent men from their families. Rehabilitating children's loving relationship with their mother—once their violent father had been removed—was presented as the key conduit for healing.

The assumption in the mid-1970s that family violence was solely perpetrated by men was new. When "baby battering" was first made visible by medical professionals in the early 1960s, perpetrators initially figured as *both* parents, especially young mothers. In 1962, a decade before the "battered woman" became a feature of public discussion, the "battered child" entered the Anglo-American lexicon when US-based physician C. Henry Kempe first coined the term in a study detailing "the battered child syndrome" in the *Journal of the American Medical Association*.[66] Kempe, a Jewish German-born physician who had migrated to the United States in the 1930s to avoid Nazi persecution, had come into contact with numerous children with apparently inexplicable injuries—including shattered bones, brain damage, and serious burns—in emergency rooms across Denver, Colorado. He concluded that they pointed to a previously unrecognized "syndrome" involving a child's repeated "serious physical abuse by the parent or caretaker" that was far from exclusively confined to the poorest socio-economic classes.[67] While the problem of parent-inflicted child abuse had been mentioned as early as 1888 in the *BMJ*, and tentatively rediscovered by US pediatric radiologist John Caffey in 1946, it was not until more extensive research was published by pediatric radiologists Frederic Silverman in 1953 and P.V. Wooley in 1955 that the reality of children abused at home began to be more unequivocally accepted within the US medical community.[68]

The British medical community was slower to accept that some parents routinely abused their own children. It was not until 1963, when British orthopedic surgeons Lloyd Griffiths and F.J. Moynihan publicized several cases of infants with multiple non-accidental injuries, that "battered baby syndrome" became more widely acknowledged among British physicians.[69] In response, general practitioner Eric Turner wrote that he was "relieved" to see their *BMJ* piece as many general practitioners were aware of the problem, but felt constrained by the questionable ethics of policing patients and violating confidentiality. In the years that followed, physicians' neglect in reporting child abuse was criticized in medical journals. A 1971 *Lancet* editorial reprimanded physicians for under-reporting child abuse. *Lancet* readers were told that, "it should be axiomatic that *any* injury (other than a road traffic accident) to a child of under two *must* be considered to be an instance of the battered-baby syndrome": the "correct diagnosis [was] often missed because medical and paramedical workers still [had] too low an index of suspicion."[70] Over-reporting was argued to be far preferable to under-reporting, despite concerns about infringement on patient privacy.

Throughout the 1960s, when parent-inflicted violence against children surfaced in medical and popular news reports, the abuser was typically identified as both parents—rather than primarily the father, as would become common later—and mothers often held a place of special responsibility. As emphasized in *The Lancet* in 1971, child victims of abuse often had a low weight for their age, which was interpreted as "the result of long separation of mother and child at an early and crucial 'learning' stage."[71] Sociologist Patricia Morgan similarly placed special blame on new mothers, despite her strong refutation of "Bowlbyism," and explained the rising incidence of "battered children" as resulting from new mothers' despair that having a child was not as enjoyable as media representations often portrayed it to be. The taxing work of childcare was out of sync with widely circulating images of effortlessly happy mothers caring for their children published in women's magazine and shown in television advertising.[72]

Morgan argued that the gap between expectation and reality could prove far too onerous for the inexperienced mother to bear. She warned that since "reality is different: harder, dirtier, noisier":

> We need to be a little cooler and more formal, and to emphasise to prospective parents the necessity for a serious commitment to the care and future of a child: obligations that cannot always rely on emotion for their support.[73]

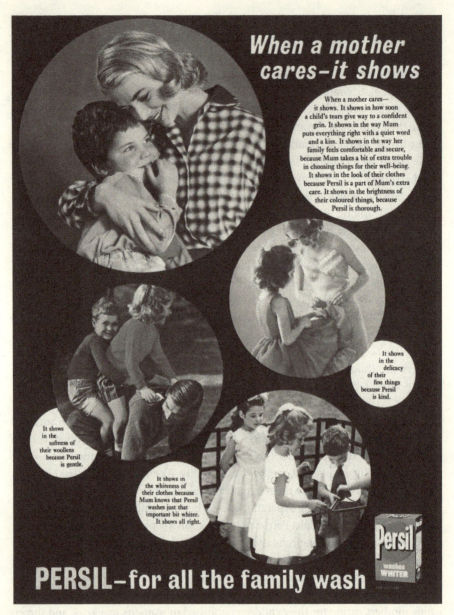

Figure 7.1. 1960 UK advertisement for Persil soap powder.
Source: Neil Baylis/Alamy Stock Photo.

In Morgan's view, any emphasis on pleasurable emotions as the basis for responsible childcare was doomed to fail. For children to be cared for properly—and without enflaming negative emotions like explosive anger—women's rationality rather than their emotions needed to be centrally involved.

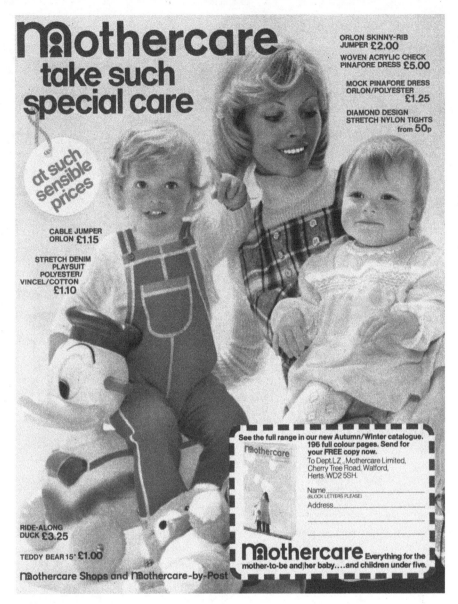

Figure 7.2. 1970s UK Mothercare advertisement.
Source: Retro AdArchives/Alamy Stock Photo.

Like many who would address family violence in the 1960s and first half of the 1970s, Morgan focused on violent mothers, identifying them as typically young and emotionally immature. Similarly, when Bowlby addressed family violence—which was seldom—the perpetrator was female. Discussing the problem late in his career in a 1983 lecture, he described parental violence against children as "maladaptive."[74]

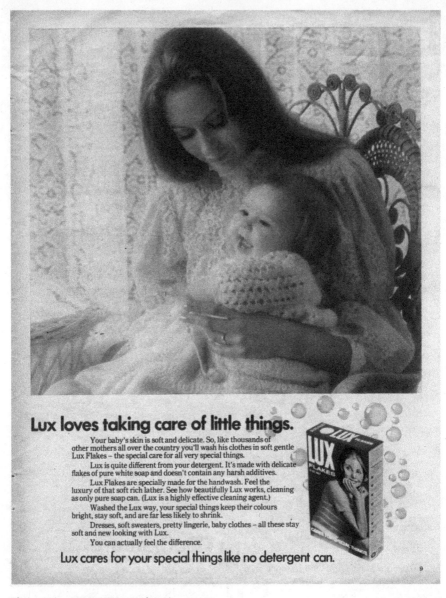

Figure 7.3. 1970s UK Lux advertisement.
Source: Retro AdArchives/Alamy Stock Photo.

He saw violence in families as a "melodramatic" exaggeration of normal familial emotion. In his view, the propensity for violence might implicate anyone—regardless of race or class—since its causes were emotional. Unsurprisingly, he identified it as most commonly the outcome of emotional immaturity, and often implicated individuals who had experienced prolonged disruptions in the maternal care they had received as children.

Consistent with Bowlby's interests, his attention to family violence was largely restricted to mothers whom he saw as having the potential for violence toward their babies. He claimed to have never encountered a violent mother in his career, however he had once treated a woman, identified as "Mrs. Q," who had come very close to intentionally hurting her young son, but had only gotten as far as hitting his crib and toys. The reason for this lay with her own childhood insecurities about her mother:

> The picture she gave me of her childhood... was one I now know to be typical. She recalled bitter quarrels between her parents in which they assaulted one another and threatened murder, and how her mother would repeatedly bring pressure on the family by threatening to desert. On two occasions Mrs. Q had returned from school to find her mother with her head in the gas oven... Mrs. Q grew up terrified that if she did anything wrong her mother would go.[75]

Bowlby focused on prevention rather than treatment, which he doubted was possible once violence had become habitual. In addition to psychotherapy, he advocated voluntary services focused on establishing mentorship connections between experienced mothers and families at risk.[76] His ideal model for prevention was Home-Start, a community project run by married middle-class women that provided "support, friendship and practical assistance"[77] to low-income mothers.[78] The support scheme aligned with Bowlby's sense of how wayward mothers should be rehabilitated—that is, by being themselves "mothered" to maturity. Willem Van der Eyken, who researched Home-Start's work since its founding in 1974, also saw it as primarily a psychotherapeutic enterprise. He described the women who volunteered for Home-Start as "mothers" (in Winnicott's meaning of the word) to the disadvantaged women that they befriended: the "'good mothering" that they practiced had "strong affinities with the functions of psychotherapy."[79]

An exclusive focus, such as Bowlby's, on female perpetrators of family violence had become largely anomalous by the early 1980s. In 1971, Erin Pizzey changed conversations about family violence when she ended the silence that had previously surrounded the "battered woman" and founded CWA. Within months of opening a women's community center in Chiswick, West London, that had been intended to help ease urban social isolation, Pizzey was visited by Kathy, a middle-aged woman who was looking for short-term housing so that she and her children could escape her violent husband. As she and Pizzey talked, Kathy removed the outer layer of her clothing to reveal dark bruises from being beaten with a chair leg:

> I could see livid purple bruises from her neck to her waist. "No one will help me," she said, and I felt such a jolt of rage that it was as though I had been electrocuted.[80]

Pizzey's life would be changed forever from this moment. She discussed her encounter with Kathy with several female acquaintances in the weeks that followed and concluded that domestic violence occurred with far more frequency in non-immigrant middle-class homes than was typically assumed. Many women who experienced spousal violence found it impossible to leave their relationship since they had nowhere to go. The matrimonial home was typically registered under their husband's name, their families were often unwilling to take them in, and state-provided temporary housing was not available for married women since they did not—because they were married—fall under the designation of "homeless." Both police and social services were reluctant to become involved in what they saw as private disputes. They usually responded by advising women to return to their husbands and resolve their disagreement.[81]

Pizzey immediately felt called to help abused women leave their violent relationships. She had witnessed domestic violence first-hand in her own family as a child and was very familiar with the psychological toll that it took on both mother and children. Having grown up in a respectable middle-class family with a father in the diplomatic service, Pizzey's socio-economic background was not the kind usually associated with domestic abuse. She had grown up in many parts of the world—China, Lebanon, Canada, the United States, and England—and her parents were financially well-off and outwardly appeared content in their marriage. Yet, despite the veneer of propriety, she had seen her mother receive regular, sometimes very severe, beatings from her father. On numerous occasions, she had herself received excessive physical punishment from both of her parents.

Pizzey wanted to expose the truth about domestic violence and overturn prevailing assumptions that it occurred most often in patriarchal immigrant (especially South Asian) families and among families struggling with financial hardship and alcohol abuse. Such perceptions were not only inaccurate, she argued, but dangerously concealed the white middle-classness of much domestic violence in Britain. She not only drew upon her own family experiences, but also pointed out that "a high percentage" of the women she helped came from higher income groups.[82] Pizzey deliberately shifted attention away from ethnic and socio-economic explanations for domestic abuse and focused on the underlying psychological causes that cut across race and class lines. She consistently pointed to emotional immaturity as common in both violent husbands *and* those wives who found it difficult to sever ties with them:

> Many of the women who come to us married soon after they left school. Most married before they were twenty-four... Usually the first beating occurs on the honeymoon because the man is still an immature, damaged child who reacts to any stress with total explosion, and what was a temper tantrum at five is a lethal act of aggression at twenty-one.[83]

For spousal relationships that were only occasionally violent, Pizzey recommended seeking out a marriage therapist to help the couple learn to manage their frustration levels. Early in her work sheltering women, she speculated that when violence had always been regularly present in a relationship and had escalated over time to life-threatening abuse, the husband's pathology was most likely beyond hope of cure. The only solution was for him to be removed from his family.

From the beginning of her work with CWA, Pizzey was intent on illuminating the serious, often lasting, emotional impact of family violence. Many of the women who were offered temporary housing in the small dilapidated four-room house at CWA showed signs of severe emotional distress. Some turned to alcohol to cope. Pizzey thus came to view her first task as helping battered women recognize that they had been emotionally damaged so they could begin the recovery process:

> It is one of my principal jobs to teach mothers and children to accept that they have been damaged by their experiences... The bruises and bones can heal, but the internal personal damage will take years to mend... The slow corroding of a personality that occurs with unkind treatment takes a lot of healing.[84]

From an early stage, Pizzey understood refuge work as educating the women who were sheltered at CWA what it meant, from an emotional perspective, to be a victim of family violence.

Pizzey's sensitivity to the emotional and psychological aspects of family violence was extended to violent husbands within a few years of CWA's launching. She reported to the Select Committee on Violence in Marriage in February 1975 that the six thousand case histories that had been gathered at CWA over the course of three years showed that, "almost without exception," battering husbands had been "either victims or witnesses of family violence as children":

> Conditioned to violence, these unfortunate men are really suffering from a personality disorder, which means they can no more control their violent impulses than stop breathing. Prison will not reform them, legal injunctions will not daunt them, and, even if long term psychiatric help might work, it is rarely available.[85]

For Pizzey and the voluntary staff at CWA, violence was treated as primarily a male problem that stemmed from exposure to family violence in childhood:

> You've only to watch the boys in the house to see that they are the next generation's potential batterers. Many of them are extremely violent by the age of three. By eleven they are potential criminals. Where ordinary children would have a tussle or just shout in annoyance, they fight to kill. It's just as the Jesuits said, "Give us a boy until he is seven and we will give you the man." Violence goes on from generation to generation... Violence is part of their normal behaviour.[86]

In her assessment, boys learned violence from their fathers, and passed this behavior on to their sons. She concluded that men who had "been imprinted with violence from childhood, so that violence is part of their normal behaviour" were beyond hope of rehabilitation and "All the legislating and punishment in the world will not change their methods of expressing their frustration."[87]

Although Pizzey's appeal to a psychological view of spousal violence evoked the language and concepts of British marriage therapists, the subject of violence was rarely mentioned in marriage therapy literature in the early 1970s—it was seldom discussed with clients who, in turn, seldom revealed it. It was also not often raised with probation officers as a reason for seeking divorce. Evidence of spousal violence was seen in hospital emergency rooms; however even obvious signs most often went unreported out of respect for patient and family privacy. Even as late as 1982—several years after the passage of legislation making it possible for women to eject their violent husbands from the family home—a Tavistock study found that clients at marriage counseling services focused almost exclusively on threats of divorce, desertion, and adultery as "marriage-threatening events" and rarely mentioned spousal violence.

> It is interesting to note the absence of husbands' violence towards wives as an acknowledged marriage-threatening event. The still equivocal significance of such behaviour in our society is perhaps reflected in the fact that, in our study, husbands' violence was never followed by a direct approach to a marital agency such as Marriage Guidance ... in our study, violence was not seen by respondents as a sufficient and "legitimate" reason for seeking help from marital agencies. Moreover, with the exception of women's refuges, agencies do not appear to encourage women to approach them when their husbands act violently towards them.[88]

The Tavistock study ventured to explain the "equivocal significance" of spousal violence as rooted in physicians' and police officers' inattention to it as an urgent problem. It was common for police to avoid involvement in domestic disputes and instead counsel women to return home to their husbands when called upon to intervene in a violent spousal attack. When women did seek help for their marital problems, it probably did not help that marriage guidance counselors and Tavistock marital therapists never directly asked about violence and focused exclusively on events in their clients' emotional histories stemming back to early childhood.

When marriage therapists addressed the reasons for clients' silence, they assumed that it stemmed from wives' complicity in domestic violence and embarrassment about exposing this. This perspective was consistent with the prominent psychological view insisting that chronically abused women often unconsciously *wanted* to be beaten and provoked violent interactions to satisfy this longing. As evidence for this, therapists pointed out that many women who left abusive marriages either returned to their spouse or entered another violent relationship.

In response to claims of abused women's masochism, US psychologist Lenore Walker introduced the idea of the "battered woman syndrome" to explain repeated victimization. Based on the stories of hundreds of women who identified as "battered" by their spouse, Walker isolated common psychological and sociological underpinnings to get at the root cause. "Battered women," she noted, had typically experienced violence in their families as children and therefore expected this from their adult relationships with men. Observing that abuse was much more common in married than unmarried heterosexual relationships, she noted important sociological causes as well. Describing the marriage license as a "license to violence" in patriarchal societies, Walker argued that women in violent marriages were manifesting an extreme version of a more widely experienced social sickness rooted in male-female inequality.[89] As she saw it:

> I believe that only where there is true equality between males and females can there be a society that is free from violence. Although I believe that aggressiveness is not an innate trait but one which is learned early in life, I do not believe we can eliminate violence from our world without also eliminating discrimination on the basis of sex.[90]

Walker estimated that "as many as 50% of all women" would "be battering victims at some point in their lives."[91]

Walker was not alone in identifying spousal violence as connected to a wider set of social problems. Sociological research in both the United States and Britain presented family violence as symptomatic of societies that were themselves increasingly violent.[92] In the era of the Vietnam war and concern over the impact of violence in the media on children's impressionable minds, domestic violence was embedded in broader concerns about the inherent violence of human nature. Some commentators went so far as to argue that if modern Western families had become violent, it was clear that these cultures needed to be examined and their values scrutinized. Feminists and sociologists of violence alike argued that domestic violence could not be solved on an ad hoc basis—there were clearly important systemic issues at work.

CWA, alongside the feminist refuge association National Women's Aid Federation (later renamed Women's Aid)—which established shelters across the UK beginning in 1974—brought public awareness to the great frequency of domestic violence in Britain. The growing movement to assist "battered women" and ultimately end family violence played a crucial role in influencing the British government to act. In response to repeated demands, in 1974 the House of Commons appointed a Select Committee on Violence in Marriage to investigate solutions. The committee met over five months in 1974–1975 and produced a report in July 1975 that included not only detailed minutes of meetings but all the evidence presented and arguments heard during the final month of the inquiry. Erin Pizzey was the first person interviewed by the committee, followed by psychiatrist John Gayford, who had studied the psychological effects of domestic violence on women at CWA. Interviewed next were staff and several women housed at CWA. Clearly showing the influence that CWA held over public opinion on family violence, it was only after interviews with Pizzey and other CWA affiliates that Jo Sutton, the National Coordinator of National Women's Aid Federation, was interviewed, followed by legal experts, members of the Department of Health and

Social Services, and marriage guidance counselors. Aside from considerations of the problem's scale, discussions focused on illuminating what spousal violence typically involved: how long it went on, how severe the injuries, whether wives participated in violence, and whether children were also abused. The committee wanted to understand the underlying causes of violence in marriage to decide whether its resolution should primarily happen through government channels or through the work of voluntary organizations like Women's Aid.

Based on their research, the committee made three suggestions for government action, all focused on preventing family violence. First, the committee called for young people's compulsory education concerning the emotional realities of marriage and parenthood. They recommended expanding the sex education curriculum at secondary schools to focus more on educating young people about healthy spousal and parent-child relationships. Second, the committee emphasized the need for services aimed at preventing alcohol abuse. Although committee members had debated the recurring preoccupation with alcoholism as an outdated Victorian holdover, it nonetheless made its way into their final recommendations. Third, in keeping with up-to-date research on family violence, the committee stressed the overwhelming importance of a collaborative effort among statutory and voluntary social services to end to the "cycle of violence." Most discussion and evidence presented in the meetings' minutes focused on this last, and most ambitious, recommendation. All committee members agreed with Pizzey and Gayford's recommendation that children be removed from violent homes so that they did not learn, and later repeat, their violent parent's behavior. Although it was acknowledged that there was not yet decisive proof of a "cycle of violence," committee members concluded that existing evidence indicated that it was most likely correct.

The report's focus on violence prevention was certainly influenced by several members' staunch political anti-violence commitment. Most were Labour MPs. Many, including feminists Audrey Wise and Lena Jeger, who wrote for *The Guardian* and adamantly defended retaining an entirely public NHS, had been involved in anti-war activism. The report stated at the outset that all committee members were "disappointed and alarmed by the ignorance and apparent apathy of some Government Departments and individual ministers towards the extent of marital violence."[93] The committee expressed deep concern for the physical injuries—some fatal—inflicted on women in their families, which also extended to pronounced sensitivity to long-term psychological damage. They were especially impressed by John Gayford's study of close to one hundred battered women housed at CWA—described as "particularly moving and persuasive"—which they saw as providing key evidence of the damaging emotional impact of spousal abuse.[94]

Children, however, were the committee's primary concern, even in instances where they had not been subjected to physical attack. Committee members saw children as fundamental to the prevention of future abuse. The report emphasized the future impact of marital violence, which went far beyond "the plight of a particular category of unhappy women" to shape "the future of families, involving men, women and—most important of all—their children."[95] The "cycle of family violence" was described as passed down from fathers to sons, while girls were consistently noted as responding to violence by becoming passive and self-undermining. Recent studies had warned that since boys mimicked their fathers' behavior, they were destined to become violent themselves, whereas girls identified with their mothers' victimhood and were likely to choose violent partners as adults.

The first step toward ending the "cycle of violence" was to enable women to leave the family home with their children. Both CWA and the Committee on Violence in Marriage prioritized alternative housing for abused women and their children. This immediately posed a problem, not only because local housing authorities were reluctant to view "battered women" as "homeless"—and thus qualifying for state-provided temporary housing—but because government services had long focused on keeping married couples together rather than encouraging women to leave their husbands. One of the most prominent points of contention was whether services for battered women should be state run or provided by voluntary organizations like CWA and the National Women's Aid Federation. Although the committee favored state services to guarantee that rising demand was sufficiently met, representatives from both CWA and National Women's Aid were opposed to this. They convinced the committee that the best immediate measure for helping battered women lay in providing regular funding for CWA and Women's Aid to create more refuges. In both organizations' view, the state's explicit support for the two-parent heterosexual nuclear family made it impossible for conflict not to arise were they to assume responsibility for women abused by their husbands. For these women to be protected, the agency offering help needed to be indifferent to the potential dissolution of their marriages, and even, in many cases, actively supportive of this outcome. As one refuge staff member pointed out, social workers experienced conflict between their commitment to keeping families together and their duty to meet the actual needs of abused women and their children. The two positions were inescapably opposed.

Although committee members were overwhelmingly preoccupied with the prevention of future violence, they did not give serious consideration to entrenched sexism in British society. Feminist readings of spousal violence—although a feature of public conversation by 1974—were left out of committee discussions despite the inclusion of Women's Aid. Government participation in creating a less violent society was focused on improving children's surroundings and emotional care.

Pizzey went even further than the committee to disavow feminist analyses of domestic violence. While feminists approached spousal abuse as a window into the truth about *all* intimate heterosexual relationships—with Jill Tweedie declaring that battered women made "the position of all women within marriage and society... crystal clear"—Pizzey was unrelenting in insisting that spousal violence was a psychological aberration.[96] In aiming to end the cycle of violence, she wanted to help the children of the women temporarily housed in refuges grow up to become loving non-violent spouses: "if her son and daughter grow up to make a warm and happy marriage, we will have broken generations of violence."[97] In her view, refuges served an important purpose in removing children from violent environments, not only because their lives might be in danger, but also because children were emotionally at risk of becoming future perpetrators of violence:

> The child that is the most able survivor is the potential batterer in the next generation. This child learns to cut off from both parents and look after himself. He becomes "affectionless." He relates to everyone. He is popular, cheerful, and cheeky while he is young. When he gets older his cheek turns to aggressive rudeness. His gregarious nature irritates because he uses it to manipulate and he usually sides with his father and despises his mother. He begins to treat his mother like his father does.[98]

Drawing upon Bowlby's vision of child development, Pizzey did not call for structural change, but instead treated each violent family as its own individual space for reform. Like Bowlby, she saw the emotional education that children received in their families as the basis for them becoming loving (and non-violent) spouses and nurturing parents.

Influenced by therapeutic community experiments launched since the end of WWII, Pizzey drew upon this social psychiatric model of care as a means for re-socializing women and children, and, by 1976, violent men as well.[99] Although she initially saw violent husbands as intractable to change—as her 1974 international bestselling *Scream Quietly or the Neighbours Will Hear* argued—she always held out hope that the damage that women and children experienced in violent families could be overcome. To this end, she sought to create spaces where women and children could be freed from their habituation to violence. The refuge was meant to function as much more than a common living space. It was meant to be a community where women, "support[ed] each other emotionally, regulat[ed] each other's treatment of the children, rebuil[t] shattered self-confidence, and [took] jobs and mix[ed] with the world outside from a secure base."[100] Residents had much greater value to one another than mental health professionals since they had directly experienced family violence and could fully understand its impact on body and mind.

Pizzey's social therapy approach to battered women's refuges became the model of protection and rehabilitation most studied and most often written about in the media. Even feminist observers reported positively on CWA as a non-violent haven that gave children the opportunity to develop into emotionally secure adults. Jill Tweedie, for example, was emphatic that CWA residents "never hit their own children," and that, although many were "used to a very rough life, all goes smoothly": "They live together, twenty or so women in a house built for a couple and one baby, they clean, they cook, they pool their monies and there are no quarrels, no aggression."[101] Tweedie concluded that, "Violence is a male problem."[102] The overwhelming response to Women's Aid shelters and community homes for women and children was very optimistic. Since family violence was so often presented as a problem created by men, violence in future generations was seen as avoidable only through the ejection of the adult male family member.

The *Report of the Select Committee on Violence in Marriage*—the drafting of which strongly bore the mark of Erin Pizzey, John Gayford, and other witnesses associated with CWA—paved the way for several legislative reforms in favor of helping battered women escape their violent marriages. In 1976, the Domestic Violence and Matrimonial Proceedings Act gave women the right to occupy the matrimonial home regardless of whether it was in their husband's name, and in 1977 the Homeless Person's Act was passed, giving battered wives priority in obtaining social housing.[103] Government research into family violence showed that in 1977, 11,400 women and 20,850 children had been sheltered in temporary refuges.[104] Changes in housing provisions for women in abusive relationships were intended to make the dissolution of violent marriages easier to obtain, while they also endorsed the one-parent family as necessary in extreme cases. Such families—with the help of supplementary benefits from the state—were seen as adequately meeting children's needs. With their material requirements met, children could be fully provided their mother's love.[105] Here was a radical reformulation of the post-WWII ideal of the loving family: it was reduced to its most basic form in the mother-child relationship. However inconclusive studies of the "cycle of violence" were, the widely invoked possibility of emotional harm and mental impressionability rendered the provision of housing and state benefits to one-parent families not only acceptable but, in some cases, the best possible arrangement.

The spotlighting of white middle-class family violence in the 1970s presented a compelling challenge to the notion that the two-parent heterosexual nuclear family could reliably function as a bulwark for emotional health. For some, doubt was assuaged by the assurances of Erin Pizzey and others who passed through the doors of CWA that communities made up of mothers and children could successfully direct female relationality toward preventing future violence. Women's own potential for violence toward family members was little discussed in the early years of the refuge movement, leaving open the possibility that women's and men's psychological natures were different from one another.

Most participants in discussions of family violence in the 1970s focused on children's emotional wellbeing and favored preventing future violence through child rearing in conflict-free environments rather than attempting to keep the family together at all costs. Identifying both husbands and wives in violent relationships as having themselves been "emotionally deprived" as children, much of the evidence presented to the Select Committee on Violence in Marriage emphasized the unstable and immature personalities of *both* spouses and underscored the often premature and sexually unfettered nature of such relationships. Many were noted to have had only very brief courtships that had resulted in pregnancy.[106] Violence was thus treated as yet another outcome of emotional deprivation stemming from children's poor relationships with their mothers. Government response to violent homes was underwritten by a commitment to rehabilitating female relationality—but here extending beyond the mother-child to female relationships formed at refuges across

Violent Women: Unthinkable in 1970s Britain?

Pizzey had started her career as an internationally renowned pioneer of "battered women's" refuges by emphasizing that psychologically immature men were entirely responsible for family violence.[107] However, by 1981, in an article published in *New Society*, Pizzey would dispute the notion that men were the sole instigators of family violence, arguing that many women in abusive relationships were "prone to violence" and unconsciously *chose* violent relationships. As she and her and co-author (and second husband) Jeff Shapiro explained, such women were not purely victims of circumstance, but rather "for deep psychological reasons of [their] own, [they] sought] out a violent relationship or a series of violent relationships, with no intention of leaving."[108] The article was immediately criticized, with letters to the editor at *New Society* arguing that Pizzey had "invented a class of deviants ('violence-prone women'),"[109] an idea that was "*not* shared by the great majority of those who live or work in refuges."[110] Some additionally felt betrayed by Pizzey's disavowal of statements she had made earlier, notably in her 1974 book that had brought the problem of domestic abuse to international attention, *Scream Quietly or the Neighbours Will Hear*.[111]

The *New Society* article would further strain Pizzey's relationship with women's aid organizations across the UK. There had already been tension resulting from the frequent media attention that Pizzey received and tendency for the refuge movement to be associated with her non-feminist view of family violence. There would be a more decisive rupture in 1982 following the publication of *Prone to Violence*, her book-length treatment of the psychology of "battered women" (the title of which summarized the book's argument). Leaders of refuge organizations across the UK condemned Pizzey's book as inaccurate. Sociologist Rebecca Dobash described Pizzey's assessment as "saying that battered wives are basically masochists."[112] Morna Burdon, of Scottish Women's Aid (SWA), was emphatic about SWA's "dissociat[ion] ... from Erin Pizzey," stressing the socio-economic reasons why women were often unable to leave, or returned to, abusive relationships:

> There are many reasons for a woman to return to the home where she has been beaten. Not one of the 10,000 or more women we have dealt with has ever acted in a way that would suggest that they in any way need or are addicted to violence. In our experience, such women simply do not exist.[113]

Women housed at shelters across Britain also publicly denounced Pizzey. Many were adamant that her characterization of the "violence prone" woman could not have been further from their own experiences.

Feminists and others associated with the refuge movement saw Pizzey's ideas as dangerous because they could be used to support the long-standing view that abused women had instigated their violent treatment. Pizzey, however, did not believe that complicity in violence meant that a woman deserved her abuse. If anything, what she interpreted as a gravitational pull toward violent relationships made outside intervention even more necessary. Drawing on her own childhood experiences—described in her 1978 memoir *Infernal Child: World Without Love*—she presented her awareness of violence addiction as beginning with witnessing her mother's inability to leave her violent father, a scenario that she saw repeated when she met Kate in 1971. Kate was the first woman that Pizzey took in, and she returned to her husband only three days after fleeing the relationship, her injuries still visible.

Pizzey's thoughts on the "violence prone" were left out of her early publications. She would later explain that this was strategic since she did not want to divert attention from the immediate need to obtain enough shelter to satisfy demand. Although she publicly presented family violence as caused by severely disturbed men, her early awareness of what she would later call "violence addiction" in certain women—increasingly how she came to view her own mother—fueled her desire to help women in violent relationships un-learn this pattern (which, she argued, would one day preside over their own children's lives if the "cycle" were not interrupted). She saw the difficulty of re-socializing abused women as contributing, above all, to its urgency.

In the decades that followed, Pizzey would repeatedly experience the disavowal of activists in the refuge movement. She, in turn, became less sympathetic to the complexity of female victimhood and more focused on exposing women's equal participation in family violence. She came to argue that "violence prone" women enacted forms of psychological manipulation, or "emotional violence," that gravely injured the psyches of their partners and children. Drawing on her own childhood experiences of maternal abuse, she argued that women in violent relationships were often as brutal as the men they married:

> Indeed, my mother's explosive temper and abusive behaviour shaped the person I later became like no other event in my life. Thirty years later, when feminism exploded onto the scene, I was often mistaken for a supporter of the movement. But I have never been a feminist, because, having experienced my mother's violence, I always knew that women can be as vicious and irresponsible as men.[114]

Although she had played a powerful role in popularizing the idea of the "cycle of violence" in the 1970s, Pizzey ultimately did not, by the end of the decade, view it as a wholly male phenomenon. By 1998, she had come to view "violence prone" women as themselves violent. Describing such women as "emotional terrorists" in their families, Pizzey argued that they perpetuated violence in the home:

> In my work with family violence, I have come to recognize that there are women involved in emotionally and/or physically violent relationships who express and

enact disturbance beyond the expected (and acceptable) scope of distress. Such individuals, spurred on by deep feelings of vengefulness, vindictiveness, and animosity, behave in a manner that is singularly destructive; destructive to themselves as well as to some or all of the other family members, making an already bad family situation worse. These women I have found it useful to describe as "family terrorists."[115]

Pizzey's theory of "violence addiction" was much derided by the early 1980s. By 1998, she had great difficulty finding a publisher who would be associated with her view on the "emotional terrorist" in the home. She had, by then, been sidelined not only by feminists but even by members of her own organization. Renamed Refuge in 1993—following an earlier change of name to Chiswick Family Rescue in 1979, around the time that Pizzey had taken an active interest in helping rehabilitate violent men in addition to their partners and children—the nonprofit does not currently acknowledge her involvement in their founding. Pizzey's name is not even mentioned in the organization's history provided on their website.[116]

By 1998, Pizzey would largely be forgotten by the world. However, in the early 1980s, the notion that women played a central role in creating family violence was seen as a serious threat to the refuge movement, which presented violence as flowing in one direction, from the abuser to the abused. The reasons an abused person might stay in a violent relationship were understood as structural: in a sexist society, economically organized around male breadwinning and female caretaking, it could be impossible to leave.

Pizzey's views on female participation in domestic violence might indeed have been rooted in her retrospective understanding of her parents' relationship when she was a child. However, despite this, the response to her insistence on mutual complicity in intimate partner violence and ultimate refusal of passive female victimhood is illuminating. She was banished from public conversation rather than engaged with by advocates of the refuge movement.[117] Why was her thesis that women participated in their violent relationships so controversial? Psychological explanations of family violence were appealing when they focused on men. The proposal that violence might be relational at its core, and therefore genderless, was difficult to square with the contemporary idealization of mother love, and female relationality more broadly. Britain's gender-differentiated social order was maintained in no small part through appeals to emotional difference, founded upon the presumption of female adeptness in matters of the heart. That violence could come about because of early exposure to violence shed light on the potential relational nature and origins of violence. That this implicated women in family violence—as psychologically capable of making violence happen, even intensifying it—was, for many, beyond the pale.

Conclusion

From the schizophrenia-inducing impact of possessive parenting to the patriarchal stunting of girls' psychological development to the generational transmission of family violence, 1970s family reform efforts focused on the pathological relational dynamics inherent to middle-class nuclear families. Although concern for the impact of family dysfunction on emotional health was by then longstanding, these critical reform movements worked to prevent very different kinds of outcomes. While the postwar welfare state had focused on preventing delinquency, divorce, and neurosis, the intellectuals and activists featured in this chapter instead fought against systemic gender inequalities, the abuses of institutional psychiatry, and violence in British society. However radical were their ambitions for change, their demands were rooted in the prevalent belief that intimate childhood relationships were a crucial source of love for the world and the most promising antidote to violence, both physical *and* emotional.

Throughout the 1970s, family emotion held an important place in the social imaginary as the foundation for intimacy and basis for creating healthy relational subjectivities. In all the social movements explored in this chapter, mothers played an important role in producing emotionally mature and independent, yet highly socially attuned, non-violent people. Although the mother-child relationship had for decades been seen as playing a central role in subjectivity formation, by the 1970s subjectivity-making had itself become invested with even higher social value. The more that British people came to expect of adult maturity, the more that was expected of women as relational experts. Since the end of WWII, children had become both the inspiration and practical foundation for a politics that linked psychological well-being to social harmony. Queer theorist Lee Edelman has argued that the figure of the child has served politically "as a pledge of a covenant that shields us against the persistent threat of apocalypse now—or later."[118] In the case of Britain between 1945 and 1979, the future rested with the figure of an inherently relational child. To women's liberation feminists, radical psychiatrists, fathers' rights' activists, and anti-family-violence reformers alike, decisions to create a better future appeared to rest not with the child as an autonomous subject but with the child's relationship to their emotional caretaker(s).

Family life was politicized in new ways from the late 1960s on, as adult men and women asserted their right to have not only *a* family but an emotionally fulfilling family, whether through access to birth control to prevent unplanned children, ease in ending dysfunctional marriages, or an end to the stigma surrounding queer relationships. As family life was politicized in the 1960s and 1970s and revealed to be often violent and psychologically damaging to those involved in it, mothers became even further enmeshed in the politics of future-making in the present.

Freedom and privacy had been increasingly elided since the end of WWII, and this was especially clear in the 1970s. With privacy now associated with sexuality and romantic love—and, in turn, the gateway to liberated self-expression—advocates for changes to laws surrounding sexuality and family life focused on protecting individuals' right to privacy. As discussed in chapter 5, this was at the forefront of the decriminalization of homosexuality. The private lives of consenting adults were presented as beyond the legislative dominion of the state. The capacity to accept the responsibilities that accompanied this freedom were, however, predicated on an individual's close relationship with their mother in childhood. The ability not only to choose but to sustain harmonious intimacy developed out of this important first relationship. Lauren Berlant and Michael Warner have argued that intimacy's appearance as a wholly private affair serves political ends. Emotional intimacy has, since the 1960s, increasingly been widely seen as both defining and guaranteeing the privacy of acceptable adult sexuality. Heteronormative culture's "metacultural intelligibility" rests upon the "ideologies and institutions of intimacy."[119] But why does intimacy in its ideal form so often assume the appearance of the mother-child relationship, and female-engineered relationality more broadly? What work went into making this impervious to challenge despite the many compelling criticisms levelled against the white middle-class family in the 1960s and 70s?

Although the politics of intimacy are largely concealed in the twentieth and twenty-first centuries, in the decades after WWII the public benefits of emotional intimacy between spouses and their children were more clearly spelled out. Concern that Britain's state-supported health and social services would infringe upon citizens' private lives and interfere with the cultivation of intimacy, affection, and friendship haunted their development in the decades after WWII. The state's cold and impersonal mechanics were frequently raised as a threat to relationships based on love. As a result, the state funding of grassroots voluntary organizations was preferred to state-run organizations providing marriage counseling, housing for "battered women," and support for struggling lower-income mothers (of the kind provided by Home-Start). Their community-based voluntary orientation appeared better equipped at protecting citizens' privacy from the intrusions of an expanding welfare state.

In the 1970s, intimate relationships were believed to play a crucial (and irreplaceable) role in men and women's development toward emotionally mature adulthood. When divorced fathers spoke out in the mid-1970s about the emotional importance of children's relationship with their fathers, they presented fathers as performing the same emotional function as mothers. They campaigned for equal parental rights and simply changed the word "mother" to "parent" in their discussions of children's emotional needs.[120] Keith Parkin's manifesto, published in *The Guardian* on June 12, 1974, began by appealing to the equal importance of both parents: "It is time society decided that children need two parents, irrespective of whether the natural parents are married, separated or divorced."[121] In support of Parkin, *Times* reporter Maureen Green lamented the tendency to ignore "the claims of the paternal instinct" as the outcome of women's dominance over domestic life. Proclaiming that, "Today's game of Happy Families seems to be more than ever run by the mother," both FNF and its supporters focused their criticisms on a perceived collusion of women, psychologists, and the courts in preventing men from performing their rightful (and socially necessary) emotional role in the family:

> If the family becomes unhappy, if separation and divorce follow, the father is simply discarded. Mother and children continue as a family, but he is sent into a

sort of exile, from which he finds it difficult to continue to know, love and express his interest in his children ... Families Need Fathers is concerned to present father as a more significant figure in family life. They are asking whether the mother-child seam has not been overmined by psychologists. Maybe it is now time to investigate father love ... Paternal deprivation can exist, too; children can love and miss their fathers.[122]

Framing the need for fathers within the psychological language of maternal deprivation theory, FNF leadership focused on the emotional consequences of "paternal deprivation" following divorce. Children, they argued, suffered negative consequences to their emotional development when separated from their fathers. It was therefore time to consider the full emotional scope of family life and move away from an exclusive focus on the mother-child relationship.

FNF's insistence on children's emotional need for their fathers was hotly contested. "Grey-haired [male] judges" repudiated FNF, arguing that men seeking custody of their children needed to stop behaving like women, while many feminists maintained that fathers seeking custody should not dismiss generations of women's expertise in childcare methods. Women, unlike men, had painstakingly devoted themselves to practicing the recommendations of child experts like Bowlby, Winnicott, and Spock. As much as men might long for equality in childcare, it could not instantly be made into reality. As a result, FNF critics argued that children were better off with their mothers than their fathers in the event of divorce. As Jill Tweedie put it:

> Until men take a far more active interest ... in what happens to their children at home, women must keep their children ... Until there is equal pay and equal job opportunities and men show themselves as dedicated as women to bringing about good and extensive crèches and nursery schools, women must keep their children.[123]

Although Tweedie was sensitive to the complex historical conditions that had caused men to become ineffectual parents, her comments were reminiscent of the chastising guidance offered by the *Daily Herald*'s advice columnist in 1952 to a disgruntled divorced father seeking custody of his child: "the baby needs his mother more than anyone else in the world ... one thing is certain. To wrest a child from its mother is the cruelest wrong that selfishness ever prompted."[124]

Women occupied a central place in the expanding value of relational intimacy in the mid-twentieth-century decades. They were essential to maintaining the emotional norms and values that were at the heart of white middle-class heterosexual culture. Even the nuclear family's detractors often upheld women's greater capacity for stable non-violent relationality. As early as 1937, Edward Griffith noted that modern women, unlike their mothers, began to "want more from life; more pleasures, more consideration and more understanding. They are in search of a greater ideal, and so when they marry they expect more and hope for a fuller life."[125] But, he was careful to add, this did not mean that they were less committed to child rearing. Far from it, he assured his readers. The modern woman's "chief interest in life" continued to be her children, and this was evident in the fact that she expended even more time and energy ensuring that her children were well-raised than her mother and grandmother had: "She wants the best for them."[126]

Those touting the benefits of the mother-child relationship were even less ambiguous in their idealization of modern motherhood in the 1970s, even though the social agenda that they supported was greatly transformed. While Griffith had been motivated to educate women about such biologically informed issues as birth spacing to maintain the health of both mother and child, by 1979, mothers were seen as performing their most important social task by loving their children without any self-interest and preparing them emotionally for a long process of authentic (and liberatory) self-realization, one that would ideally be completed by early adulthood. Alongside the 1970s backlash against the male-breadwinning, female-homemaking middle-class family, mothers' responsibilities were expanded by radical psychiatrists, feminists, and leaders of the refuge movement to include helping her children become more relational, peace-loving, psychologically free men and women. Far from being liberated by the critical backlash of the 1970s, British mothers had been given a new and more ambitious set of emotional responsibilities.

Epilogue: Intimacy in the Age of the Individual

> The breakdown of family life is a huge social and economic, as well as moral, evil. The foot-soldiers in every inner city riot are those who have never known a proper home ... A child deprived of a normal family life is far less likely to grow up educated, employable and law-abiding. The weakness in family life in Britain is probably the biggest single cause, not merely of habitual crime, but also of poor educational standards and so of chronic unemployment. All these evils are interconnected. The financial and economic cost is incalculable. The cost in human misery doesn't bear thinking about.
> —Paul Johnson, *The Guardian*, January 12, 1987

> Love demands expression. It will not stay still, stay silent, be good, be modest, be seen and not heard, no. It will break out in tongues of praise, the high note that smashes the glass and spills the liquid. It is no conservationist love. It is a big game hunter and you are the game.
> —Jeanette Winterson, *Written on the Body*, 1992

By the fall of 1987, when Margaret Thatcher uttered the infamous statement "there is no such thing as society," Britain had in many ways entered a different era than the one described in this book. Intimate relationships had come to be seen as incommensurable with the dealings of the state. In British neoliberal discourse, private life stood as the place where the state emphatically did not belong, signifying—at a resolutely anti-statist moment—the limits of government authority. Although radical psychiatrists and second-wave feminists argued that the personal was political, Britain's Conservative government disavowed the personal and private as having anything to do with the functions of the state. The family had become both an emblem of privacy as well as a refuge from the market's unpredictability. It was the domain over which individuals could both assert responsibility and turn for support in times of trouble. Nonetheless, despite its ostensible positioning outside the state's operations, the nuclear family retained tremendous political importance in Thatcher's Britain. It was seen as providing necessary protection for children and ensuring that they would grow into adults who could manage their own freedom. From Thatcher's perspective in 1987, the family was both the goal of privacy and that which made privacy possible in the first place.

Anti-statism did not become a political priority overnight. Government funded services had, since the end of WWII, borne the taint associated with the state's impersonal bureaucratic operations. In the 1960s, however, anxieties about state intervention, especially its connection to dehumanizing institutionalization, increasingly made their way into critiques of Britain's welfare services. As the *Glasgow Herald*'s Molly Plowright put it in 1965, the "trained welfare worker" put "human being[s] into categor[ies]."[1] On the other hand, the selfless volunteer who served people in need was an "individual, making her own gesture of love," and "one of the Welfare State's biggest anachronisms."[2]

State-supported psychiatry came under especially harsh criticism as an insidious moralizing tool, an extension of the power abuses perpetrated by the family, and a mechanism for suppressing difference and making people governable. The once powerful myth of the classless "people's war," which had never truly described reality on the ground, no longer captured the public imagination as a basis for understanding the role and functions of the state. As radical psychiatrist David Cooper would proclaim at the Congress for the Dialectics of Liberation in 1967, the Soviet Union's failure lay in its neglect of individuals' "micro-social" landscapes. Socialist societies more generally, he argued, had dangerously overlooked "liberation on the level of the individual and the concrete groups in which he is directly engaged."[3] Cooper's emphasis on the importance of "inner reality" and the "micro-social" was echoed in the contemporary practices of marriage therapists and psychiatric social workers who emphasized the far-reaching social consequences of intimate relationships alongside their promises of individual fulfillment. Unlike their earlier post-war predecessors, this generation of mental health professionals put primary emphasis on the psychological benefits of intimate relationships for individuals' self-realization rather than their contributions to stabilizing public life. In other words, what began as a collectivist-inspired endeavor became an individualist one.

Although the social democratic spirit of the immediate postwar moment may have largely been displaced by a renewed commitment to individualism by the early 1980s, the nuclear family—and particularly the threat of its disappearance—retained immense political significance. Teenage mothers, single-parent families, and unemployed fathers—grouped together within the capacious category of Britain's "underclass" as recipients of welfare and symbols of family decay—came to be associated with the disappearance of the entrepreneurial spirit and a perceived growing nationwide incapacity for self-governance.[4] Rather than undermining the Conservative government's commitment to limiting government intervention, the growth of the police force was rationalized as necessary for managing citizens who were incapable of responsibly protecting their children from harm. A new emphasis on law and order also coincided with cutbacks in public spending on marriage and family services by the end of the decade. Although the late 1980s still preceded the most strident reactions to Britain's "therapy culture," there was a growing expectation that spouses and parents should be capable of maintaining stable relationships without the help of psychological experts.[5]

There was much public support throughout the 1980s for the neoliberal conflation of economic and social problems and accompanying law and order approach to preventing family breakdown. However, this view also inspired significant opposition. Although Conservatives were the self-described "party of the family," by the middle of the decade Thatcher was criticized for having failed the family through cuts to child and housing benefits, reductions in nursery schools, and decreased funding for health and social services.[6] And by 1989, population statistics showed that one out of every four children was born outside of marriage, one out of every five pregnancies was aborted, and teenage abortions had risen from 9% of conceptions in 1969 to 36% in 1989:

> All this under a Prime Minister who placed restoration of traditional family values at the heart of the new moral crusade … In the last decade, children born out of wedlock have doubled, cohabitation has trebled, and divorce touches nearly four out of ten marriages.[7]

Thatcher had recently unveiled a plan to "save the family," which targeted fathers who had shirked on child support payments. In response, she was widely panned in the press for misunderstanding the real challenges involved in raising a family.

At a moment when the Conservative focus on the family appeared to amount to nothing more than rhetoric, the Labour Party, under Neil Kinnock's leadership, promised to restore funding to social and voluntary services that directly supported mothers and their children. Public support for Labour's promise to re-establish comprehensive family services undoubtedly helped boost the party's lead in public opinion polls in 1990. However, this did not signal a desire to return to the family welfare politics of the post-WWII decades. Following the change of Conservative leadership in November 1990, and John Major's victory in 1992 (capturing a record number of popular votes since 1951), the voting public revealed that a change in mood had taken place since Thatcher was elected in 1979. British political priorities had changed, and it would take much more than the threat of family decline to steer it off its new course.[8]

Within this new neoliberal climate, intimate relationality was still highly sought after. Intimacy continued to hold powerful associations with the most meaningful kind of life. As Lauren Berlant has pointed out, "People consent to trust their desire for 'a life' to institutions of intimacy; and it is hoped that the relations formed within those frames will turn out beautifully, lasting over the long duration, perhaps across generations."[9] Only a few months after Thatcher had declared that there was "no such thing as society," emotional intimacy was presented in *The Guardian* as the necessary prerequisite for "supersex" and the gateway to a lasting, mutually fulfilling marriage.[10] The article discussed the recent blockbuster *Super Marital Sex* by Kinsey Institute sex researcher Paul Pearsall, who had coined the hyperbolic terms "supersex" and "psychasm" to describe the elevated sexual experience that committed monogamous relationships could provide when emotional intimacy was fully engaged. Pearsall, and his devoted following of readers in the late 1980s, saw 1960s free love as both unfulfilling and unerotic in comparison to intimate marital sex. *The Guardian* reporter saw the popularity of Pearsall's book as showing that when it came to sex "the moral majority has won. You need to be doting a husband to join the game."[11]

Sex was not the only—or even for some, primary—component of much-sought-after marital intimacy in this moment. Self-help articles in women's magazines stressed intimacy's many facets and sought to teach readers how to create it in their own marriages. For example, Leo Buscaglia noted that intimacy had sexual and verbal components, but insisted that compassion was also an important ingredient.[12] Intimacy advisors also frequently emphasized the benefits of undisturbed time spent together. Women's magazines and mainstream newspapers alike advised couples to dispense with all "distractions from intimacy," like computers, televisions, and phones, and put on some candles along with their favorite music.[13] Others, like University of Sussex psychologist Maryon Tysoe, took a different approach and suggested that shared interests be added to the mix to produce "a more sustaining bond than passion."[14] She advised couples that, "Mixing romantic dinners with ferreting together in supermarket freezers appears to have a better prognosis than endless eye contact in flickering restaurant candlelight."[15] Whatever the precise practices attached to intimacy, there was no question that it was seen as an important foundation for both lasting marriage and personal happiness.

Although intimacy continued to stand as a virtue, it had also taken on new associations with danger in the 1980s and 1990s. Fear of intimacy was highlighted in sex and marriage publications, advice columns, and magazine articles as something that many people (particularly women) suffered from. Many who were vocal about this fear described intimacy as triggering a distressing dissolution of personal boundaries. Intimacy thus did not stand as a straightforward gateway to harmonious bonding and end to loneliness and alienation. Novelist Jeannette Winterson described romantic love as "terrifying" and a source of unending (even self-annihilating) distraction.[16] Psychotherapist Susie Orbach, who would later become Winterson's wife, described intimacy as often experienced as a threat to "personal boundaries and separateness."[17] Psychoanalyst Rosalind Coward declared kissing, the most emblematic act of intimacy and an activity that many married women avoided, as it "evoke[d] the fear of being destroyed and devoured."[18] Intimacy for many women was, at its core, emotional chaos. It did not build a solid foundation (as 1940s marriage improvement literature had proclaimed).[19] Rather, it disrupted. In this individualistic neoliberal age, romantic intimacy had to be carefully monitored lest it upend the status quo and bring about the death of the personal self.

Amid discussion of intimacy avoidance, in the 1980s and 1990s there was also ongoing public conversation among feminists as to whether a more authentic form of loving might emerge in the wake of greater gender equality and LGBTQ+ social and self-acceptance—a form of loving that people would not feel deep ambivalence toward. Contributors to *Spare Rib* in 1991 declared their ongoing desire—against the evidence of their own lived experiences—for a committed mutually fulfilling romantic relationship: "how could we find this new kind of loving? ... We can't live without it, so we've got to make it good."[20] Assuming that successful love lasted a lifetime, contributors described themselves as bad at relationships because each had had so many. Maria, a forty-year-old Polish lesbian living in the UK, began her contribution by declaring that she did not have "any answers" since she had had more relationships "than the average dyke's had hair-cuts."[21] She described the "kind of loving" worth aspiring to as allowing the individual to have "everything":

> Quite simply, I want it all. To stay an individual in my own right and to find deep and lasting love... To settle down and to be free. In the meantime there's that lifelong task of loving myself. Loving myself against the odds, despite the stereotypes (lonely lesbian, suffering writer, victim Pole etc. etc.) and finding the confidence within, from which commitment is possible.[22]

Thirty-nine-year-old Cathy, identified as a Black heterosexual British woman, described her lack of faith in the existence of the kind of love that she wanted—one in which the woman in the relationship did not feel exploited and emotionally unsatisfied. Her "twenty-five years experience of men" had made her want to entirely abandon romantic relationships and focus only on herself. Yet, despite this—comparing her desire for love with a man to a smoker's desire for cigarettes—she confessed that she would "probably never quit the habit."[23]

As impossible as it may have seemed given the many serious obstacles—not least gender inequality and internalized homophobia and racism—lasting intimacy remained for many in Britain firmly attached to the aspirational ideal of a fully lived life. Despite decades of evidence attesting to the rarity of permanent sexually monogamous love relationships, this was the kind of relationship most associated with emotional intimacy. The notion that some emotional connections (stable, monogamous) are by nature more emotionally intimate than others (queer, fleeting, anonymous) has been remarkably durable. In the US context, legal scholar Kenji Yoshino has pointed out that bisexual erasure has arisen out of the value ascribed to monogamy and its presumed connection to "monosexuality," whether hetero or homo.[24] Intimacy aspirations, performance, and policing have become unquestioned, and seemingly apolitical, means for establishing clear boundaries around what does and does not stand as acceptable sexuality and "healthy" forms of relationship.

As this book has shown, intimacy found a home in the male-breadwinning, female-homemaking family, most especially in the mother-child relationship. This two-parent child-producing version of the family may have become an object of critique, but the value attached to intimacy weathered the last half of the twentieth century largely unscathed. This is not to say, however, that the two-parent, child-producing family has been ejected from associations with the "good," or right, kind of emotional life. Intimacy remains, for many, quintessentially tied to the family, and not only for supporters of "family values." Demands for equal access to marriage, adoption, and reproductive technologies aimed at creating new kinds of families (including single-parent families and same-sex parent families) also mobilize the language of access to emotional fulfillment and wellbeing.[25] Removing social and political barriers to having a life partner and becoming a parent are now widely seen as human rights issues in Britain and beyond.[26]

In exploring the psychopolitics of emotional life in the decades following WWII, this book has highlighted the social and political value attached to intimate relationships between 1945 and 1979, decades associated with the rise and fall of social democracy in Britain. These decades have traditionally been the focus of studies of the "classic welfare state" and postwar political consensus on the one hand and, on the other, explorations of the "sexual revolution" and the expansion of private freedoms. This book moves the historical focus onto the underlying preoccupation with intimate relationality, understood in developmental and therapeutic terms as a necessary precondition for emotional health. I argue that the decades that preceded the shift toward neoliberal values in the 1980s were marked by "consensus" that close personal relationships played a determining role in ensuring the wellbeing of both individual citizens and the political communities to which they belonged. The many compelling and diverse associations made between emotional "health" and citizenship in the decades after WWII are what endowed intimate relationships with consequential political value and thus made emotional life political in Britain after 1945.

Just as we see the social currency of intimacy persist into the present day, mental health has taken on even broader everyday significance than it held in the 1950s, 1960s, and 1970s. The ascendance of psychopharmacology's profitability since the 1990s has owed much to the popularity of depression as a diagnosis, widely described as psychiatry's "common cold." It now seems increasingly possible, as pharmaceutical advertisements have often implied and consumers appear to agree (given skyrocketing prescriptions for SSRIs), that no one is immune to severe mental suffering. Alongside this, growing awareness at the end of the twentieth century of the expansiveness and potential irreversibility of trauma further confirmed the suspected fragility of mental and emotional health. With the growth of interdisciplinary trauma studies since the 1990s, there is also a sense that trauma's origins and boundaries are far more capacious and lasting (even transmitted through generations) than previously understood.[27] More recently, sensitivity to the pervasiveness of trauma has included "trigger warnings" in educational contexts and greater attention to the long-term psychological damage caused by racism, sexism, homophobia, and transphobia. And so, during roughly the same moment that Thatcher expressed the neoliberal view that "changing the economics" would ultimately "change the heart and soul," we also see a rising belief that people are even more vulnerable to lasting emotional harm than earlier believed.[28] Illuminations of the ubiquity of trauma and mental affliction counter Thatcher's confident late-twentieth-century predictions about the widespread ascendance of resilient self-supporting entrepreneurship.

This book has uncovered an overlooked, yet deeply important, transformation in Britain during the second half of the twentieth century toward the widespread belief that both society and selves primarily develop out of intimate relationships between mothers and their children, as well as between spouses, lovers, and friends. As a consequence of this view during these decades, citizens' degree of emotional wellbeing (or "deprivation") was taken to be an indicator of potential power abuses and social injustices that, for this reason, became a compelling spur for political action. At the same time, the notion that people, events, and collectively held values were produced through close interpersonal relationships (rather than naturally given) also inspired hope. Futures that appeared worrying or uncertain might conceivably be brought within direct human control.

While the social reforms and political movements discussed in this book belonged to a specific moment in British history, the concerns they reflected are in many ways still very current on both sides of the Atlantic. As Britons and North Americans alike confront serious and escalating challenges around inclusion, we may need now, more than ever, far more openness toward what Michel Foucault aptly described as "relations not resembling those that are institutionalized."[29] In acting as deliberate, inventive alternatives, "non-institutionalized" relations can help illuminate how normalizing relational structures and dynamics at all scales limit the political futures of currently marginalized groups and negatively impact individual emotional destinies. And, if approached in a way that explicitly resists replicating homogenizing and exclusionary relational norms and values, attempts at "non-institutional" relationality (including, but not limited to, childfree partnerships, single-parent families, non-monogamous romance, and non-heteronormative family structures) can potentially provide a basis for configuring anti-oppressive, anti-violent forms of interpersonal life and, if truly mutually negotiated and created, allow for genuinely inclusive social realities.

Notes

Introduction

1. John Bowlby, *Maternal Care and Mental Health: A Report Prepared on Behalf of the World Health Organization* (Geneva, 1951).
2. John Bowlby, *Child Care and the Growth of Love* (London, 1953).
3. Henry Dicks, *Marital Tensions: Clinical Studies towards a Psychological Theory of Interaction* (New York, 1967), 45.
4. Antony Grey, "Towards a Sexually Sane Society," in *Speaking for Our Lives: Historic Speeches and Rhetoric for Gay and Lesbian Rights (1892–2000)*, ed. Robert Ridinger (New York, 2004).
5. David Cooper, *To Free a Generation: The Dialectics of Liberation* (New York, 1968), 10.
6. See Marga Vicedo, *The Nature and Nurture of Love: From Imprinting to Attachment in Cold War America* (Chicago, 2013); Frank C.P. van der Horst, *John Bowlby: From Psychoanalysis to Ethology* (Chichester, 2011).
7. Mathew Thomson, *Lost Freedom: The Landscape of the Child and the British Postwar Settlement* (Oxford, 2014).
8. The child also took on new political significance in the international arena in this moment. In 1946, the UN created the UN International Children's Emergency Fund (UNICEF). The creation of this specialized agency for the protection and wellbeing of children followed from a recognition that the dangers facing children had not ended with the war. The special entitlements of children and families still needed to be articulated and defended in peacetime. Article 16.3 of the Universal Declaration of Human Rights recognized that "the family is the natural and fundamental group unit of society and is entitled to protection by the society and the State." Article 25, which recognized an individual's and a family's right to health and wellbeing, was explicit about the protection of mother and child: "Motherhood and childhood are entitled to special care and assistance." Cited in Mark Ensalaco, "The Right of the Child to Development," in *Children's Human Rights: Progress and Challenges for Children Worldwide*, eds. Mark Ensalaco and Linda C. Majka (Lanham, 2005), 11.
9. Michèle Barrett and Mary McIntosh, *The Anti-Social Family* (London, 1982), 32–33. Lee Comer similarly noted in 1974 that "less than 10% of the population have (or will ever achieve) such a lifestyle." Lee Comer, *Wedlocked Women* (London, 1974), 210.
10. Michel Foucault, "Friendship as a Way of Life," April 1981 interview, in *Michel Foucault: Ethics, Subjectivity, and Truth, volume 1*, ed. Paul Rabinow (New York, 1994).
11. See Elaine Tyler May, *Homeward Bound: American Families in the Cold War Era* (New York, 1988); Deborah Weinstein, *The Pathological Family: Postwar America and the Rise of Family Therapy* (Ithaca, 2013).
12. During the depression years in Britain as much as a quarter of the working aged population (in aggregate nationally) was unemployed.
13. Rhodri Hayward, "The Pursuit of Serenity," in *History and Psyche: Culture, Psychoanalysis and the Past*, eds. Sally Alexander and Barbara Taylor (London, 2012), 284; Rhodri

Hayward, "Busman's Stomach and the Embodiment of Modernity," *Contemporary British History* 31, no. 1 (2017), 1–23.

14. Derek Fraser, *The Evolution of the British Welfare State: A History of Social Policy since the Industrial Revolution* (London, 1973); David Gladstone, *The Twentieth-Century Welfare State* (London, 1999); Pat Thane, *Foundations of the Welfare State* (London, 1982); Gøsta Esping-Anderson, *The Three Worlds of Welfare Capitalism* (Cambridge, 1990); Susan Pedersen, *Family, Dependence, and the Origins of the Welfare State: Britain and France, 1914–1945* (Cambridge, 1993); Jose Harris, "Political Thought and the Welfare State 1870–1940: An Intellectual Framework for British Social Policy," *Past & Present* 135 (May 1992), 116–141; Ann Shola Orloff, "Gendering the Comparative Analysis of Welfare States: An Unfinished Agenda," *Sociological Theory* 27, no. 3 (September 2009), 317–343; Seth Koven and Sonya Michel, "Womanly Duties: Maternalist Politics and the Origins of Welfare States in France, Germany, Great Britain, and the United States, 1880–1920," *The American Historical Review* 95, no. 4 (October 1990), 1076–1108; Sonya Michel and Rianne Mahon, *Child Care Policy at the Crossroads: Gender and Welfare State Restructuring* (London, 2002).

15. Fraser, *The Evolution of the British Welfare State*.

16. See Bruno Latour, *Reassembling the Social: An Introduction to Actor-Network-Theory* (Oxford, 2008).

17. "Five Questions: Professor Dame Elizabeth Anionwu," https://peopleshistorynhs.org/videos/five-questions-elizabeth-anionwu/.

18. "Five Questions: Alan Bennett," https://peopleshistorynhs.org/videos/five-questions-alan-bennett/.

19. "Five Questions: Joe O'Donaghue's First Memory," https://peopleshistorynhs.org/videos/five-questions-joe-odonaghues-first-memory/.

20. For example, Frank Mort, *Dangerous Sexualities: Medico-Moral Politics in England Since 1830* (London: Routledge, 2000).

21. For discussion of how this developed in the United States, see Kathleen Jones, *Taming the Troublesome Child: American Families, Child Guidance, and the Limits of Psychiatric Authority* (Cambridge, 2002); Elizabeth Lunbeck, *The Psychiatric Persuasion: Knowledge, Gender, and Power in Modern America* (Princeton, 1994).

22. National Association for Mental Health, *1968 Annual Report* (London, 1968), 4.

23. Michal Shapira, *The War Inside: Psychoanalysis, Total War, and the Making of the Democratic Self in Postwar Britain* (Cambridge, 2013); Jonathan Toms, *Mental Hygiene and Psychiatry in Modern Britain* (Basingstoke, 2013); Rhodri Hayward, "The Invention of the Psychosocial: An Introduction," *History of the Human Sciences* 25, no. 5 (2012), 3–12; Michael E. Staub, *Madness is Civilization: When the Diagnosis Was Social, 1948–1980* (Chicago, 2011); Suzanne Stewart-Steinberg, *Impious Fidelity: Anna Freud, Psychoanalysis, Politics* (Ithaca, 2011); Jamie Cohen-Cole, *The Open Mind: Cold War Politics and the Sciences of Human Nature* (Chicago, 2014) Tom Harrison, *Bion, Rickman, Foulkes, and the Northfield Experiments: Advancing on a Different Front* (London, 1999); Eric Rayner, *The Independent Mind in British Psychoanalysis* (Northvale, 1991).

24. See Michel Foucault, *Madness and Civilization: A History of Insanity in the Age of Reason* (London, 1961); Jan Goldstein, *The Post-Revolutionary Self: Politics and Psyche in France, 1750–1850* (Cambridge, 2005); Erving Goffman, *Asylums: Essays on the Social Situation*

of Mental Patients and Other Inmates (Chicago, 1961); Norbert Finzsch and Robert Jutte, eds., *Institutions of Confinement* (Cambridge, 1996); Andrew Scull, *Museums of Madness: The Social Organization of Insanity in Nineteenth-Century England* (New York, 1979); Diana Gittens, *Madness in Its Place: Narratives of Severalls Hospital, 1913–1997* (London, 1998). Nikolas Rose has not worked on asylums, however his examinations of the development of the "psy" sciences are deeply indebted to Foucault. See Nikolas Rose, *The Psychological Complex* (London, 1985); Nikolas Rose, *Inventing Our Selves: Psychology, Power and Personhood* (Cambridge, 1996); Nikolas Rose, *Governing the Soul: The Shaping of the Private Self* (London, 1990).

25. Hannah Arendt, "What is Authority?" in *Between Past and Future: Eight Exercises in Political Thought* (New York, 1961).
26. See Philip Rieff, *Freud: The Mind of the Moralist* (New York, 1959); Christopher Lasch, *Haven in a Heartless World: The Family Besieged* (New York, 1977); Carl Schorske, *Fin-de-siècle Vienna: Politics and Culture* (New York, 1979); Eli Zaretsky, *Secrets of the Soul: A Social and Cultural History of Psychoanalysis* (New York, 2004).
27. Viviana Zelizer, *Pricing the Priceless Child: The Changing Social Value of Children* (New York, 1985).
28. Cathy Unwin and Elaine Sharland, "From Bodies to Minds in Childcare Literature: Advice to Parents in Inter-war Britain," in *In the Name of the Child: Health and Welfare, 1880–1940*, ed. Roger Cooter (London, 1992), 174–199; Deborah Thom, "Wishes, Anxieties, Play and Gestures: Child Guidance in Inter-War England," in *In the Name of the Child: Health and Welfare, 1880–1940*, ed. Roger Cooter (London, 1992), 200–220.
29. Ellen Key, *The Century of the Child* (London, 1909), 4–5.
30. John Bowlby, "Psychology and Democracy," *The Political Quarterly* 17, no. 1 (January 1946), 61–75: 65.
31. D.W. Winnicott, *The Child, the Family and the Outside World* (London, 1957); John Bowlby, *Maternal Care and Mental Health* (Geneva, 1951); Anna Freud and Dorothy Burlingham, *Young Children in War-Time* (London, 1949).
32. This did not mean that some feminists, like Lee Comer, did not support men honing their capacity for more effective childcare. See Lee Comer, "The Motherhood Myth," *Australian Left Review* (March 1972), 28–34.
33. Jack Halberstam, *In a Queer Time and Place: Transgender Bodies, Subcultural Lives* (New York, 2005), 10.
34. Halberstam, *In a Queer Time and Place*, 10.
35. Ian Hacking, "Kinds of People: Moving Targets," *Proceedings of the British Academy* 151 (2007), 285–318.
36. Henry Dicks, *Marital Tensions: Clinical Studies towards a Psychological Theory of Interaction* (New York, 1967).
37. Friend, "Counselling Correspondence," 1979, HCA/Friend/3/3, London: Hall-Carpenter Archives.
38. For discussions of this in the United States, see Kristin Celello, *Making Marriage Work: A History of Marriage and Divorce in the Twentieth-Century United States* (Chapel Hill, 2009); Molly Ladd-Taylor, *Mother Work: Women, Child Welfare, and the State, 1890–1930* (Urbana, 1994).
39. See Kathleen Lynch, "Love Labour as a Distinct and Non-Commodifiable Form of Care Labour," *The Sociological Review* 55, no. 3 (2007), 550–570.

40. Donald W. Winnicott, "A Man Looks at Motherhood," in *The Child, the Family, and the Outside World* (Harmondsworth, 1964), 17 [my emphasis].
41. Lauren Berlant, *Compassion: The Culture and Politics of an Emotion* (London, 2014).
42. See Jean Duncombe and Dennis Marsden, "Whose Orgasm is this Anyway? 'Sex Work' in Long-term Heterosexual Couple Relationships," in *Sexual Cultures*, eds. Jeffrey Weeks and Janet Holland (New York, 1996), 220–238; Lauren Berlant and Michael Warner, "Sex in Public," in *Intimacy*, ed. Lauren Berlant (Chicago, 2000), 311–330; Laura Kipnis, "Adultery," in *Intimacy*, ed. Lauren Berlant (Chicago, 2000), 9–47; Gayle Rubin, "Thinking Sex: Notes for a Radical Theory of the Politics of Sexuality," in *Pleasure and Danger: Exploring Female Sexuality*, ed. Carole S. Vance (London, 1992), 267–293.
43. Rubin, "Thinking Sex," 279.
44. Geoffrey Gorer, *Sex and Marriage in England Today: A Study of the Views and Experience of the Under-45s* (London, 1971).
45. Policy Advisory Committee on Sexual Offences, *Working Paper on the Age of Consent in Relation to Sexual Offences* (London, 1979), 7. Evidence submitted by the Royal College of Psychiatrists.
46. Policy Advisory Committee on Sexual Offences, *Working Paper*, 7.
47. See Alex Owen, *The Place of Enchantment: British Occultism and the Culture of the Modern* (Chicago, 2004); Alison Winter, *Mesmerized: Powers of Mind in Victorian Britain* (Chicago, 1998); Joy Dixon, *Divine Feminine: Theosophy and Feminism in England* (Baltimore, 2001). These studies have challenged the utility of conventional characterizations of modernity—especially those derived from Marx and Weber—and have highlighted the diverse range of new, highly rationalized, self-consciously "modern" forms of social and moral meaning in Britain in the nineteenth and twentieth centuries (including individuals and groups that targeted the irrational, the emotional, and the spiritual as integral features of Western modernity).
48. Ian Hacking, *Historical Ontology* (Cambridge, 2004), 99–109.
49. E.P. Thompson, *The Making of the English Working Class* (London, 1963); Joan Wallach Scott, "The Evidence of Experience," in *Questions of Evidence: Proof, Practice, and Persuasion across the Disciplines*, eds. James Chandler, Arnold I. Davidson, and Harry Harootunian (Chicago, 1994), 363–387; Michel de Certeau, *The Practice of Everyday Life* (Berkeley, 1984).
50. For discussions of the disputed chronology of Britain's "sexual revolution," see Hera Cook, *The Long Sexual Revolution* (Oxford, 2004); Kate Fisher, *Sex Before the Sexual Revolution* (Cambridge, 2010); Claire Langhamer, *The English in Love* (Oxford, 2013).

Chapter 1

1. H.V. Dicks, *The Psychological Foundations of the Wehrmacht* (War Office, 1944), 1, WO 241/1, National Archives.
2. J.R. Rees, ed., *The Case of Rudolf Hess: A Problem of Diagnosis in Forensic Psychiatry* (London, 1947), 195.
3. H.V. Dicks, "Personality Traits and National Socialist Ideology," *Human Relations* 3, no. 2 (June 1950), 111–155: 111.
4. Dicks, *The Psychological Foundations of the Wehrmacht*, 8.
5. Dicks, *The Psychological Foundations of the Wehrmacht*, 9.

6. See Peter Mandler, *Return from the Natives: How Margaret Mead Won the Second World War and Lost the Cold War* (New Haven, 2013); Daniel Pick, *The Pursuit of the Nazi Mind: Hitler, Hess, and the Analysts* (Oxford, 2014).
7. Dicks, *The Psychological Foundations of the Wehrmacht*, 6.
8. Joanne Meyerowitz, "'How Common Culture Shapes Separate Lives': Sexuality, Race, and Mid-Twentieth-Century Social Constructionist Thought," *The Journal of American History* 96, no. 4 (March 2010), 1057–1084: 1059.
9. See Chris Renwick, *British Sociology's Lost Biological Roots: A History of Futures Past* (Basingstoke, 2012).
10. For example, Joshua Bierer, the first editor of the *International Journal of Social Psychiatry*, saw the kibbutz as the healthiest social form.
11. Gustave Le Bon, *The Crowd: A Study of the Popular Mind* (London, 1896).
12. Wilfred Trotter, *Instincts of the Herd in Peace and War* (London, 1916).
13. Sigmund Freud, *Massenpsychologie und Ich-Analyse* (Vienna, 1921).
14. See Edward Glover, *War, Sadism and Pacifism; Three Essays* (London, 1933).
15. P03-B-B-02, Papers of John Rickman, British Psycho-Analytical Society Archives.
16. R.H. Curtis explained that after-care was intended for patients whose breakdown was caused by "an unsuitable environment." R.H. Curtis, "Some Developments, Legal and Administrative, in Mental Treatment," *Journal of Mental Science* (January 1938), 195–196.
17. "The First 'Mental Hospital,'" *The Lancet* 1, no. 5209 (June 30, 1923), 1339–1304: 1339.
18. "A Hospital for Mental Diseases," *British Medical Journal* 1, no. 2460 (February 22, 1908), 457.
19. "Treatment of Temporary Mental Disorder in General Hospitals," *The Lancet* 2, no. 4344 (December 1, 1906), 1525–1526: 1526.
20. Stephen Taylor, "The Suburban Neurosis," *The Lancet* 1, no. 5978 (March 26, 1938), 759–761: 761. See also, Rhodri Hayward, "Desperate Housewives and Model Amoebae: The Invention of Suburban Neurosis in Inter-War Britain," in *Health and the Modern Home*, ed. Mark Jackson (London, 2007), 42–62.
21. Henry L. Wilson, "The Treatment of the Voluntary Boarder, The Retreat, York, 1891–1930," *Journal of Mental Science* 79 (January 1933), 105; Curtis, "Some Developments, Legal and Administrative, in Mental Treatment," 193; "Our Mental Hospitals: Report of the Board of Control for 1945," *The Lancet* 2, no. 6428 (November 9, 1946), 691.
22. Helen Boyle, "Watchman, What of the Night?" *Journal of Mental Science* 85, no. 358 (September 1939), 867.
23. Curtis, "Some Developments, Legal and Administrative, in Mental Treatment," 200.
24. Cited in "Britons Need 'Mind Doctoring,'" *Daily Mail*, May 10, 1938.
25. Pioneer Health Centre Annual Report (1935), 3, SA/PHC/A.2, Wellcome Library.
26. John Comerford, *Health the Unknown: The Story of the Peckham Experiment* (London, 1947), 14.
27. "Pioneers in Peckham: 'Health Before Disease,'" *The Observer*, March 31, 1935, 25.
28. "Manalive, A New Biological Study, The Pioneer Health Centre," *The Times*, June 24, 1939, 13.
29. Innes Pearse and Lucy H. Crocker, *The Peckham Experiment: A Study in the Living Structure of Society* (London, 1943).
30. Innes Pearse and G. Scott Williamson, *Biologists in Search of Material* (London, 1938), 39.

31. Cited in Innes Hope Pearse, *The Quality of Life: The Peckham Approach to Human Ethology* (Edinburgh, 1979), 27–28.
32. Cited in Pearse, *The Quality of Life*, 28.
33. Cited in Pearse, *The Quality of Life*, 27–28.
34. Pearse, *The Peckham Experiment*, 10 [her emphasis].
35. "Health Centres of Today," *The Lancet* 1, no. 6394 (March 16, 1946), 391.
36. Pearse, *The Peckham Experiment*, 10.
37. They were the first to offer complete health "overhauls" in Britain. Their only forerunner was the Metropolitan Life Insurance Co. in the United States, and these were voluntary for subscribers.
38. Pearse, *The Quality of Life*, 41.
39. Innes Pearse and G. Scott Williamson, *The Case for Action: A Survey of Everyday Life under Modern Industrial Conditions, with Special Reference to the Question of Health* (London, 1931), 30.
40. Pearse and Williamson, *The Case for Action*, 30.
41. Pearse and Williamson, *The Case for Action*, 46.
42. Alison Stallibrass, *Being Me and Also Us: Lessons from the Peckham Experiment* (Edinburgh, 1989), 24.
43. Cited in the Pioneer Health Centre Annual Report (1935), 6.
44. Cited in the Pioneer Health Centre Annual Report (1935), 8.
45. Comerford, *Health the Unknown*, 27.
46. Pearse, *The Quality of Life*, 9.
47. Pearse, *The Quality of Life*, 11.
48. J.M. Richards, "The Pioneer Health Centre: Analysis," *The Architectural Review* 77, no. 462 (May 1, 1935), 208–216: 208.
49. Pearse and Williamson, *The Case for Action*, 140.
50. Pearse and Williamson, *The Case for Action*, 140.
51. Pearse and Williamson, *The Case for Action*, 144.
52. Close to 900 families had joined the center by then, many of whom re-enrolled after it reopened in 1946.
53. The new and improved battle schools focused more on morale building. They also needed to train non-professional civilian soldiers as the British Army grew.
54. Ben Shephard, *A War of Nerves: Soldiers and Psychiatrists in the Twentieth Century* (Cambridge, MA, 2001), 257.
55. W.R. Bion and John Rickman, "Intra-Group Tensions in Therapy," *The Lancet* 2, no. 6274 (November 27, 1943), 678–682: 678.
56. Bion and Rickman, "Intra-Group Tensions in Therapy," 678.
57. Thomas F. Main, "The Concept of the Therapeutic Community," in *The Ailment and Other Psychoanalytic Essays*, ed. Jennifer Johns (London, 1989), 123–141: 130.
58. Main, "The Concept of the Therapeutic Community," 131.
59. Harold Bridger, "The Discovery of the Therapeutic Community: The Northfield Experiments," in *The Social Engagement of Social Science*, eds. Eric Trist and Hugh Murray (London, 1990), 68–87: 76.
60. Bridger, "The Discovery of the Therapeutic Community," 76.
61. Bridger, "The Discovery of the Therapeutic Community," 78.
62. Bridger, "The Discovery of the Therapeutic Community," 78.

63. "War in the Head: How the Army Dealt with Some of Its Psychiatric Casualties during the Second World War," BBC Radio 4, 1994, Wellcome Library.
64. Harold Bridger, "Groups in Open and Closed Systems," paper presented at the Therapeutic Communities Today Conference, August 1984, 54–68: 63, Harold Bridger Papers, Planned Environment Therapy Trust (PETT) Archive [uncatalogued].
65. Harold Bridger, "Group Discussion," (Undated), 1. Harold Bridger Papers, PETT Archive [uncatalogued].
66. Bridger, "The Discovery of the Therapeutic Community," 82.
67. Maxwell Jones and Aubrey Lewis, "Effort Syndrome," *The Lancet* 1, no. 6148 (June 28, 1941), 813–818: 818.
68. Patients suffered from "breathlessness, palpitations, left chest pain, postural giddiness, occasional fainting attacks and fatigue." Maxwell Jones, *Social Psychiatry: A Study of Therapeutic Communities* (London, 1952), 2.
69. Jones, *Social Psychiatry*, 3–4.
70. Jones, *Social Psychiatry*, 13.
71. A.T.M. Wilson, "Group Techniques in a Transitional Community," *The Lancet* 1, no. 6457 (May 31, 1947), 735–738.
72. Wilson, "Group Techniques in a Transitional Community," 735.
73. Major A. Curle and Lt.-Col. E.L. Trist, cited in Robert Ahrenfeldt, *Psychiatry in the British Army in the Second World War* (London, 1958), 234–235.
74. Main, "The Concept of the Therapeutic Community," 128; Clare Makepeace, *Captives of War: British Prisoners of War in Europe in the Second World War* (Cambridge, 2017).
75. Wilson, "Group Techniques in a Transitional Community," 737.
76. Wilson, "Group Techniques in a Transitional Community," 736.
77. Wilson, "Group Techniques in a Transitional Community," 738.
78. Wilson, "Group Techniques in a Transitional Community," 737: "The increasing rate of the demand for psychiatric help is shown by the following figures: during the first month about 5% of the repatriates were seen, all referred through a medical or other officer; whereas in the third and fourth months some 60% were spontaneously seeking advice."
79. Wilson, "Group Techniques in a Transitional Community," 736.
80. Robert N. Rapoport, *Community as Doctor: New Perspectives on a Therapeutic Community* (London, 1960), 10.
81. D.W. Winnicott, "Thoughts on the Meaning of the Word Democracy," *Human Relations* 4 (1950), 171–185: 176; Russell Barton, *Institutional Neurosis* (Bristol, 1959).
82. Rees, *The Case of Rudolf Hess*, 203.
83. Rees, *The Case of Rudolf Hess*, 195.
84. Henry Dicks, "Reports and Analysis of 167 Cases: A Psychiatric Investigation Carried Out in 1943-44," PP/HVD/A/2/7, Wellcome Archives.
85. Caroline Playne, *The Neuroses of the Nations* (London, 1925).
86. Dicks, "Reports and Analysis of 167 Cases."
87. Dicks, *The Psychological Foundations of the Wehrmacht*, 8.
88. Dicks, *The Psychological Foundations of the Wehrmacht*, 9.
89. Dicks, *The Psychological Foundations of the Wehrmacht*, 8.
90. Dicks, *The Psychological Foundations of the Wehrmacht*, 8.
91. Dicks, *The Psychological Foundations of the Wehrmacht*, 9.
92. Dicks, *The Psychological Foundations of the Wehrmacht*, 11.

93. H.V. Dicks, "National Socialism as a Psychological Problem," PP/HVD/A/3/24, Wellcome Archives.
94. H.V. Dicks, "Answers to a Questionnaire from the Hoover Institute and Library on Psychological Warfare, January 18 1948," PP/HVD/B/1/23, Wellcome Archives.
95. J. Cohen, from correspondence between H.V. Dicks, G.R. Hargreaves, and J. Cohen, dated March 5 and 7, 1945, PP/HVD/B/1/11, Wellcome Archives.
96. Dicks, "Answers to a Questionnaire from the Hoover Institute and Library on Psychological Warfare."
97. Philippe Pinel's late-eighteenth-century introduction of "moral treatment" constituted the "first revolution" and Freud introduced the "second." See Rudolf Dreikurs, "Group Psychotherapy and the Third Revolution in Psychiatry," *International Journal of Social Psychiatry* 1, no. 3 (1955), 23–32; Rapoport, *Community as Doctor*.
98. "The Peckham Experiment," *The Lancet* 1, no. 6286 (February 19, 1944), 259–260: 259.
99. "The Peckham Experiment," *The Lancet*, 259.
100. See Nikolas Rose, *Governing the Soul: The Shaping of the Private Self* (London, 1999), 156.
101. William Beveridge, *Social Insurance and the Allied Services* (London, 1942). See also Susan Pedersen, *Family, Dependence, and the Origins of the Welfare State: Britain and France, 1914–1945* (Cambridge, 1993).
102. Richard Titmuss, *Essays on the Welfare State* (London, 1958).
103. J.R. Rees, "Experiences of Neurosis and Backwardness in the War-Time Army: Can They Help with Civilian Problems?" National Association for Mental Health Conference Report (1946), PP/ADD/D.3, Wellcome Archives.
104. James Spence, *The Purpose of the Family: A Guide to the Care of Children* (London, 1947), 34.
105. Spence, *The Purpose of the Family*, 34.

Chapter 2

1. Tom Main, "Clinical Problem of Repatriates," in *The Ailment and Other Psychoanalytic Essays*, ed. Jennifer Johns (London, 1989), 144–155: 151.
2. Lady Allen of Hurtwood, "Children in 'Homes,'" *The Times*, July 15, 1944, 5.
3. Main, "Clinical Problem of Repatriates," 151.
4. Susan Isaacs, Letter to *The Times*, July 18, 1944, 5.
5. Anonymous Letter to *The Times*, July 31, 1944, 5.
6. Allen, "Children in 'Homes,'" 5.
7. See, for example, Russell Barton, *Institutional Neurosis* (Bristol, 1959); T.F. Main, "The Sociatry of a Neurosis Hospital," 1949, P07-A, British Psycho-Analytical Society Archives.
8. National character studies produced during the war also presented similar arguments. See Ruth Benedict, *The Chrysanthemum and the Sword* (Boston, 1946); Margaret Mead, *And Keep Your Powder Dry* (New York, 1942).
9. Hilda Lewis, *Deprived Children: The Mersham Experiment, A Social and Clinical Study* (London, 1954); Donald Ford, *The Deprived Child and the Community* (London, 1955); John Bowlby and James Robertson, "A Two-Year-Old Goes to Hospital," *Proceedings of the Royal Society of Medicine* 46, no. 426 (1952), 425–427; B.M. Spinley, *The Deprived and the Privileged: Personality Development in English Society* (London, 1953); René Spitz, "Hospitalism: An Inquiry in the Genesis of Psychiatric Conditions in Early Childhood,"

Psychoanalytic Study of the Child 1 (1945), 53–74; Frank Bodman, "The Social Adaptation of Institution Children," *The Lancet* 1, no. 7170 (January 28 1950), 173–176; John Rickman and Geoffrey Gorer, *The People of Great Russia* (London, 1949); Anna Freud and Dorothy Burlingame, *Infants Without Families: The Case For and Against Residential Nurseries* (London, 1947); Myra Curtis, *Report of the Care of Children Committee* (London, 1946).

10. William Beveridge, *Social Insurance and Allied Services* (New York, 1942).
11. On WWII's importance in introducing a new British preoccupation with security, see Mathew Thomson, *Lost Freedom: The Landscape of the Child and the British Post-War Settlement* (Oxford, 2014).
12. This was also a problem in the United States. See Mical Raz, *What's Wrong with the Poor? Psychiatry, Race, and the War on Poverty* (Chapel Hill, 2013).
13. See Lionel Rose, *Erosion of Childhood* (London, 1991), 153; Carolyn Steedman, *Childhood, Culture, and Class in Britain: Margaret McMillan, 1860–1931* (New Brunswick, 1990).
14. Harry Hendrick, *Child Welfare: Historical Dimensions, Contemporary Debate* (Bristol, 2003); Denise Riley, *War in the Nursery: Theories of Child and Mother* (London, 1983); Michal Shapira, *The War Inside: Psychoanalysis, Total War, and the Making of the Democratic Self in Postwar Britain* (Cambridge, 2013); Thomson, *Lost Freedom*; John Stewart, *Child Guidance in Britain, 1918–1955: The Dangerous Age of Childhood* (London, 2013); Nikolas Rose, *Inventing Our Selves: Psychology, Power, and Personhood* (Cambridge, 1996).
15. In particular, Shapira, *The War Inside*, and Thomson, *Lost Freedom*, demonstrate how children became the focal point of transformative social and political changes in Britain after WWII.
16. Kathleen Jones, *Taming the Troublesome Child: American Families, Child Guidance, and the Limits of Psychiatric Authority* (Cambridge, 2002), 59.
17. Cited in Stewart, *Child Guidance in Britain*, 1.
18. Jones, *Taming the Troublesome Child*, 93.
19. Feversham Committee, *The Voluntary Mental Health Services: The Report of the Feversham Committee* (London, 1939), 150; Commonwealth Fund, *The Commonwealth Fund: Historical Sketch, 1918–1962* (New York, 1963), 28–29.
20. Stewart, *Child Guidance in Britain*, 5. There were over three hundred clinics in operation in Britain by 1955.
21. See Charles L.C. Burns, *Maladjusted Children* (London, 1955). See also Sarah Hayes, "Rabbits and Rebels: The Medicalisation of Maladjusted Children in Mid-Twentieth Century Britain," in *Health in the Modern Home*, ed. Mark Jackson (London, 2007), 128–152.
22. Burns, *Maladjusted Children*, 15.
23. Burns, *Maladjusted Children*, 49–50 [my emphasis].
24. Robert Skidelsky, *English Progressive Schools* (Harmondsworth, 1969), 137.
25. Labour politics became increasingly interested in working-class life conditions in this period. Steedman, *Childhood, Culture, and Class in Britain*, 8.
26. *The Times*, July 28, 1939, 15. The report was produced by several of Britain's leading mental health organizations.
27. The 1908 Children Act focused on preventing infant mortality and cruelty to children, juvenile smoking, and the treatment of juvenile offenders.

28. Hendrick, *Child Welfare*, 157.
29. Department of Education and Science, *Report of the Committee on Maladjusted Children*, 3
30. Burns, *Maladjusted Children*, 1
31. Schools for "maladjusted" children—unlike schools for deaf or blind children—were expected to make treatment part of their educational goal. See David Wills, *Throw Away Thy Rod* (London, 1960), 12.
32. Lady Allen of Hurtwood, *Whose Children?* (London, 1945), 14.
33. Allen, *Whose Children?*, 10.
34. Allen, *Whose Children?*, 9.
35. See Laura Lee Downs, *Childhood in the Promised Land: Working-Class Movements and the Colonies de Vacances in France 1880–1960* (Durham, 2002).
36. Amy St. Loe Strachey, *Borrowed Children: A Popular Account of Some Evacuation Problems and Their Remedies* (New York, 1940), 4–5.
37. Strachey, *Borrowed Children*, 4–5.
38. Cited in a letter dated November 18, 1939. Amy St. Loe Strachey, *These Two Strange Years: Letters from England, October 1939–September 1941* (New York, 1942), 10.
39. Strachey, *These Two Strange Years*, 10–11.
40. Katherine Wolf, "Evacuation of Children in Wartime," *Psychoanalytic Study of the Child* (1945), 389–404: 389.
41. Susan Isaacs, ed., *The Cambridge Evacuation Survey: A Wartime Study in Social Welfare and Education* (London, 1941), 52.
42. Anna Freud and Dorothy Burlingham, *Young Children in War-Time* (London, 1949); Isaacs, ed., *The Cambridge Evacuation Survey*; Richard Padley and Margaret Cole, eds., *Evacuation Survey: A Report to the Fabian Society* (London, 1940).
43. Isaacs, ed., *The Cambridge Evacuation Survey*, 7.
44. Isaacs, ed., *The Cambridge Evacuation Survey*, 9.
45. "Children in 'Homes,'" Letters to *The Times*, July 25, 1944, 6.
46. "Children in 'Homes,'" *The Times*, July 31, 1944, 5.
47. E. Moberly Bell, "Children in 'Homes,'" Letter to *The Times*, August 15, 1944, 6.
48. "Children in 'Homes': How the Inquiry Will Be Carried Out," *The Times*, October 7, 1944, 5.
49. Bodman, "The Social Adaptation of Institution Children," 173–176.
50. Bodman, "The Social Adaptation of Institution Children," 173.
51. Hendrick, *Child Welfare*, 133; Gordon Lynch, "Pathways to the 1946 Curtis Report and the Post-War Reconstruction of Children's Out of Home Care," *Contemporary British History* (April 2019), 22–43.
52. Cited in Agatha H. Bowley, *Child Care: A Handbook on the Care of the Child Deprived of a Normal Home Life* (Edinburgh, 1951), 47.
53. *Children Act 1948*, 859.
54. Great Britain, *Children Act 1948*, 859.
55. House of Commons Debate, "Mary Ford," 20 March 1959, vol. 602 col. 874.
56. House of Commons Debate, "Mary Ford," 20 March 1959, vol. 602 col. 874.
57. Bowley, *Child Care*, 47.
58. Jean S. Heywood, *The Deprived Child and the Nation* (London, 1964).

59. See Myra Curtis, *Report of the Care of Children Committee: Presented to the Secretary of State for the Home Department, the Minister of Health, and the Minister of Education* (London, 1946), 11.
60. Stephen Cretney, *Law, Law Reform and the Family* (Oxford, 1998), 185.
61. Cretney, *Law, Law Reform and the Family*, 194.
62. Riley, *War in the Nursery*.
63. John Bowlby "Research Application to the Ford Foundation," 1955, PP/BOW/D.5/1, Wellcome Archives.
64. John Bowlby, *Maternal Care and Mental Health* (Geneva, 1951), 12.
65. Tara Zahra, "Lost Children: Displacement, Family, and Nation in Postwar Europe," *Journal of Modern History* (March 2009), 45–86: 46–47.
66. Bowlby, *Maternal Care and Mental Health*, 6.
67. Bowlby, *Maternal Care and Mental Health*, 6.
68. Bowlby, *Maternal Care and Mental Health*, 15.
69. John Bowlby, *Child Care and the Growth of Love* (London, 1953), 157.
70. Bowlby, *Maternal Care and Mental Health*, 82–83.
71. League of Nations, *The Placing of Children in Families* (Geneva, 1938).
72. Bowlby, *Child Care and the Growth of Love*, 106.
73. Bowlby, *Child Care and the Growth of Love*, 107.
74. Bowlby et al, *Protest, Detachment, and Despair*, Chapter 8, 2–15. PP/BOW/D.3/35, Wellcome Archives.
75. Bowlby et al, *Protest, Detachment, and Despair*, Chapter 1, 5.
76. Bowlby et al, *Protest, Detachment, and Despair*, Chapter 1, 5.
77. James Robertson, *A Two-Year-Old Goes to Hospital, A Guide to the Film* (London, 1953), 1.
78. James Robertson and John Bowlby, *A Two-Year-Old Goes to Hospital* (London, 1952).
79. Robertson, *A Two-Year-Old Goes to Hospital, A Guide to the Film*, 5.
80. Robertson, *A Two-Year-Old Goes to Hospital, A Guide to the Film*, 3.
81. John Bowlby and James Robertson, "A Two-Year-Old Goes to Hospital," *Proceedings of the Royal Society of Medicine* 46, no. 426 (1952), 425–427: 426.
82. John Bowlby et al, "The Effects of Mother-Child Separation: A Follow-Up Study," *British Journal of Medical Psychology* 29, no. 3–4 (1956), 211–247: 242.
83. See Marga Vicedo, *The Nature and Nurture of Love: From Imprinting to Attachment in Cold War America* (Chicago, 2013); Frank C.P. van der Horst, *John Bowlby: From Psychoanalysis to Ethology* (Chichester, 2011).
84. John Bowlby, "Separation Anxiety," *International Journal of Psycho-Analysis* 41, no. 2–3 (1960), 89–133: 96.
85. Robertson, *A Two-Year-Old Goes to Hospital, A Guide to the Film*, iii.
86. James Robertson, *Hospitals and Children: A Parent's-Eye View* (London, 1962), 20.
87. See also Shapira, *The War Inside*, 198–238.
88. "Going to Hospital," *Nursery World*, June 12, 1958, 23.
89. James Robertson, *Going to Hospital with Mother, A Guide to the Documentary Film* (London, 1958), 7: "During the past five years, more than 400 mothers have come into residence."
90. Hugh McLeave, "Hospitals Should Be Just Like Home," *Year Chronicle*, April 19, 1958.
91. See Shapira, *The War Inside*, 229–235.
92. McLeave, "Hospitals Should be Just Like Home."

93. Harry Platt, *The Welfare of Children in Hospital: Report of the Committee* (London, 1959), 17. In 1959, Robertson compiled a list of hospitals in Britain that would allow mothers to reside alongside their hospitalized children. He found that sixty-eight hospitals provided accommodation for between two and twelve mothers at a time. While just under a third were in London, such hospital accommodation existed throughout the country. "Hospitals Where Mothers Can Be Admitted with Their Children," MH 52/497, National Archives.
94. "Children in Hospital," *The Observer*, February 15, 1959, 14.
95. John Bowlby, "The Influence of Early Environment in the Development of Neurosis and Neurotic Character," *The International Journal of Psychoanalysis* 21 (1940), 154–178: 175.
96. J.G. Howells, "Separation of Mother and Child," *The Lancet* 1, no. 7022 (March 1958), 691.
97. Margaret Mead, "Some Theoretical Considerations on the Problem of Mother-Child Separation," *American Journal of Orthopsychiatry* 24, no. 3 (July 1954): 471–483.
98. See Marga Vicedo, "Mothers, Machines and Morals: Harry Harlow's Work on Primate Love from Lab to Legend," *Journal of the History of the Behavioral Sciences* 45, no. 3 (Summer 2009), 193–218.
99. Henry Cass (director), *No Place for Jennifer* (UK: 1950).
100. The 1956 film *Child in the House* (directed by Cy Endfield) showed a girl's struggle to cope with uncaring relatives who kept her from seeing her father. Her mother's long hospitalization had prompted her family's breakup.
101. Mary Burbury, "Mental Health and Personal Responsibility," NAMH 1956 Annual Meeting (London, 1956), 34.
102. Notable examples include Phyllis Hambledon's novel *No Difference to Me*, later made into the film *No Place for Jennifer*; the films *Twice Upon a Time* and *Background*, both released in 1953; and *Child in the House* (1956) based on a 1955 novel by the same name by Janet McNeill.
103. Lee Edelman, *No Future: Queer Theory and the Death Drive* (Durham, 2004).
104. Carolyn Steedman, *Strange Dislocations: Childhood and the Idea of Human Interiority, 1780–1930* (Cambridge, 1995), 5.
105. Viviana Zelizer, *The Purchase of Intimacy* (Princeton, 2009); Eva Illouz, *Cold Intimacies and the Making of Emotional Capitalism* (Cambridge, 2017); Arlie Hochschild, *The Managed Heart: Commercialization of Human Feeling* (Berkeley, 2012).
106. See Denise Riley, "War in the Nursery," *Feminist Review* 2 (1979), 82–108: 106.
107. Edelman, *No Future*, 2.
108. E.F.M. Durbin and John Bowlby, "Personal Aggressiveness and War," in *War and Democracy: Essays on the Causes and Prevention of War* (London, 1938), 49.
109. Durbin and Bowlby, "Personal Aggressiveness and War," 49 [my emphasis].

Chapter 3

1. Elaine Grand, "Miserable Married Women," *The Observer*, May 7, 1961, 34.
2. Grand, "Miserable Married Women," 34.
3. Grand, "Miserable Married Women," 34.
4. Grand, "Miserable Married Women," 34.
5. Grand, "Miserable Married Women," 34.
6. Grand, "Miserable Married Women," 34.

7. Merrell P. Middlemore, *The Nursing Couple* (London, 1941), 111.
8. Donald W. Winnicott, *The Child, the Family and the Outside World* (Harmondsworth, 1964), 45.
9. Doris Odlum, *You and Your Children: BBC Talks by a Woman Medical Psychologist* (London, 1946), 27-8.
10. "Should Mothers of Young Children Work?" *Ladies Home Journal* 75 (November 1958), 158.
11. Jerry J. Bigner, "Parent Education in Popular Literature: 1950-1970," *The Family Coordinator* 21, no. 3 (1972), 313-319.
12. Donald W. Winnicott, *Getting to Know Your Baby* (London, 1945); Benjamin Spock, *Baby and Child Care* (New York, 1946).
13. Arlie Russell Hochschild, *The Managed Heart: Commercialization of Human Feeling* (Berkeley, 2012); Jean Duncombe and Dennis Marsden, "Love and Intimacy: The Gender Division of Emotion and 'Emotion Work,'" *Sociology* 27, no. 2 (May 1993), 221-241; Kathleen Lynch, "Love Labour as a Distinct and Non-Commodifiable Form of Care Labour," *The Sociological Review* 55, no. 3 (2007), 550-570; Eva Illouz, *Cold Intimacies and the Making of Emotional Capitalism* (Cambridge, 2017); Viviana Zelizer, *The Purchase of Intimacy* (Princeton, 2009).
14. Duncombe and Marsden, "Love and Intimacy," 221.
15. Lynch, "Love Labour as a Distinct and Non-Commodifiable Form of Care Labour," 551.
16. Especially movements like the Wages for Housework Campaign. See Selma James, *Women, the Unions and Work, or ... What is Not to Be Done* (London, 1975).
17. For discussion of this in the US context, see Rebecca Jo Plant, *Mom: The Transformation of Motherhood in Modern America* (Chicago, 2010); Anne Harrington, "Mother Love and Mental Illness: An Emotional History," *Osiris* 31 (2016), 94-115; Molly Ladd-Taylor, *Mother-Work: Women, Child Welfare, and the State, 1890-1930* (Urbana, 1994); Sonya Michel, *Children's Interests/Mother's Rights: The Shaping of America's Child Care Policy* (New Haven, 1999); Molly Ladd-Taylor and Lauri Umansky, eds., *"Bad" Mothers: The Politics of Blame in Twentieth-Century America* (New York, 1998).
18. Betty Friedan noted in *The Feminine Mystique* (New York, 1963) that middle-class housewives increasingly turned to tranquilizers in response to their dissatisfaction. Five years later, sociologist Hugh Parry published a study confirming what Friedan had suspected: women were twice as likely to use tranquilizers as men. See Andrea Tone, *The Age of Anxiety: A History of America's Turbulent Affair with Tranquilizers* (New York, 2008); Jonathan Metzl, "'Mother's Little Helper': The Crisis of Psychoanalysis and the Miltown Resolution," *Gender and History* 15, no. 3 (August 2003), 240-267.
19. Donald W. Winnicott, "A Man Looks at Motherhood," in *The Child, the Family, and the Outside World*, 17 [my emphasis].
20. See Women's Group on Public Welfare, *Our Towns: A Close Up, A Study Made in 1939-1942* (Oxford, 1943).
21. Women's Group on Public Welfare, *The Neglected Child and his Family: A Study made in 1946-7 of the Problem of the Child Neglected in His Own Home* (Oxford, 1948), 16.
22. Women's Group on Public Welfare, *The Neglected Child and his Family*, 16.
23. Women's Group on Public Welfare, *The Neglected Child and his Family*, 23.
24. Women's Group on Public Welfare, *The Neglected Child and his Family*, 22-23
25. Eva Hubback, "Children in Distress," Letter to the Editor, *The Times*, July 14, 1948, 5.

26. Eva Hubback, "Children Neglected in their Own Homes," *The Times*, July 6, 1949, 5.
27. Hubback, "Children Neglected in their Own Homes," 5.
28. Hubback, "Children in Distress," 5.
29. Hubback, "Children Neglected in Their Own Homes," 5.
30. Women's Group on Public Welfare, *The Neglected Child and His Family*, 22. "It is she who stands out eminently as the person who gives the 'temper' to the household. It is her caliber which matters."
31. Women's Group on Public Welfare, *The Neglected Child and His Family*, 16.
32. Women's Group on Public Welfare, *The Neglected Child and His Family*, 106.
33. See John Welshman, "Recuperation, Rehabilitation and the Residential Option: The Brentwood Centre for Mothers and Children," *Twentieth Century British History* 19, no. 4 (2008), 502–529: 522.
34. Doris Abraham, "Brentwood Recuperative Centre: Home for Problem Mothers," *Medical World* 90 (1959), 251–254: 252.
35. Joint Committee of the British Medical Association and the Magistrates' Association, *Cruelty to and Neglect of Children* (London, 1956), 49. Social work was presented as the other solution to child neglect.
36. Abraham, "Brentwood Recuperative Centre," 253.
37. Abraham, "Brentwood Recuperative Centre," 253.
38. Mary D. Sheridan, "The Intelligence of 100 Neglectful Mothers," *British Medical Journal* 1, no. 4959 (January 14 1956), 91–93.
39. Mary D. Sheridan, "Neglectful Mothers," *The Lancet* 1, no. 7075 (April 4, 1959), 722–725.
40. See James Hamilton, "Introduction," in *The New Mother Syndrome: Coping with Stress and Depression*, ed. Carol Dix (Garden City, 1985), xi.
41. T.F. Main, "Mothers with Children on a Psychiatric Unit," in *Psychosocial Nursing*, ed. Elizabeth Barnes (London, 1968), 119–136.
42. Cases of severe psychosis were not admitted at the Cassel because the therapy provided was considered inappropriate to their level of need.
43. T.F. Main et al, *The Cassel Hospital: Reports for the Five Years, 1953–1958* (Surrey, 1958); Doreen Weddell, "Family-Centred Nursing," in *Psychosocial Nursing*, ed. Elizabeth Barnes (London, 1968), 137–142.
44. Main, "Mothers with Children on a Psychiatric Unit," 122.
45. Main, "Mothers with Children on a Psychiatric Unit," 125.
46. Main, "Mothers with Children on a Psychiatric Unit," 122.
47. Ann Oakley, *Housewife* (London, 1974).
48. Tom Main, "A Fragment on Mothering," in *Psychosocial Nursing: Studies from the Cassel Hospital*, ed. Elizabeth Barnes (London, 1968), 147.
49. Main, "A Fragment on Mothering," 148.
50. Imrich Gluck and Margaret Wrenn, "Contribution to the Understanding of the Disturbances of Mothering," *British Journal of Medical Psychology* (September 1959), 171–182: 173.
51. Main, "A Fragment on Mothering," 148–149.
52. Gluck and Wrenn, "Disturbances of Mothering," 171.
53. Main, "A Fragment on Mothering," 147.
54. Main, "A Fragment on Mothering," 154 [my emphasis].

55. Doreen Weddell, "Change of Approach," in *Psychosocial Nursing: Studies from the Cassel Hospital*, ed. Elizabeth Barnes (London, 1968), 61–72: 65.
56. Doreen Weddell, "Outline of Nurse Training," in *Psychosocial Nursing: Studies from the Cassel Hospital*, ed. Elizabeth Barnes (London, 1968), 16–23: 21.
57. Gluck and Wrenn, "Disturbances of Mothering," 171–182.
58. Gluck and Wrenn, "Disturbances of Mothering," 173.
59. Gluck and Wrenn, "Disturbances of Mothering," 173.
60. Gluck and Wrenn, "Disturbances of Mothering," 174.
61. Gluck and Wrenn, "Disturbances of Mothering," 173.
62. Gluck and Wrenn, "Disturbances of Mothering," 178.
63. Gluck and Wrenn, "Disturbances of Mothering," 171.
64. Anne Zachary, "A New Look at the Vulnerability of Puerperal Mothers," *The Family as In-Patient: Families and Adolescents at the Cassel Hospital* (London, 1987), 184–207: 185.
65. R.E. Hemphill, "Incidence and Nature of Puerperal Psychiatric Illness," *BMJ* 2, no. 4796 (December 6, 1952), 1232–1235: 1232.
66. "Puerperal Psychoses," *BMJ* 2, no. 5526 (December 3, 1966), 1342–1343: 1342.
67. Mary Martin, "Puerperal Mental Illness: A Follow-up Study of 75 Cases," *BMJ* 2, no. 5099 (September 27, 1958), 773–777: 773.
68. D. Bardon et al, "Mother and Baby Unit: Psychiatric Survey and 115 Cases," *BMJ* 2, no. 5607 (June 22, 1968), 755–758: 758.
69. T.F. Main, "Cassel Hospital for Functional Nervous Disorders," in "The Expanding Field of Mental Health in England and Wales, ed. Doris Odlum (London, 1968), 6, MS 7913/41, Wellcome Library.
70. "The Hospital with Double Beds," *Evening News*, August 26, 1975.
71. Winnicott, *The Child, the Family and the Outside World*, 26.
72. Arnold Gesell and Frances Ilg, *Infant and Child in the Culture of Today* (New York, 1943), 273.
73. E. James Anthony and Therese Benedek, *Parenthood: Its Psychology and Psychopathology* (Boston, 1970), 179.
74. Winnicott, *The Child, the Family and the Outside World*, 26.
75. Doreen Weddell, "Psychology and Nursing," *Nursing Times*, 51 (1955), 63.
76. Weddell, "Psychology and Nursing," 65.
77. Joint Committee of the British Medical Association and the Magistrates' Association, *Cruelty to and Neglect of Children*, 53.
78. William Beveridge, *Social Insurance and the Allied Services* (London, 1942), 53 [my emphasis].
79. Beveridge, *Social Insurance and the Allied Services*, 49–52.
80. Beveridge, *Social Insurance and the Allied Services*, 52.
81. William Beveridge, *Voluntary Action: A Report on Methods of Social Advance* (London, 1948), 264–265.
82. Pat Thane notes that unmarried mothers, on the other hand, benefited from the welfare state. See Pat Thane and Tanya Evans, *Sinners? Scroungers? Saints?: Unmarried Motherhood in Twentieth-Century England* (Oxford, 2012), 107.
83. Susan Pedersen, *Family, Dependence, and the Origins of the Welfare State: Britain and France, 1914–1945* (Cambridge, 1993).
84. See Riley, *War in the Nursery*, 154.

85. Married Women's Association, "Lobbying Activities," 5MWA/6, Married Women's Association Papers, Women's Library.
86. Married Women's Association, "Lobbying Activities," 5MWA/6, Women's Library.
87. Married Women's Property Act 1964, Chapter 19, https://www.legislation.gov.uk/ukpga/1964/19/pdfs/ukpga_19640019_en.pdf?view=extent.
88. Krista Cowman, *Women in British Politics, c.1689–1979* (Basingstoke, 2010), 167.
89. Talcott Parsons and Robert F. Bales, *Family Socialization and Interaction Process* (Glencoe IL, 1955), 51.
90. "Should Mothers of Young Children Work?" *Ladies Home Journal*, November 1958, 159.
91. "Should Mothers of Young Children Work?" 159.
92. "Should Mothers of Young Children Work?" 159.
93. "Should Mothers of Young Children Work?" 159.
94. "Should Mothers of Young Children Work?" 160.
95. "Should Mothers of Young Children Work?" 159.
96. John Newson and Elizabeth Newson, *Infant Care in an Urban Community* (London, 1963), 49–50: 210. Peter Willmott and Michael Young similarly found "Mum" to have a strong presence in all her extended family's lives in the working-class London borough of Bethnal Green. See Michael Young and Peter Willmott, *Family and Kinship in East London* (London, 1957); Lise Butler, "Michael Young, the Institute of Community Studies, and the Politics of Kinship," *Twentieth Century British History* 26, no. 2 (May 2015), 203–224.
97. Newson and Newson, *Infant Care in an Urban Community*, 209–210.
98. Young and Willmott, *Family and Kinship in East London*, 190–191.
99. Young and Willmott, *Family and Kinship in East London*, 61.
100. Peter Lomas, "The Husband-Wife Relationship in Cases of Puerperal Breakdown," *British Journal of Medical Psychology* 32, no. 2 (1959), 117–123: 117.
101. Alva Myrdal and Viola Klein, *Women's Two Roles* (London, 1956).
102. Duncombe and Marsden, "Love and Intimacy." See also Jane Lewis, ed., *Gender, Social Care and Welfare State Restructuring in Europe* (Aldershot, 1998).
103. Lynch, "Love Labour as a Distinct and Non-Commodifiable Form of Care Labour," 550.
104. Notable examples include Eileen Skellern, Doreen Weddell, Gillian Elles, Elizabeth Barnes, Dame Elizabeth Cockayne, and J.R. Rees.
105. Olga Franklin, *Daily Mail*, November 4, 1958, 5.
106. *The Woman's Mirror*, July 22, 1960. Similarly, an article in *The Evening News* (August 26, 1975) noted the homely feel of the Cassel hospital and its grounds: "The site of the hospital is a beautiful spot. There are tennis courts and workrooms for pottery and painting. There is a rumpus room for small children. 'We try to make it seem more like home than an institution,' said a sister, apologising for toys not tidied away and a child's bed unmade. The fathers have made a small children's playground with swings and a sand pit. Other patients have taken over the painting and decor." "Newspaper cuttings," Cassel Hospital Papers [uncatalogued], PETT.
107. Franklin, *Daily Mail*, 6.
108. Franklin, *Daily Mail*, 6.
109. Departmental Committee on Human Artificial Insemination, *Report of the Departmental Committee on Human Artificial Insemination* (London, 1960), 39.

Chapter 4

1. E.F. Griffith, *International Congress on Mental Health, London 1948, volume 4* (London, 1948), 172.
2. Griffith, *International Congress on Mental Health*, 172.
3. Griffith, *International Congress on Mental Health*, 173.
4. The Feversham Committee, *The Voluntary Mental Health Services: The Report of the Feversham Committee* (London, 1939), 53–54.
5. The term "depth psychology" refers to all forms of psychological therapy and research that posit the existence of an unconscious mind.
6. National Marriage Guidance Council, *Counsellor Basic Training Prospectus* (London, 1985).
7. William Beveridge, *Social Insurance and Allied Services* (London, 1942) 8; T.H. Marshall, *Citizenship and Social Class* (Cambridge, 1950).
8. See Claire Langhamer, *The English in Love: The Intimate Story of an Emotional Revolution* (Oxford, 2013); Anthony Giddens, *The Transformation of Intimacy: Sexuality, Love, and Eroticism in Modern Societies* (Stanford, 1992).
9. Shaul Bar-Haim, *The Maternalists: Psychoanalysis, Motherhood, and the British Welfare State* (Philadelphia, 2021); Jonathan Toms, "Political Dimensions of 'the Psychosocial': The 1948 International Congress on Mental Health and the Mental Hygiene Movement," *History of the Human Sciences* 25, no. 5 (2012), 91–106; Rhodri Hayward, "The Invention of the Psychosocial: An Introduction," *History of the Human Sciences* 25, no. 5 (2012), 3–12; Michael E. Staub, *Madness Is Civilization: When the Diagnosis Was Social, 1948–1980* (Chicago, 2011); Suzanne Stewart-Steinberg, *Impious Fidelity: Anna Freud, Psychoanalysis, Politics* (Ithaca, 2011); Michal Shapira, *The War Inside: Psychoanalysis, Total War, and the Making of the Democratic Self in Postwar Britain* (Cambridge, 2013); Denise Riley, *War in the Nursery: Theories of the Child and Mother* (London, 1983); Mathew Thomson, *Psychological Subjects: Identity, Culture, and Health in Twentieth-Century Britain* (Oxford, 2006); Camille Robcis, *The Law of Kinship: Anthropology, Psychoanalysis, and the Family in France* (Ithaca, 2013); Dagmar Herzog, *Cold War Freud: Psychoanalysis in an Age of Catastrophes* (Cambridge, 2017); Eli Zaretsky, *Political Freud: A History* (New York, 2015); Ellen Herman, *The Romance of American Psychology: Political Culture in the Age of Experts* (Berkeley, 1995).
10. Hera Cook, *The Long Sexual Revolution: English Women, Sex and Contraception, 1800–1975* (Oxford, 2004); Janet Finch, "The State and the Family," in *Families and the State: Changing Relationships*, eds. Sarah Cunningham-Burley and Lynn Jamieson (London, 2003), 29–45; Jane Lewis, *The End of Marriage? Individualism and Intimate Relations* (Cheltenham, 2001); Langhamer, *The English in Love*; Giddens, *The Transformation of Intimacy*, 184–204.
11. Eva Illouz, *Saving the Modern Soul: Therapy, Emotions, and the Culture of Self-Help* (Berkeley, 2008).
12. See, for example, Illouz, *Saving the Modern Soul*; Laura Kipnis, *Against Love: A Polemic* (New York, 2003); Wendy Langford, *Revolutions of the Heart: Gender, Power, and the Delusions of Love* (London, 2002); Lauren Berlant and Michael Warner, "Sex in Public," in *Intimacy*, ed. Lauren Berlant (Chicago, 2000), 311–330.
13. For example, Helena Wright, *The Sex Factor in Marriage: A Book For Those Who Are or Are About to Be Married* (London, 1932); Marie Carmichael Stopes, *Married Love: A New Contribution to the Solution of Sex Difficulties* (London, 1918); Marie Carmichael Stopes, *Marriage in My Time* (London, 1935).

14. Stopes, *Married Love*, xvii.
15. Stopes, *Married Love*, 68–70.
16. Edward Fyfe Griffith, *A Sex Guide to Happy Marriage* (New York, 1952) [1935], 46.
17. Edward Fyfe Griffith, *Sex and Citizenship* (London, 1941), 202–203.
18. Alexander C. T. Geppert, "Divine Sex, Happy Marriage, Regenerated Nation: Marie Stopes' Marital Manual Married Love and the Making of a Best-Seller, 1918–1955," *Journal of the History of Sexuality* 8, no. 3 (1998), 389–433: 396.
19. Edward Fyfe Griffith, *Modern Marriage*, 19th edition (London, 1946).
20. Barbara Evans, *Freedom to Choose: The Life and Work of Dr. Helena Wright, Pioneer of Contraception* (London, 1984), 154.
21. Edward F. Griffith, *The Pioneer Spirit* (Upton Grey, 1981), 75–77.
22. See Edward F. Griffith, *Modern Marriage and Birth Control* (London, 1937); Edward F. Griffith, *Voluntary Parenthood* (London, 1937).
23. Stopes, *Married Love*, vii.
24. Wendy Kline describes similar developments in the United States in the 1930s, noting that Paul Popenoe incorporated marriage counseling as part of a eugenic program focused on family stability. Wendy Kline, *Building a Better Race: Gender, Sexuality, and Eugenics from the Turn of the Century to the Baby Boom* (Berkeley, 2001). See also Kristin Celello, *Making Marriage Work: A History of Marriage and Divorce in the Twentieth-Century United States* (Chapel Hill, 2009); Rebecca Davis, *More Perfect Unions: The American Search for Marital Bliss* (Cambridge, 2010).
25. "Memorandum on the work of the Marriage Guidance Council," PP/EFG/A.10, Wellcome Library.
26. Marriage Guidance Council, "To Those About to Marry," 1938, PP/EFG/A.12, Wellcome Library.
27. Marriage Guidance Council, "1938 Annual Report," 4, PP/EFG/A.8, Wellcome Library.
28. Marriage Guidance Council, "1938 Annual Report," 4.
29. David Mace, *Marriage Counselling* (London, 1948).
30. Marriage Guidance Council, "1943 Annual Report," 4, PP/EFG/A.12, Wellcome Library.
31. Marriage Guidance Council, "1943 Annual Report," 4.
32. David Mace, "Marriage Guidance in England," *Marriage and Family Living* 7, no.1 (February 1945), 1–5: 2.
33. "Marriage Guidance Council correspondence 1942," PP/EFG/A.10.
34. "Proposed Institute of Marriage and Parenthood," September 1941, PP/EFG/A.8.
35. In 1947, the expanding network of local councils was centralized under the National Marriage Guidance Council. J.H. Wallis and H.S. Booker, *Marriage Counselling: A Description and Analysis of the Remedial Work of the National Marriage Guidance Council* (London, 1958), 6.
36. In 1940, 25,633 out-of-wedlock births had been registered; 55,173 were registered in 1944. While 39,350 infants were born within the first seven months of marriage in 1940, four years later this number had fallen to 27,966. See Kathleen Kiernan, Hilary Land, and Jane Lewis, *Lone Motherhood in Twentieth-Century Britain* (Oxford, 1998), 27–28.
37. "A Welfare Service Proposed," *The Guardian*, February 6, 1947, 5.
38. Lord Denning, *Final Report of the Committee on Procedure in Matrimonial Causes* (London, 1947), 12.
39. Denning, *Final Report of the Committee on Procedure in Matrimonial Causes*, 13.

40. Denning, *Final Report of the Committee on Procedure in Matrimonial Causes*, 13 [my emphasis].
41. See Anna Freud and Dorothy Burlingham, *Infants without Families: The Case for and Against Residential Nurseries* (London, 1943); Susan Isaacs, ed., *The Cambridge Evacuation Survey* (London, 1941); Richard Padley and Margaret Cole, eds., *Evacuation Survey: A Report to the Fabian Society* (London, 1940); Katherine Wolf, "Evacuation of Children in Wartime," *Psychoanalytic Study of the Child* 1 (1945), 389–404.
42. Denning, *Final Report of the Committee on Procedure in Matrimonial Causes*, 5.
43. Sir Sidney Harris, *Report of the Departmental Committee on Grants for the Development of Marriage Guidance* (London, 1948), 5.
44. See Rudolf Dreikurs, "Group Psychotherapy and the Third Revolution in Psychiatry," *International Journal of Social Psychiatry* 1, no. 3 (1955), 23–32.
45. Robert N. Rapoport, *Community as Doctor: New Perspectives on a Therapeutic Community* (London, 1960).
46. A national Marriage Guidance Training Board was also formed in 1949. Harris, *Report of the Departmental Committee on Grants for the Development of Marriage Guidance*, 11.
47. Harris, *Report of the Departmental Committee on Grants for the Development of Marriage Guidance*, 10.
48. Henry V. Dicks, "The Mental Hygiene of Married Life" (1950), PP/HVD/D/1/2, Wellcome Library. See also Henry V. Dicks, "Clinical Studies in Marriage and the Family: A Symposium on Methods," *The British Journal of Medical Psychology* 26, no. 3 (1953), 181–196.
49. Henry Dicks, *Marital Tensions: Clinical Studies towards a Psychological Theory of Interaction* (New York, 1967), 45.
50. Christopher Clulow, "Enid Balint obituary," TCCR Archives [uncatalogued]. Eichholtz married Tavistock psychoanalyst Michael Balint in 1953, and the bulk of her work was published under Enid Balint.
51. Clulow, "Enid Balint obituary."
52. Enid Balint, "The Nature of an Effective Marriage Counselling Service," January 25, 1955, TCCR Archives [uncatalogued].
53. Kathleen Bannister, Alison Lyons, Lily Pincus, James Robb, Antonia Shooter, and Judith Stephens, *Social Casework in Marital Problems: The Development of a Psychodynamic Approach* (London, 1955), 83–93.
54. Dicks, *Marital Tensions*, 86–88.
55. Bannister et al, *Social Casework in Marital Problems*, 89.
56. Bannister et al, *Social Casework in Marital Problems*, 91.
57. Bannister et al, *Social Casework in Marital Problems*, 78.
58. Lily Pincus, ed. *Marriage: Studies in Emotional Conflict and Growth* (London, 1960), 5.
59. Joan King, *The Probation Service* (London, 1958), 47.
60. The cross-class phenomenon of marriage breakdown had also been noticed by many during the war, when financial provisions for divorce proceedings were made available to members of the armed forces. See House of Lords Debate, "Legal Aid and Advice Bill," 27 June 1949, vol. 163 col. 304–342.
61. Dicks, *Marital Tensions*, 68.
62. King, *The Probation Service*, 122–127.
63. King, *The Probation Service*, 68.

64. Mace, *Marriage Counselling*, 10 [emphasis is mine].
65. Mace, *Marriage Counselling*, 10.
66. Mace, *Marriage Counselling*, 23.
67. NMGC counselors were typically middle-aged, married housewives. Many had received a university education in social work or an allied field before marriage.
68. See, for example, David Mace, "What I Have Learned about Family Life," *The Family Coordinator* (April 1974), 189.
69. Family Planning Association (FPA), *Family Planning in the Sixties: Report of the Family Planning Association Working Party*, chapter 7, page 24. PP/AWD/H/7/8, Wellcome Library.
70. FPA, *Family Planning in the Sixties*, chapter 1, page 7.
71. FPA, *Family Planning in the Sixties*, chapter 7, page 24.
72. J.D. Sutherland, "Introduction," in *Social Casework in Marital Problems: The Development of a Psychodynamic Approach*, eds. Kathleen Bannister et al (London, 1955), ix.
73. Wallis and Booker, *Marriage Counselling*, 138.
74. Wallis and Booker, *Marriage Counselling*, 138.
75. Jan Goldstein, *The Post-Revolutionary Self: Politics and Psyche in France, 1750–1850* (Cambridge, 2005), 4.
76. Goldstein, *The Post-Revolutionary Self*, 7.
77. Pincus, *Marriage: Studies in Emotional Conflict and Growth*, 34.
78. Pincus, *Marriage: Studies in Emotional Conflict and Growth*, vii.
79. T.F. Main, "Mutual Projection in a Marriage," *Comprehensive Psychiatry* 7, no. 5 (1966), 445.
80. Pincus, *Marriage: Studies in Emotional Conflict and Growth*, 17.
81. Pincus, *Marriage: Studies in Emotional Conflict and Growth*, 17.
82. T.F. Main, "A Theory of Marriage and Its Technical Applications," in Jennifer Johns ed., *The Ailment and Other Psychoanalytic Essays* (London, 1989), 77. Mr. and Mrs. Adams were pseudonyms given to the couple.
83. Main, "Mutual Projection in a Marriage," 447.
84. Main, "Mutual Projection in a Marriage," 444–445.
85. Main, "Mutual Projection in a Marriage," 452.
86. Pincus, *Marriage: Studies in Emotional Conflict and Growth*, 121.
87. Pincus, *Marriage: Studies in Emotional Conflict and Growth*, 113.
88. Pincus, *Marriage: Studies in Emotional Conflict and Growth*, 137.
89. Pincus, *Marriage: Studies in Emotional Conflict and Growth*, 55.
90. Bannister et al, *Social Casework in Marital Problems*, 82.
91. Nancy Holt, *Counselling in Marriage Problems* (London, 1971), 74.
92. Drusilla Beyfus, *The English Marriage* (London, 1968).
93. Holt, *Counselling in Marriage Problems*, 6.
94. For example, David Mace, "An English Advice Column," *Marriage and Family Living* 12, no. 3 (August 1950): 100–102; David Mace, *Coming Home: A Series of Five Broadcast Talks* (London, 1946).
95. A.P. Herbert, *Holy Deadlock* (London, 1934).
96. "Divorce," *The Guardian*, November 24, 1950, 8.
97. Elaine Grand, "Miserable Married Women," *Observer*, May 7, 1961, 34 [original emphasis].
98. "What Makes Marriage Sacred," *The Guardian*, May 2, 1964, 3.
99. Gillian Tindall, "A Shoulder to Cry On," *The Guardian*, August 1, 1968, 7.

100. Tindall, "A Shoulder to Cry On," 7.
101. Tindall, "A Shoulder to Cry On," 7.
102. Ann Shearer, "Analysing the Answers," *The Guardian*, February 7, 1968, 7.
103. "Mr. Abse Bows to Divorce Storm: 7 Year Clause Goes," *The Guardian*, May 4, 1963, 2.
104. Leo Abse, *Private Member* (London, 1973), 161–162.
105. Abse, *Private Member*, 162.
106. "The Churches and Divorce," *The Times*, April 3, 1963.
107. House of Lords Debate, 22 May 1963, "Matrimonial Causes and Reconciliation Bill," vol. 250 col. 389.
108. House of Commons Debate, "Matrimonial Proceedings Bill," 23 March 1960, vol. 620 col. 525.
109. House of Commons Debate, "Matrimonial Proceedings Bill," 23 March 1960, vol. 620 col. 525.
110. O.R. McGregor, "Towards Divorce Law Reform," *British Journal of Sociology* 18 (1967): 91–99.
111. Archbishop of Canterbury's Group on the Divorce Law, *Putting Asunder: A Divorce Law for Contemporary Society* (London, 1966), 142.
112. Archbishop of Canterbury's Group on the Divorce Law, *Putting Asunder*, 142.
113. House of Commons Debate, "Divorce Reform Bill," 9 February 1968, vol. 758 col. 810.
114. House of Commons Debate, "Divorce Reform Bill," 9 February 1968, vol. 758 col. 812.
115. "First Divorce Law Change in 30 Years?" *The Guardian*, April 5, 1969, 3.
116. House of Lords Debate, "Matrimonial Causes and Reconciliation Bill," 22 May 1963, vol. 250 col. 397.
117. "Reply to Church Critics," *The Guardian*, May 23, 1963, 2.
118. "Bishops Split over Divorce Bill," *The Guardian*, July 1, 1969, 1.
119. "Protecting First Wives' Pensions," *The Guardian*, January 17, 1969, 20.
120. "Bishops Split over Divorce Bill," 1.
121. Abse, *Private Member*, 180.
122. In his memoir, *Private Member*, Abse invoked Freud when describing this phase of his political career as his "tryst with Eros."
123. Mary Stott, "Looking Back on 10 years of Liberal Divorce Laws," *The Guardian*, September 26, 1979, 10.
124. Geoffrey Gorer, *Sex and Marriage in England Today: A Study of the Views and Experience of the Under-45s* (London, 1971), 84–85.
125. Gorer, *Sex and Marriage in England Today*, 2.
126. Gorer, *Sex and Marriage in England Today*, 149.
127. Pat Thane, "The 'Scandal' of Women's Pensions in Britain: How Did It Come About?" in *Britain's Pensions Crisis History and Policy*, eds. Hugh Pemberton et al (Oxford, 2006), 76–90.
128. "Woman's Guardian," *The Guardian*, July 16, 1973, 9.
129. Institute of Marital Studies, "Marriage Study," 1971, TCCR Archives [uncatalogued].
130. This phrasing was first used in Ernest W. Burgess and Harvey V. Locke, *The Family, from Institution to Companionship* (New York, 1945).
131. Kiernan, Land, and Lewis, *Lone Motherhood in Twentieth-Century Britain*, 63.

132. Michel Foucault, *Discipline and Punish: The Birth of the Prison* (New York, 1977); Michel Foucault, *Madness and Civilization: A History of Insanity in the Age of Reason* (London, 1961).
133. Giddens, *The Transformation of Intimacy*, 58.
134. See Cook, *The Long Sexual Revolution*; Langhamer, *The English in Love*; Jeffrey Weeks, *The World We Have Won: The Remaking of Erotic and Intimate Life* (London, 2007).
135. "Marriage À La Mode," *The Guardian*, 20 August 20, 1987, 8.
136. See Davis, *More Perfect Unions*.
137. Susan Pedersen, *Family Dependence and the Origins of the Welfare State* (Cambridge, 1993); Sarah Cunningham-Burley and Lynn Jamieson, eds., *Families and the State* (London, 2003).

Chapter 5

1. House of Lords Debate, "Homosexual Offences and Prostitution," 4 December 1957, vol. 206 col. 764.
2. Antony Grey, *Quest for Justice: Towards Homosexual Emancipation* (London, 1992), 31–32.
3. "Homosexual Says 'Sense of Shame' is Lifted," *The Guardian*, September 16 1967, 3.
4. "Homosexual Says 'Sense of Shame' is Lifted," 3.
5. "Senior Counsellor's Correspondence," HCA/AT/7/165, Hall-Carpenter Archives.
6. A total of 301,939 calls received since March 4, 1974.
7. "Friend Pamphlet," 1978, HCA/Lewisham Friend/2, Hall-Carpenter Archives.
8. See, for example, Jeffrey Weeks *Coming Out: Homosexual Politics in Britain from the Nineteenth Century to the Present* (London, 1977); Jeffrey Weeks, *The World That We Have Won: The Remaking of Erotic and Intimate Life* (London, 2007); Grey, *Quest for Justice*; Tommy Avicolli Mecca, *Smash the Church, Smash the State! The Early Years of Gay Liberation* (San Francisco, 2009).
9. Weeks, *Coming Out*, 158: "In 1938 there were 134 cases of sodomy and bestiality known to the police in England and Wales, in 1952, 670, and in 1954, 1,043. For indecent assault, the increase was from 822 cases in 1938 to 3,305 in 1953, while for 'gross indecency' (the Labouchere offence) the rise was from 316 in 1938 to 2,322 in 1955." There was thus a seven-fold increase for "gross indecency" in contrast to the four-fold increase in the number of sexual crimes that were not specifically homosexual in nature.
10. Frank Mort, "Mapping Sexual London: The Wolfenden Committee on Homosexual Offences and Prostitution," *New Formations* 37 (1999): 92–113.
11. Committee on Homosexual Offences and Prostitution, *Report of the Committee on Homosexual Offenses and Prostitution* (London, 1957), 42–43.
12. See Callum Brown, *The Death of Christian Britain: Understanding Secularisation, 1800–2000* (London, 2009).
13. House of Lords Debate, "Homosexual Offences and Prostitution," 4 December 1957, vol. 206 col. 753.
14. Patrick Devlin, *The Enforcement of Morals*. 1959 Maccabean Lecture in Jurisprudence (Oxford, 1959).
15. John Wolfenden, *Turning Points: The Memoirs of Lord Wolfenden* (London, 1976), 131.
16. Harry Cocks, "Conspiracy to Corrupt Public Morals and the 'Unlawful' Status of Homosexuality in Britain after 1967," *Social History* 41, no. 3 (2016): 267–284.

17. See J.E. Hall Williams, "The Ladies' Directory and Criminal Conspiracy the Judge as *Custos Morum,*" *The Modern Law Review* 24, no. 5 (September 1961), 626–631.
18. H.L.A. Hart, *Law, Liberty and Morality* (Stanford, 1963), 22.
19. Hart, *Law, Liberty and Morality*, 22 [my emphasis].
20. See Cathy Gere, *Pain, Pleasure, and the Greater Good: From the Panopticon to the Skinner Box and Beyond* (Chicago, 2017).
21. Cited in Grey, *Quest for Justice*, 125–126.
22. Published discussions of the Hart-Devlin debate overwhelmingly sided with Hart. Alexander Irvine, "Homosexuality," *Spectator*, August 7, 1964, 181–182; Alan Ryan, "Judges, Stick to Your Bench," *New Society* March 25, 1965, 25–26; Richard Wollheim, "The Case of the Ladies Directory," *New Statesman*, June 28, 1963, 976.
23. Grey, *Quest for Justice*, 38–39.
24. Weeks, *Coming Out*, 176.
25. "Church Assembly Split on Homosexuality: Debate on Wolfenden Report," *The Guardian*, November 15, 1957, 14.
26. House of Lords Debate, "Homosexual Offences and Prostitution," 4 December 1957, vol. 206 col. 764. Available at: https://api.parliament.uk/historic-hansard/lords/1957/dec/04/homosexual-offences-and-prostitution-1.
27. Sarah Igo, *The Known Citizen: A History of Privacy in Modern America* (Cambridge MA, 2018), 3.
28. "Homosexual Acts: Call to Reform Law," *The Times*, March 7, 1958, 11.
29. "Homosexual Acts: Call to Reform Law," 11.
30. Antony Grey, "English Attitudes to Homosexuality," in *Speaking Out: Writings on Sex, Law, Politics, and Society* (London, 1997), 75 [originally a talk given to the Dutch Cultuur en Ontspanningscentrum (COC) in April 1963].
31. Grey, "English Attitudes to Homosexuality," 75.
32. Albany Trust, "Homosexuality: Proposals for Social Action," HCA/AT/10/3, Hall-Carpenter Archives.
33. See Tommy Dickinson, *"Curing Queers": Mental Nurses and Their Patients, 1935–74* (Manchester, 2015).
34. Grey, *Quest for Justice*, 65.
35. Antony Grey, *The Albany Trust and Its Work* (London, 1971).
36. Antony Grey, "Albany Trust: Casework," 1966, HCA/Grey/2/5, London: Hall-Carpenter Archives.
37. See Henry Minton, *Departing from Deviance: A History of Homosexual Rights and Emancipatory Science in America* (Chicago, 2002); Harry Oosterhuis, *Stepchildren of Nature: Krafft-Ebing, Psychiatry, and the Making of Sexual Identity* (Chicago, 2000).
38. Committee on Homosexual Offences and Prostitution, *Report of the Committee on Homosexual Offenses and Prostitution*, 109.
39. Albany Trust, "Malik Survey," 1963–64, HCA/AT/10/3, Hall-Carpenter Archives.
40. Albany Trust, "Malik Survey."
41. David Mace, *Marriage Counselling* (London, 1948).
42. Grey, "English Attitudes to Homosexuality," 78.
43. Albany Trust, "Homosexuality: Proposals for Social Action," HCA/AT/10/3.
44. Grey, *Quest for Justice*, 2

45. Chris Waters, "The Homosexual as a Social Being in Britain, 1945–1968," *Journal of British Studies* 51, no. 3 (December 2012), 705.
46. Michael Schofield, *Sociological Aspects of Homosexuality* (London, 1965).
47. Schofield, *Sociological Aspects of Homosexuality*, 175.
48. Schofield, *Sociological Aspects of Homosexuality*, 173.
49. Albany Trust, "Enquiries," 1966, HCA/AT/15/7, Hall-Carpenter Archives.
50. Clients and counselors have been given pseudonyms to protect their identities.
51. Grey, "Albany Trust: Casework."
52. Grey, "Albany Trust: Casework."
53. Grey, *Quest for Justice*, 147.
54. Grey, *Quest for Justice*, 147.
55. Albany Trust, "Trustees Meeting, 25 May 1976," HCA/AT/10/10, Hall-Carpenter Archives.
56. Albany Trust, "British Sex Research Institute Correspondence," 1969–70, HCA/AT/7/65, Hall-Carpenter Archives.
57. Albany Trust, "1968 Proposal for £100,000 for a Three-year Sex Programme of Research, Education and Social Action," HCA/AT/7/52, Hall-Carpenter Archives.
58. Like the trust's proposed psychosexual out-patient clinic (1964), its proposed British Sex Research Institute (1968–69) never received the funding needed for it to be launched.
59. Albany Trust, "Research Projects," 1968–70, HCA/AT/7/52, Hall-Carpenter Archives.
60. This grant was set at £10,000 for 1974 and 1975 and then increased to £12,000 per year until it was revoked by Prime Minister Margaret Thatcher in 1978–1979 following a controversy—initiated by Mary Whitehouse—over the Albany Trust's alleged support of pedophiles.
61. The CHE, unlike the GLF, has been described as an "organization" rather than a "movement" (see Weeks, *Coming Out*). Politically situated mid-way between the Albany Trust and the GLF, which was radically democratic and anti-establishment, the CHE, from its origins in 1964, wanted to see more social facilities and meeting places for queer men (primarily) and women. In the 1970s, the CHE was the largest and longest running activist organization campaigning for social change for queer men and women.
62. Friend, "Friend Advertising," HCA/Friend/3/1, Hall-Carpenter Archives.
63. Friend, "Friend Advertising."
64. Friend, "Counselling," HCA/Friend/3/2, Hall-Carpenter Archives.
65. Homosexuality would not be removed from the *Diagnostic and Statistical Manual of Mental Disorders* until 1973.
66. Weeks, *Coming Out*, 180 [my emphasis].
67. Lauren Berlant, "Intimacy: A Special Issue," in *Intimacy*, ed. Lauren Berlant (Chicago, 2000), 2.
68. Friend, "Counselling," 1971–79, HCA/Friend/3/2.
69. Friend, "Counselling," HCA/Friend/3/2.
70. Friend, "Counselling Correspondence," 1979, HCA/Friend/3/3, Hall-Carpenter Archives.
71. Friend, "Counselling Correspondence," 1980, HCA/Friend/3/5, Hall-Carpenter Archives.
72. Friend, "Counselling Correspondence," 1980–82, HCA/Friend/3/5.
73. Friend, "Counselling Correspondence," 1980–82, HCA/Friend/3/5.
74. Friend, "Counselling," 1979, HCA/Friend/3/2.
75. Friend, "Counselling," 1979, HCA/Friend/3/2.
76. Friend, "Counselling," 1979, HCA/Friend/3/2.

77. Friend, "Counselling," 1979, HCA/Friend/3/2.
78. Friend, "Counselling," 1979, HCA/Friend/3/2.
79. David Halperin, *How to Be Gay* (Cambridge, 2012), 5–6.
80. Halperin, *How to Be Gay*, 13.
81. Friend, "Counselling," 1971–79, HCA/Friend/3/2.
82. Friend, "Counselling Correspondence," 1980–82, HCA/Friend/3/5.
83. Friend, "Counselling Correspondence," 1980, HCA/Friend/3/5.
84. Friend, "Counselling Correspondence," 1980, HCA/Friend/3/5.
85. Friend, "Counselling Correspondence," 1980, HCA/Friend/3/5.
86. Friend, "Counselling Correspondence," 1980, HCA/Friend/3/5.
87. Friend, "Counselling Correspondence," 1978, HCA/Friend/3/2.
88. "Correspondence regarding Albany Trust Opposition to Evangelical Christian Counselling," HCA/AT/7/149, 1977–84, Hall-Carpenter Archives.
89. T.D. Vaughan, "Concepts (I)," in *Concepts of Counselling*, ed. T.D. Vaughan (London, 1975), 10–22: 14.
90. Bill Logan, "Weaving New Stories Over the Phone: A Narrative Approach to a Gay Switchboard," in *Queer Counselling and Narrative Practice*, ed. D. Denborough (Adelaide, 2002), 138–159: 140.
91. Christopher Behan, "A Reflection," in *Queer Counselling and Narrative Practice*, ed. D. Denborough (Adelaide, 2002), 162–166: 163.
92. For a broader discussion of how counselors might use counseling for social change, see Vaughan, *Concepts of Counselling*, 17–18.

Chapter 6

1. "For the Protection of Adolescents," *The Times*, March 10, 1976, 15.
2. "For the Protection of Adolescents," 15.
3. "For the Protection of Adolescents," 15.
4. P.E. Brown and P.K. Poppleton, "Age of Consent," *The Times*, March 20, 1976, 15.
5. K.M. Fox, "Age of Consent," *The Times*, April 1, 1976, 17.
6. Helen Waldax, "Age of Consent, *The Times*, June 26, 1976, 15.
7. See J.M. Tanner, *Growth at Adolescence* (Oxford, 1962).
8. Policy Advisory Committee on Sexual Offences, *Working Paper* on the Age of Consent in Relation to Sexual Offences. London, 1979, 7.
9. Committee on Homosexual Offences and Prostitution, *Report of the Committee on Homosexual Offences and Prostitution* (London, 1957), 24.
10. Lord Chancellor Gerald Gardiner, "Age of Majority: Memo by Lord Chancellor," 23 October 1967, CAB/129/133, The National Archives, UK.
11. G. Stanley Hall, *Adolescence: Its Psychology and Its Relation to Physiology, Anthropology, Sociology, Sex, Crime, Religion, and Education* (New York, 1904), xiii; Sigmund Freud, "The Transformation of Puberty," in *Three Essays on the Theory of Sexuality*, translated by James Strachey (London, 1905), 73–96.
12. Freud, *Three Essays on the Theory of Sexuality*, 73–96.
13. Jeffrey P. Moran, *Teaching Sex: The Shaping of Adolescence in the 20th Century* (Cambridge, 2000); Pamela Horn, *Young Offenders: Juvenile Delinquency, 1700–2000* (Stroud, 2010).

14. See John Stewart, *Child Guidance in Britain* (London, 2013); Michal Shapira, *The War Inside: Psychoanalysis, Total War, and the Making of the Democratic Self in Postwar Britain* (Cambridge, 2013).
15. Horn, *Young Offenders*, 183–184; Melanie Tebbutt, *Making Youth: A History of Youth in Modern Britain* (London, 2016), 61.
16. Horn, *Young Offenders*, 183.
17. Sidney F. Hatton, *London's Bad Boys* (London, 1931), 29.
18. Basil Henriques, *The Indiscretions of a Warden* (London, 1950), 180.
19. Henry Wilson, "The Early Diagnosis of Schizophrenia," *BMJ* 1, no. 4721 (June 30 1951), 1502–1504; "Problems of Adolescence," *BMJ* 1, no. 5168 (January 23, 1960), 26–28; Doris Odlum, *Journey Through Adolescence* (London, 1957), 27.
20. "Crisis at Adolescence," *The Lancet* 1, no. 7488 (March 4, 1967), 486.
21. Anna Freud, "Adolescence," *The Psychoanalytic Study of the Child* 13 (1958), 255–278: 261; Moses Laufer, "A Psychoanalytical Approach to Work with Adolescents," *Psychotherapy and Psychosomatics* 12 (1965), 294.
22. John Evans, "Psychotherapy for Adolescents," February 15, 1977, HCA/JCGT/1/1, Hall-Carpenter Archives.
23. Michael Staub, *Madness Is Civilization: When the Diagnosis Was Social, 1948–1980* (Chicago, 2011).
24. Laufer, "A Psychoanalytical Approach to Work with Adolescents"; Doreen Martin, "The Beginnings of the Growth and Development of an Adolescent Unit in the Cassel Hospital," *Psychotherapy and Psychosomatics* 13, no. 4 (1965): 309–313.
25. Anne Jones, *Counselling Adolescents: School and After* (London, 1984), 17–18.
26. Anne Jones, *School Counselling in Practice* (London, 1970), 102.
27. Gordon Stewart Prince, *Teenagers Today* (London, 1968).
28. Odlum, *Journey Through Adolescence*, 8.
29. Prince, *Teenagers Today*.
30. See National Marriage Guidance Council, *Your Teenagers: Help with Parents' Problems* (London, 1965); Odlum, *Journey Through Adolescence*; Prince, *Teenagers Today*.
31. Freud, "Adolescence," 266. Michael Rutter, *Changing Youth in a Changing Society: Patterns of Adolescent Development and Disorder* (London, 1979), 43.
32. Odlum, *Journey Through Adolescence*, 85.
33. Odlum, *Journey Through Adolescence*, 92.
34. Tanner, *Growth at Adolescence*.
35. National Marriage Guidance Council, *Your Teenagers: Help with Parents' Problems*, 10.
36. Margaret White and Jennet Kidd, *Sound Sex Education: A Handbook for Parents, Teachers, and Education Authorities* (London, 1976), 21.
37. Odlum, *Journey Through Adolescence*, 142–144; Alan H.B. Ingleby, *Learning to Love: A Wider View of Sex Education* (London, 1961), 109.
38. Marion Hilliard, *Problems of Adolescence: A Woman Doctor's Advice on Growing Up* (London, 1958), 10–11.
39. Ingleby, *Learning to Love*, 108–109.
40. Ingleby, *Learning to Love*, 108–109.
41. Odlum, *Journey Through Adolescence*, 125.
42. Odlum, *Journey Through Adolescence*, 125.

43. See Michael Schofield, *The Sexual Behaviour of Young People* (London, 1965); Royal Society of Health, *Sex Education of School Children* (London, 1971); Nicholas Tyndall, ed., *Sex Education in Perspective* (London, 1972).
44. Sheila Rowbotham, *Promise of a Dream: Remembering the Sixties* (London, 2000), 38.
45. See, for example, "Adolescent, Teenager, or Human Being?" *The Lancet* 1, no. 7180 (April 8, 1961), 757–758: 757.
46. British Medical Association, *Venereal Disease and Young People: A Report* (London, 1964), 7. The number of births among unmarried girls under twenty had risen from 52,000 in 1960 to more than 81,000 in 1965. See Schofield, *The Sexual Behaviour of Young People*, 6.
47. See National Marriage Guidance Council, *Sex Education in Perspective: A Symposium on Work in Progress* (London, 1972); Royal Society for the Promotion of Health, *Sex Education of Schoolchildren* (London, 1971); Haim Ginnott, *Between Teenager and Parent* (London, 1973).
48. International Planned Parenthood Federation, *A Survey on the Status of Sex Education in European Member Countries* (London, 1975); Dorothy M. Dallas, *Exploring Sex Education in School and Society* (Slough, 1972); White and Kidd, *Sound Sex Education*.
49. White and Kidd, *Sound Sex Education*, 8
50. See Ken Fogelman, *Growing Up in Great Britain: Papers from the National Child Development Study* (London, 1983), 287–299.
51. Nancy Zinkin Papers, SA/HVA/G.7/6/2, Wellcome Library.
52. Nancy Zinkin Papers, SA/HVA/G.7/6/2, Wellcome Library.
53. Responsible Society Research and Education Trust, *Sex Education in Schools—What Every Parent Should Know* (Milton Keynes, 1982).
54. Martin Cole (director), Global Films in association with The Institute for Sex Education and Research (UK, 1971).
55. Oliver Pritchett, "Mixed Reception for Sex Film," *The Guardian*, April 17, 1971, 7.
56. Pritchett, "Mixed Reception for Sex Film," 7.
57. Basil Gingell, "Archbishop of Canterbury Says Sex Education Film Is Unsuitable for Use in Schools," *The Times*, April 29, 1971, 2.
58. "Inquiry Sought on Sex Lessons," *The Guardian*, April 22, 1971, 5.
59. "Britain's Week," *The Listener*, April 29, 1971, 541.
60. "The Joy of Sex Education" (London: British Film Institute, 2009), 31 [booklet accompanying DVD].
61. The usual demand was that there should be no sex education instruction outside of biology classes, or if there were to be such instruction, parents should be informed of the precise content of the course or lecture and their consent required for their child to attend.
62. "The Responsible Society," Letter to the Editor of *The Times*, June 14, 1971, 13.
63. "Bulletin of the Responsible Society," 3AMS/B/15/06, Women's Library.
64. "The Responsible Society," *The Times*, 13
65. Volunteers were sent to cafes and discos in London to teach young people how to use forms of contraception. "Volunteers to Explain Birth Control," *The Times*, May 23, 1972, 4.
66. A.S. Wigfield, "Birth Control," *The Times*, April 23, 1973, 13.
67. "Pill Secrecy Gets Official Backing," *The Guardian*, May 15, 1974, 6.
68. Sir Keith Joseph, "Edgbaston Speech," October 19, 1974. Available at: http://www.margarettthatcher.org/document/101830.
69. Joseph, "Edgbaston Speech."

70. Joseph, "Edgbaston Speech."
71. House of Lords Debate, "Address in Reply to Her Majesty's Most Gracious Speech," 30 October 1974, vol. 354 col. 35–156
72. Antony Grey, "Problem of Birth Control," *The Times*, October 25, 1974, 17.
73. Joseph, "Edgbaston Speech."
74. See Rose Hacker, *Telling the Teenagers: A Guide for Parents, Teachers and Youth Leaders* (London, 1966); Robert Chartham, *You, Your Children and Sex: What to Tell Them, How, and When* (London, 1973); Family Planning Association, *Learning to Live with Sex: A Handbook of Sex Education for Teenagers* (London, 1972); Mary Beauchamp Lane, *Learning About Life: A Child-Centred Approach to Sex Education* (London, 1973); Royal Society for the Promotion of Health, *Sex Education of Schoolchildren* (London, 1971); Alan Harris, *Questions About Sex* (London, 1968).
75. See, for example, Odlum, *Journey Through Adolescence*, 147–148. Alan Harris's treatment of homosexuality in his 1968 sex advice book *Questions about Sex* was not typical in that he described homosexuality as a benign variation and a potentially lifelong sexual orientation.
76. Many European countries, including Austria, the Federal Republic of Germany, Norway, Sweden, and Denmark had developed sex education curricula, and that the Ministry of Education was actively involved in ensuring that sex education was available at schools nationwide. See International Planned Parenthood Federation, *A Survey on the Status of Sex Education in European Member Countries*.
77. The number of live births to girls under sixteen in 1957 was 924. The number rose to 2,870 by 1962. See Donald Gough, *Schoolgirl Unmarried Mothers* (London, 1967), 3.
78. Mary Whitehouse, *Cleaning Up TV: From Protest to Participation* (London, 1967), 16.
79. Jeremy Thorpe's political career ended when Norman Scott publicly claimed to have had a homosexual relationship with him between 1961 and 1963, when homosexual acts were still illegal.
80. "Liberals Are Lukewarm on Gay Rights Appeal," *The Guardian*, June 28, 1974, 10.
81. British Medical Association, *Venereal Disease and Young People*.
82. Sexual Law Reform Society, *Report of the Working Party on the Law in Relation to Sexual Behaviour* (London, September 1974). The report took four years to produce.
83. Michael De-la-Noy, "Rights and Wrongs," *The Guardian*, September 5, 1974, 11.
84. "Dr. Robinson Puts Case for Age of Consent to Be 14," *The Times*, July 6, 1972, 3.
85. "Report Calls for Age of Consent to Be 14," *The Times*, September 6, 1974, 3.
86. Mary Whitehouse, "No Compassion from Sex Law Reformers," *The Guardian*, September 11, 1974, 14.
87. Whitehouse, "No Compassion from Sex Law Reformers" [original emphasis].
88. Marjorie Jones, "Age of Consent," *The Times*, March 5, 1973, 13.
89. D. Ambrose King, "Sex and Morality," *The Times*, July 11, 1972, 15.
90. Policy Advisory Committee, *Working Paper*, 1.
91. Ronald Butt, "Who Really Wants a Change in the Age of Consent?" *The Times*, January 22, 1976, 14.
92. Tim Beaumont, "Age of Consent," *The Times*, January 26, 1976, 13.
93. Beaumont, "Age of Consent," *The Times*, 13.
94. Tim Beaumont, "Dissent: Do We Need an 'Age of Consent Law'?" *Observer Magazine*, May 20, 1977.

95. Beaumont, "Dissent: Do We Need an 'Age of Consent Law?'"
96. Josephine Butler successfully campaigned to have the age of sexual consent for girls raised from thirteen to sixteen in 1885. In response to W.T. Stead's highly sensationalized reporting of "white slavery" in the 1880s, Butler, Stead, and many others argued that girls needed to be protected from the male sexual appetite. The law was a tool for dissuading sexual predators from acting.
97. For instance, a campaign launched in Liverpool during WWII was dismissed from Parliament out of fear that it might incite an angry reaction from women's groups. HO 45/19637, The National Archives.
98. Giles Knight, "Stop this Crime Wave NOW," *Daily Mirror*, January 25, 1949. The *Daily Mirror* indicated that the number amounted to "nearly two known crimes" committed "for every day of the year," while Basil Henriques warned *Observer* readers that "many more" remained unreported. Basil Henriques, "Sex Crimes and the Law," *The Observer*, March 20, 1949.
99. "Attacks on Girls—Women Urge New Law," *Daily Mirror*, March 11, 1949.
100. Arthur Eperon, "No Child Is Safe from This Evil," *Daily Herald*, February 23, 1953.
101. Committee on Homosexual Offences and Prostitution, *Report of the Committee on Homosexual Offences and Prostitution*, 50–51.
102. Latey Committee on the Age of Majority, *Report of the Latey Committee on the Age of Majority* (London, 1967). Men and women between the ages of 18 and 21 were judged capable of entering binding contracts, buying and selling property, consenting to medical treatment, and marrying without parental consent.
103. Committee on Homosexual Offences and Prostitution, *Report of the Committee on Homosexual Offences and Prostitution*, 50.
104. Rev. Dr. John R. Meeres, letter to the editor, *The Guardian*, September 11, 1974, 14.
105. "Think Before We Lower the Age of Consent," *Welwyn Times and Hatfield Times*, June 3, 1977.
106. "Think Before We Lower the Age of Consent," *Welwyn Times and Hatfield Times*.
107. In J.M. Tanner, *Education and Physical Growth* (London, 1961). Tanner pointed out that girls menstruated on average ten months earlier than their mothers had. Michael Schofield noted that boys were also developing earlier, completing their growth on average by age seventeen. This was compared with twenty-three years of age in 1900.
108. R.I. Mawby, "Policing the Age of Consent," *Journal of Adolescence* 2 (1979), 41–49: 45.
109. If the man in question was under the age of twenty-four and this was his first offence, the case was rarely pursued, thus making the law appear pointless. Mawby, "Policing the Age of Consent," 43.
110. Cited in Policy Advisory Committee, *Working Paper*, 10.
111. Ivor H. Mills, "Effects of Child Pornography," *The Times*, February 15 1979.
112. Mills, "Effects of Child Pornography."
113. Cited in Policy Advisory Committee, *Working Paper*, 7.
114. Cited in Policy Advisory Committee, *Working Paper*, 7.
115. House of Lords Debate, "Sexual Offences (Amendment) Bill," 14 June 1977, vol. 384, col.30–74.
116. House of Lords Debate, "Sexual Offences (Amendment) Bill," 14 June 1977, vol. 384, col.30–74.

Notes

117. Joint Council for Gay Teenagers, *I Know What I Am: Gay Teenagers and the Law* (Liverpool, 1980), 1. *I Know What I Am* was presented to the PAC in July 1979. It was printed and more widely distributed in 1980. HCA/JCGT/6/1, Hall-Carpenter Archives.
118. Those aged seventeen to nineteen accounted for 58% of the increase.
119. Even though there was no law preventing lesbians from engaging in sexual relationships from age sixteen onward, the gay youth movement had strong support from lesbians who were over sixteen.
120. Joint Council for Gay Teenagers, *I Know What I Am*, 1.
121. Joint Council for Gay Teenagers, *I Know What I Am*, 2.
122. Joint Council for Gay Teenagers, *I Know What I Am*, 16.
123. Joint Council for Gay Teenagers, *I Know What I Am*, 14.
124. Joint Council for Gay Teenagers, *Breaking the Silence* (London, 1980), HCA/JCGT/6/1, Hall-Carpenter Archives.
125. Michael Burbidge, "JCGT Press Release," January 1980, HCA/JCGT/6/4, Hall-Carpenter Archives.
126. Joint Council for Gay Teenagers, *I Know What I Am*, 7.
127. Joint Council for Gay Teenagers, *I Know What I Am*, 8.
128. Michael Burbidge, "Discussion Paper," 11 October 1979, HCA/JCGT/8/2, Hall-Carpenter Archives.
129. Joint Council for Gay Teenagers, "A Response to the Home Office Working Paper on the Age of Consent in Relation to Sexual Offences," January 1980, 9. HCA/JCGT/6/1, Hall-Carpenter Archives.
130. Joint Council for Gay Teenagers, "Conference on Young Gays—Details of Second Meeting," 25 November 1978. HCA/JCGT/8/2, Hall-Carpenter Archives.
131. Joint Council for Gay Teenagers, "Conference on Young Gays—Details of Second Meeting."
132. Cited in the NCCL's proposals to the PAC for recommended reforms. HCA/GREY/1/23, Hall-Carpenter Archives.
133. Joint Working Party on Pregnant Schoolgirls and Schoolgirl Mothers, *Pregnant at School* (London, 1979), paragraph 12.
134. Ken Plummer, *Sexual Stigma: An Interactionist Account* (London, 1975), 142.
135. Antony Grey, "Correspondence with the NCCL," HCA/GREY/1/23, Hall-Carpenter Archives.
136. Policy Advisory Committee, *Working Paper*, 8.
137. Policy Advisory Committee, *Working Paper*, 8.
138. National opinion polls showed that four people to one were opposed to lowering the age of consent to fourteen. "You, the Jury," *The Listener*, December 9, 1976, 759.
139. See Hera Cook, *The Long Sexual Revolution: English Women, Sex, and Contraception, 1800–1975* (Oxford, 2004); Callum Brown, *The Death of Christian Britain* (London, 2009).
140. See Michel Foucault, *History of Sexuality*, volume 1 (New York, 1978); Gayle Rubin, "Thinking Sex: Notes for a Radical Theory of the Politics of Sexuality," in *Pleasure and Danger: Exploring Female Sexuality*, ed. Carole S. Vance (London, 1992), 267–293; Lauren Berlant and Michael Warner, "Sex in Public," in *Intimacy*, ed. Lauren Berlant (Chicago, 2000), 311–330.
141. Shyama Perera, "Girls 'Flout the Age of Consent,'" *The Guardian*, March 25, 1982, 3.
142. Perera, "Girls 'Flout the Age of Consent,'" 3.

143. See Kaye Wellings and Roslyn Kane, "Trends in Teenage Pregnancy in England and Wales: How Can We Explain Them?" *Journal of the Royal Society of Medicine*, 92 (June 1999), 277–282: 278; Department of Health and Social Security, *Teenage Mothers and Their Partners* (London, 1986).
144. For example, both *Hi!* and *Mirabelle* had advice columns and articles that focused on sex and dating.
145. "JCGT, GYM, and CHE," HCA/JCGT/1/4, Hall-Carpenter Archives.
146. "JCGT, GYM, and CHE," HCA/JCGT/1/4.
147. Reported in "Gay Youth" (GYM Newsletter), August–September 1982. HCA/JCGT/6/2, Hall-Carpenter Archives.
148. Victoria Gillick, "Schoolgirl Promiscuity," *The Times*, December 18, 1984, 13.
149. House of Commons Debate, "Contraceptives (Children)," 24 October 1985, vol. 84 col. 225w.
150. Jane Pilcher, "Gillick and After: Children and Sex in the 1980s and 1990s," in *Thatcher's Children? Politics, Childhood and Society in the 1980s and 1990s*, eds. Jane Pilcher and Stephen Wagg (London, 1996), 77–93: 91.
151. Burbidge, "Discussion paper," 11 October 1979.
152. Burbidge, "Discussion paper," 11 October 1979.
153. Joseph, "Edgbaston Speech." See also Keith Joseph, *The Times*, October 22, 1974, 15.
154. Lorna Sage, *Bad Blood* (London, 2000), 194.
155. Pilcher, "Gillick and After: Children and Sex in the 1980s and 1990s," 82.
156. The Sexual Offences (Amendment) Act 2000 equalized the age of consent for both heterosexual and homosexual relations at age sixteen.

Chapter 7

1. Keith Parkin, "Fathers Need Their Families," *The Guardian*, June 12, 1974, 11.
2. Parkin, "Fathers Need Their Families," 11.
3. Jill Tweedie, "Father Figured," *The Guardian*, November 25, 1974, 9.
4. Tweedie, "Father Figured," 9.
5. "The Man Who Tries to be Mum," *The Guardian*, September 27, 1979, 13.
6. Lee Comer, "The Motherhood Myth," *Australian Left Review* (March 1972) [Comer is here citing R.D. Laing's *The Politics of Experience* (New York, 1967)].
7. *Edmonton Journal*, "What Price Refuge for Battered Wives?" February 10, 1978, 5.
8. Liz Kelly, "Who Needs Enemies with Friends like Erin Pizzey?" *Spare Rib*, February 1983, 39.
9. John Hills, "Open Space: Why Most Men Even More Inadequate than Women in Trying to Look After Children," *The Guardian*, October 26, 1978, 11.
10. Sheila Rowbotham, "To Be or Not to Be: The Dilemmas of Mothering," *Feminist Review* 31 (1989), 82–93: 86.
11. Rowbotham, "To Be or Not to Be: The Dilemmas of Mothering," 86.
12. The "schizophrenogenic mother" was first described by Frieda Fromm-Reichmann in 1948 and further developed by Theodore Lidz in the 1960s. See Frieda Fromm-Reichmann, "Notes on the Development of Treatment of Schizophrenics by Psychoanalytic Psychotherapy," *Psychiatry* 11, no. 3 (1948): 263–273; Theodore Lidz, *Schizophrenia and the Family* (New York, 1965).

13. Edmund Leach, *A Runaway World? The Reith Lectures 1967* (London, 1968).
14. Philip Larkin, "This Be the Verse," *New Humanist*, August 1971.
15. David Cooper, *The Grammar of Living* (London, 1974), 57.
16. "Mr. G," MIND Conference Report, 1969. PP/ADD/D.3, Wellcome Archives.
17. Loach directed both *In Two Minds* (1967) and *Family Life* (1971).
18. "Mr. G," MIND Conference Report, 1969. PP/ADD/D.3, Wellcome Archives.
19. "Mr. G," MIND Conference Report, 1969. PP/ADD/D.3, Wellcome Archives.
20. See William Sargant, "Treating Schizophrenia," *The Times*, March 8 1967, 13.
21. Lidz, *Schizophrenia and the Family*.
22. R.D. Laing, *The Divided Self* (Harmondsworth, 1965), 194.
23. R.D. Laing and Aaron Esterson, *Sanity, Madness and the Family* (London, 1964), 63.
24. Laing and Esterson, *Sanity, Madness and the Family*, 45.
25. Laing and Esterson, *Sanity, Madness and the Family*, 25.
26. Laing and Esterson, *Sanity, Madness and the Family*, 25.
27. Laing and Esterson, *Sanity, Madness and the Family*, 25.
28. Laing and Esterson, *Sanity, Madness and the Family*, 62.
29. Laing and Esterson, *Sanity, Madness and the Family*, 36.
30. Laing and Esterson, *Sanity, Madness and the Family*, 17.
31. Mary Barnes and Joseph Berke, *Two Accounts of a Journey through Madness* (London, 1971), 26.
32. Barnes and Berke, *Two Accounts of a Journey Through Madness*, 103.
33. Barnes and Berke, *Two Accounts of a Journey Through Madness*, 164.
34. Barnes and Berke, *Two Accounts of a Journey Through Madness*, 165.
35. Barnes and Berke, *Two Accounts of a Journey Through Madness*, 174.
36. Barnes and Berke, *Two Accounts of a Journey Through Madness*, 224.
37. Barnes and Berke, *Two Accounts of a Journey Through Madness*, 269.
38. Berke used the term "mother" rather than the gender-neutral term "parent" to describe how he cared for Mary.
39. For example, *The Divided Self* received positive reviews from Peter Toynbee in *The Observer* (June 12, 1960); Maurice Richardson in *New Statesman*; and Alisdair McIntyre in *The Observer*.
40. Sheila Rowbotham, *Promise of A Dream: Remembering the Sixties* (London, 2001), 126.
41. Rowbotham, *Promise of A Dream: Remembering the Sixties*, 126.
42. Dozens of articles were published each year in *The Guardian, The Observer, Spare Rib*, and *New Statesmen*.
43. R.D. Laing, *The Politics of Experience* (New York, 1967), xv.
44. Juliet Mitchell, *Woman's Estate* (Harmondsworth, 1971), 43.
45. "'I Went to Freud First of All. And Sort of Surprisingly Found His Theory Incredibly Useful for Understanding Femininity,'" *Spare Rib*, April 1974, 6–8: 6.
46. Available at: http://www.dialecticsofliberation.com/1967-dialectics/memories/.
47. Available at: http://www.dialecticsofliberation.com/1967-dialectics/memories/.
48. Mitchell, *Woman's Estate*, 13–14.
49. Hannah Gavron, *The Captive Wife* (London, 1966); Mitchell, *Woman's Estate*, 151.
50. Mitchell, *Woman's Estate*, 162.
51. Mitchell, *Woman's Estate*, 14.
52. Rowbotham, *Promise of a Dream*, 145.

53. Rowbotham, *Promise of a Dream*, 145.
54. Comer, "The Motherhood Myth," 34.
55. Comer, "The Motherhood Myth," 28–29.
56. See Mari Jo Buhle, *Feminism and Its Discontents: A Century of Struggle With Psychoanalysis* (Cambridge, 1998).
57. Michelene Wandor, "Family Everafter—how effective is the family structure today," *Spare Rib*, November 1972, 12.
58. Wandor, "Family Everafter," 13.
59. "Interview with Lee Comer," *Spare Rib*, June 1974.
60. Stella Fitzsimon, Letter to the Editor, *Spare Rib*, September 1972, 3.
61. Sheila Rowbotham, "To Be or Not to Be: The Dilemmas of Mothering," *Feminist Review* 31, no. 1 (1989), 82–93: 86–87.
62. Lee Comer, *Wedlocked Women* (Leeds, 1974), 217.
63. Erin Pizzey, *This Way to the Revolution: A Memoir* (London, 2011), 82.
64. House of Commons Select Committee on Violence in Marriage, *Report from the Select Committee on Violence in Marriage, Together with the Proceedings of the Committee, Session 1974–75* (London, 1975), v.
65. In Pizzey's memoir, *This Way to the Revolution*, she describes being aware of female perpetrators of violence as early as 1972. She later claimed that during the first year of Chiswick's operation, sixty-two out of one hundred of the women housed there had been violent toward their partners and/or children.
66. C.H. Kempe, Frederic N. Silverman, Brandt F. Steele, William Droegemuller, and Henry K. Silver, "The Battered Child Syndrome," *Journal of the American Medical Association* (1962), 181: 17–24.
67. Cited in Marie Borland, *Violence in the Family* (Manchester, 1976).
68. Samuel West, "Acute Periosteal Swellings in Several Young Infants of the Same Family, Probably Rickety in Nature," *BMJ* 1, no. 1435 (June 30, 1888) i, 856; J. Caffey, "Multiple Fracture of the Long Bones of Infants Suffering from Chronic Subdural Haematoma," *American Journal of Roentgenology*, 56 (1946), 163–73; F.N. Silverman, "Roentgen Manifestations of Unrecognized Skeletal Trauma in Infants," *American Journal of Roentgenology*, 69 (1953), 413; P.V. Wooley and W. Evans, "Significance of Skeletal Lesions in Infants Resembling Those of Traumatic Origin," *Journal of the American Medical Association*, 158 (1955), 539. Although physicians may have increasingly seen parent-inflicted violence against children as a problem, they often did not report it to police in order to maintain doctor-patient confidentiality.
69. D.L. Griffiths and F.J. Moynihan, "Multiple Ephiphysial Injuries in Babies ('Battered Baby' Syndrome)," *BMJ* 2, no. 5372 (December 21, 1963), 1558–1561.
70. "Violent Parents," *The Lancet* 2, no. 7732 (November 6, 1971), 1017–1018.
71. "Violent Parents," 1017. The article proceeded to suggest that "Increased and improved mother/baby contact during the infant's stay in special nursery may well have a beneficial effect and decrease the risk of subsequent battering."
72. Patricia Morgan, *Child Care: Sense and Fable* (London, 1975), 332.
73. Morgan, *Child Care: Sense and Fable*, 332–333.
74. John Bowlby, "Violence in the Family as a Disorder of the Attachment and Caregiving Systems: The 1983 Karen Horney Lecture," May 1983, 1. PP/BOW/K.10/59, Wellcome Archives.

75. Bowlby, "Violence in the Family as a Disorder of the Attachment and Caregiving Systems," 21.
76. Bowlby, "Violence in the Family as a Disorder of the Attachment and Caregiving Systems," 28.
77. Bowlby, "Violence in the Family as a Disorder of the Attachment and Caregiving Systems," 28.
78. Willem Van der Eyken, *Home-Start: A Four-Year Evaluation* (Leicester, 1982), 8. Ninety percent of the recipients of Home-Start's help were "struggling on a very low income," forty percent were single parents, and many lived in "poor or overcrowded housing," experiencing "physical or emotional battering (both the parents *and* the children)," and having "suffered from deprivation in their own childhood"; thirteen percent were listed as "ethnic minorities."
79. Van der Eyken, *Home-Start: A Four-Year Evaluation*, 70.
80. Pizzey, *This Way to the Revolution*, 69.
81. The lack of police intervention in domestic violence was also discussed in the *Report from the Select Committee on Violence in Marriage*.
82. Erin Pizzey, *Scream Quietly or the Neighbours Will Hear* (Harmondsworth, 1974), 70. Pizzey notes that, "One social worker we came across informed Women's Aid that wife-beating was a West Indian syndrome" since "He hadn't received and hadn't expected complaints from women of any other group" (24).
83. Pizzey, *Scream Quietly or the Neighbours will Hear*, 77.
84. Erin Pizzey, *Infernal Child: A Memoir* (London, 1978), 126.
85. House of Commons Select Committee on Violence in Marriage, *Report from the Select Committee on Violence in Marriage*, 1.
86. Pizzey, *Scream Quietly or the Neighbours will Hear*, 74.
87. House of Commons Select Committee on Violence in Marriage, *Report from the Select Committee on Violence in Marriage*, 2.
88. Julia Brannen and Jean Collard, *Marriages in Trouble: The Process of Seeking Help* (London, 1982), 80–81.
89. Lenore Walker, *The Battered Woman* (New York, 1979), xv.
90. Walker, *The Battered Woman*, x-xi.
91. Walker, *The Battered Woman*, ix-x.
92. See Richard J. Gelles, *The Violent Home: A Study of Physical Aggression Between Husbands and Wives* (New York, 1974); A.R.K. Mitchell, *Violence in the Family* (Hove, 1978); Jean Renvoize, *Web of Violence: A Study of Family Violence* (London, 1978).
93. House of Commons Select Committee on Violence in Marriage, *Report from the Select Committee on Violence in Marriage*, vi.
94. House of Commons Select Committee on Violence in Marriage, *Report from the Select Committee on Violence in Marriage*, viii.
95. House of Commons Select Committee on Violence in Marriage, *Report from the Select Committee on Violence in Marriage*, xxv.
96. Jill Tweedie, "Beaten Up Women and Their Children," *Spare Rib*, June 1973, 12.
97. House of Commons Select Committee on Violence in Marriage, *Report from the Select Committee on Violence in Marriage*, 2 [Pizzey is quoted here].
98. Pizzey, *Scream Quietly or the Neighbours will Hear*, 78.

99. "Rescuing Women and Children from Violence: London Home is Refuge for Battered Wives," *The Christian Science Monitor*, November 9, 1977, 24. "Once again, Chiswick tried to fill a vacuum by opening in 1976 a house for men. There violent men can stay if they feel the desperation of their problems overwhelming them; they can talk out their problems with experienced workers."
100. Pizzey, *Scream Quietly or the Neighbours Will Hear*, 45.
101. Tweedie, "Beaten Up Women and Their Children," 12.
102. Tweedie, "Beaten Up Women and Their Children," 12.
103. Many women had been living in refuges for up to nine months because of housing shortages.
104. Activists at National Women's Aid had lobbied the government for this research.
105. British single-parent families very often struggled with poverty. Supplementary benefits were given to families to meet their basic needs, however these were stopped if the parent went to work. It was therefore extraordinarily difficult to approach the income level of a two-parent family.
106. House of Commons Select Committee on Violence in Marriage, *Report from the Select Committee on Violence in Marriage*, 151. For example, "Mr. A had little stability as a child and appears to have been significantly emotionally deprived … Mrs. A was also a somewhat deprived child and received only limited education … She married young, and immediately after marriage her husband went to prison."
107. On Pizzey's international impact, see Zora Simic, "From Battered Wives to Domestic Violence: The Transnational Circulation of Chiswick Women's Aid and Erin Pizzey's Scream Quietly or the Neighbours Will Hear (1974)," *Australian Historical Studies* 51, no. 2 (May 2020): 107–126.
108. Erin Pizzey and Jeff Shapiro, "Choosing a Violent Relationship," *New Society*, April 23, 1981, 133–135: 133.
109. C.R. Cheeseman, "Women and Violence," Letters, *New Society* May 7, 1981, 240. Cheeseman was affiliated with Merton Women's Aid Limited.
110. Val Binney, "Women and Violence," Letters, *New Society* May 7, 1981, 240. Binney was affiliated with the Women's Aid Federation Research Team.
111. See, for example, "When Trust Takes a Cruel Beating," *The Guardian*, November 10, 1982, 12.
112. Derek Bateman, "Women Denounce Pain Addiction Book," *Glasgow Herald*, October 26, 1982, 6.
113. Bateman, "Women Denounce Pain Addiction book," 6.
114. Erin Pizzey, "Why I Loathe Feminism … and Believe It Will Ultimately Destroy the Family," *Daily Mail*, September 24, 2009.
115. Erin Pizzey, *The Emotional Terrorist and the Violence-Prone* (Ottawa, 1998).
116. Available at: https://www.refuge.org.uk/our-story/our-history/.
117. Helen Lewis, *Difficult Women: A History of Feminism in 11 Fights* (London, 2020).
118. Lee Edelman, *No Future: Queer Theory and the Death Drive* (Durham, 2004), 18.
119. Berlant and Warner, "Sex in Public," 317.
120. Parkin, "Fathers Need their Families," 11.
121. Parkin, "Fathers Need their Families," 11.
122. Maureen Green, "Recognizing the Claims of the Paternal Instinct," *The Times*, September 20, 1974, 9.

123. Tweedie, "Father Figured," 9.
124. Joseph Brayshaw, "When Parents Part..." *Daily Herald*, August 1952.
125. Edward F. Griffith, *Voluntary Parenthood* (London, 1937), 3.
126. Griffith, *Voluntary Parenthood*, 3.

Epilogue: Intimacy in the Age of the Individual

1. Molly Plowright, "Shelter," *The Guardian*, January 4, 1965, 6.
2. Plowright, "Shelter," 6.
3. David Cooper, *To Free a Generation: The Dialectics of Liberation* (New York, 1968), 10.
4. See John Macnicol, "From 'Problem Family' to 'Underclass,' 1945–95," in *Welfare Policy in Britain: The Road from 1945*, eds. Rodney Lowe and Helen Fawcett (Basingstoke, 1999), 69–93.
5. See Frank Furedi, *Therapy Culture: Cultivating Vulnerability in an Uncertain Age* (London, 2004); Jonathan B. Imber, ed. *Therapeutic Culture: Triumphs and Defeat* (New Brunswick NJ, 2004).
6. Neil Kinnock's speech at the 1985 Labour Party Conference, October 4, 1985, Bournemouth, UK. http://www.britishpoliticalspeech.org/speech-archive.htm?speech=191.
7. "Growing Strife in Family Life," *The Guardian*, September 21, 1990, 22.
8. Public support for the Conservatives appeared to demonstrate that the punitive law and order approach was preferred to the provision of services, which were seen as robbing individual families of initiative and self-responsibility.
9. Lauren Berlant, "Intimacy: A Special Issue," in *Intimacy*, ed. Lauren Berlant (Chicago, 2000), 1.
10. "Dismiss the Boring Old Orgasm with Supersex," *The Guardian*, January 19 1988, 10.
11. "Dismiss the Boring Old Orgasm with Supersex," 10.
12. Leo Buscaglia, "Mature Love and Intimacy," *Cosmopolitan* 196, no. 6 (December 1983), 222.
13. "Dismiss the Boring Old Orgasm with Supersex," 10.
14. "Love Is Not All You Need," *The Guardian*, February 14, 1992, 31.
15. "Love Is Not All You Need," 31.
16. Jeanette Winterson, *Written on the Body* (London, 1992).
17. Susie Orbach, "Home Front: You've lost that loving feeing," *The Guardian*, April 10, 1993, a25.
18. Rosalind Coward, "Sealed with a Kiss," *The Guardian*, February 14, 1984, 22.
19. See, for example, Edward Fyfe Griffith, *Sex and Citizenship* (London, 1941), 202–203.
20. "Looking for a New Kind of Loving," *Spare Rib* 223 (May 1991), 32–36: 32.
21. "Looking for a New Kind of Loving," 32.
22. "Looking for a New Kind of Loving," 33.
23. "Looking for a New Kind of Loving," 36.
24. Kenji Yoshino, "The Epistemic Contract of Bisexual Erasure," *Stanford Law Review* 52, no. 2 (January 2000), 353–461.
25. See Charis Thompson, *Making Parents: The Ontological Choreography of Reproductive Technologies* (Cambridge, 2005).
26. See, for example, Fernando Zegers-Hochschild et al, "Human Rights to In Vitro Fertilization," *International Journal of Gynaecology and Obstetrics* 123, no. 1 (October

2013), 86–89; Paula Gerber et al, "Marriage: A Human Right for All?" *The Sydney Law Review* 36, no. 4 (December 2014), 643.

27. For example, Cathy Caruth, *Unclaimed Experience: Trauma, Narrative, History* (Baltimore, 1996); Ruth Leys, *Trauma: A Genealogy* (Chicago, 2000); Roger Luckhurst, *The Trauma Question* (New York, 2008); Ogaga Ifowodo, *History, Trauma, and Healing in Postcolonial Narratives: Reconstructing Identities* (New York, 2013).

28. Margaret Thatcher interview, *Sunday Times*, 3 May 1981. Available at: https://www.margaretthatcher.org/document/104475.

29. Michel Foucault, "Friendship as a Way of Life," in *Michel Foucault: Ethics, Subjectivity, and Truth, volume 1*, ed. Paul Rabinow (New York, 1994), 138.

Select Bibliography

Primary Sources

Archives Consulted

The National Archives, Richmond, UK
Department of Health and Social Security (BN)
Home Office (HO)
Lord Chancellor's Office (LCO)
Medical Research Council (FD)
Ministry of Health (MH)
Prime Minister's Office (PREM)
Treasury (T)
War Office (WO)

Hall-Carpenter Archives and Women's Library and Archives, The London School of Economics, London, UK
Albany Trust (HCA/AT)
Antony Grey Papers (HCA/GREY)
Association of Social and Moral Hygiene Papers (3AMS)
Campaign for Homosexual Equality (HCA/CHE2)
FRIEND Papers (FRIEND)
Hackney Women's Aid (5HWA)
Joint Council for Gay Teenagers Papers (HCA/JCGT)
Lewisham FRIEND (HCA/Lewisham Friend)
Married Women's Association (5MWA)
Mothers in Action (5MIA)
Papers of the Council of Married Women of Great Britain (5CMS)

Wellcome Archives and Manuscripts, London, UK
Abortion Law Reform Association (SA/ALR)
Birth Control Campaign (SA/BCC)
British Medical Association (SA/BMA)
Carlos Paton Blacker Papers (PP/CPB)
Edward Fyfe Griffith Papers (PP/EFG/B)
"The Expanding Field of Mental Health in England and Wales, 50 years of progress, 1918–1968," edited by Doris Odlum [unpublished, 1968] (MS 7913/41)
Family Planning Association (SA/FPA)
Health Visitors' Association (SA/HVA)
Henry Dicks Papers (PP/HVD)
John Bowlby Papers (PP/BOW)
Letitia Fairfield Papers (GC/193)
Medical Women's Federation (SA/MWF)

Mental After Care Association (SA/MAC)
Noel Gordon Harris Papers (PP/NGH)
Pioneer Health Centre (SA/PHC)
Population Investigation Committee (SA/PIC)
Robina Addis Papers (PP/ADD)
S.H. Foulkes Papers (PP/SHF)
Sir Allen Daley Papers (PP/AWD)

Archive and Study Centre, Planned Environment Therapy Trust, Toddington, Gloucestershire, UK
Cassel Hospital Papers [uncatalogued]
Harold Bridger Papers [uncatalogued]
Joshua Bierer Papers [uncatalogued]

Tavistock Centre for Couple Relationships Archives, London, UK
Family Discussion Bureau [uncatalogued]
Institute of Marital Studies [uncatalogued]

British Psycho-Analytical Society Archives, London, UK
John Rickman Papers
T.F. Main Papers

Journals and Newspapers
British Journal of Medical Psychology
British Medical Journal
Daily Mail
The Guardian
Good Housekeeping
Hansard Parliamentary Debates (1938--1987)
Hi!
Housewife
International Journal of Psychoanalysis
International Journal of Social Psychiatry
Journal of Mental Science
Ladies Home Journal
The Lancet
The Listener
Mirabelle
My Home
New Society
New Stateman
The Observer
Spare Rib
The Times

Published Primary Sources
Abse, Leo. *Private Member*. London: Macdonald and Co., 1973.

Select Bibliography

Ahrenfeldt, Robert. *Psychiatry in the British Army in the Second World War*. London: Routledge & Kegan Paul, 1958.

Ahrenfeldt, Robert, and T.C.N. Gibbens. *Cultural Factors in Delinquency*. London: Tavistock Publications, 1966.

Ainsworth, Mary, ed. *Deprivation of Maternal Care: A Reassessment of Its Effects*. Geneva: World Health Organization, 1962.

Ainsworth, Mary. *Infancy in Uganda: Infant Care and the Growth of Love*. Baltimore, MA: Johns Hopkins University Press, 1967.

Ainsworth, Mary. "Object Relations, Dependency, and Attachment: A Theoretical Review of the Infant-Mother Relationship." *Child Development* 40 (1969): 969–1025.

Ainsworth, Mary, and Bowlby, John. "Research Strategy in the Study of Mother-Child Separation." *Courrier de la Centre International de l'Enfance* 4 (1954): 105–131.

Allen of Hurtwood, Lady Marjory. *Whose Children?* London: Simpkin Marshall, 1945.

Anthony, E. James, and Therese Benedek. *Parenthood: Its Psychology and Psychopathology*. Boston: Little, Brown, 1970.

Archbishop of Canterbury's Group on the Divorce Law. *Putting Asunder: A Divorce Law for Contemporary Society*. London: SPCK, 1966.

Arendt, Hannah. *Between Past and Future: Eight Exercises in Political Thought*. New York: Viking Press, 1961.

Arendt, Hannah. *The Origins of Totalitarianism*. New York: Harcourt Brace and Co., 1973.

Balint, Enid. *Before I Was I*. London: Free Association Books, 1993.

Bannister, Kathleen, Alison Lyons, Lily Pincus, James Robb, Antonia Shooter, and Judith Stephens, eds. *Social Casework in Marital Problems: The Development of a Psychodynamic Approach*. London: Tavistock Publications, 1955.

Barnes, Elizabeth. *People in Hospital*. London: Macmillan, 1961.

Barnes, Elizabeth, ed. *Psychosocial Nursing: Studies from the Cassel Hospital*. London: Tavistock Publications, 1968.

Barnes, Mary, and Joseph Berke. *Two Accounts of a Journey through Madness*. London: MacGibbon and Kee, 1971.

Barrett, Michèle, and Mary McIntosh. *The Anti-Social Family*. London: Verso, 1982.

Beale, G. Courtenay. *Wise Wedlock: The Whole Truth: A Book of Counsel and Instruction for All Who Seek for Happiness in Marriage*. London: Health Promotion Ltd, 1921.

Barton, Russell. *Institutional Neurosis*. Bristol, UK: Wright, 1959.

Benedict, Ruth. *The Chrysanthemum and the Sword*. Boston: Houghton Mifflin Harcourt, 1946.

Beveridge, William. *Social Insurance and the Allied Services*. London: HMSO, 1942.

Beveridge, William. *The Pillars of Security*. London: George Allen & Unwin, 1942.

Beveridge, William. *Voluntary Action: A Report on Methods of Social Advance*. London: Allen & Unwin, 1948.

Beyfus, Drusilla. *The English Marriage: What It Is Like to Be Married Today*. London: Weidenfeld and Nicolson, 1968.

Bierer, Joshua, ed. *Therapeutic Social Clubs*. London: H.K. Lewis and Co., 1948.

Biggs, John M. *The Concept of Matrimonial Cruelty*. London: The Athlone Press, 1962.

Bigner, Jerry J. "Parent Education in Popular Literature: 1950–1970." *The Family Coordinator* 21, no. 3 (1972): 313–319.

Bion, W.R. *Experiences in Groups*. London: Tavistock Publications, 1959.

Bion, W.R. "The Leaderless Group Project." *Bulletin of the Menninger Clinic* 10 (1946): 77–81.

Blood, Robert, and Donald M. Wolfe. *Husbands and Wives: The Dynamics of Married Living*. Glencoe, IL: The Free Press, 1960.

Borland, Marie, ed. *Violence in the Family*. Manchester, UK: Manchester University Press, 1976.

Bowlby, John. *A Two-Year-Old Goes to Hospital*. UK: Robertson Films, 1952.

Bowlby, John. *Attachment and Loss*. Vol. 1. London: Tavistock Publications, 1969.

Bowlby, John. *Child Care and the Growth of Love*. Edited by Margery Fry. London: Penguin, 1953.
Bowlby, John. "Critical Phases in the Development of the Social Responses in Man and Other Animals." *New Biology* 14 (1953): 25–32.
Bowlby, John. "Effects on Behaviour of Disruption of an Affectional Bond." Paper presented at Genetic and Environmental Influences on Behaviour: A Symposium Held by the Eugenics Society in September 1967. Proceedings edited by J.M. Thoday and A.S. Parkes, 94–108. New York: Plenum Press, 1968.
Bowlby, John. *Forty-Four Juvenile Thieves: Their Characters and Home Life*. London: Baillière, Tindall and Cox, 1946.
Bowlby, John. *Maternal Care and Mental Health: A Report Prepared on Behalf of the World Health Organization as a Contribution to the United Nations Programme for the Welfare of Homeless Children*. Geneva: WHO, 1951.
Bowlby, John. "Psychology and Democracy." *The Political Quarterly* 17, no. 1 (January 1946): 61–75.
Bowlby, John. "Substitute Homes." *Mother and Child* (April 1939): 3–7.
Bowlby, John. "The Abnormally Aggressive Child." *New Era in Home and School* (Sept–Oct 1938): 230–234.
Bowlby, John. "The Therapeutic Approach in Sociology." *Sociological Review* 39 (1947): 39–49.
Bowlby, John, and Mary Ainsworth. "Research Strategy in the Study of Mother-Child Separation." *Courrier* 4 (1953): 105–130.
Bowlby, John, and E.F.M. Durbin. "Personal Aggressiveness and War." In *War and Democracy: Essays on the Causes and Prevention of War*, edited by John Bowlby et al., 3–150. London: K. Paul, Trench, Trubner and Co., 1938.
Bowlby, John, and James Robertson. "A Two-Year-Old Goes to Hospital." *Proceedings of the Royal Society of Medicine* 46 (1952): 425–427.
Bowley, Agatha. *Child Care: A Handbook on the Care of the Child Deprived of a Normal Home Life*. Edinburgh: E&S Livingstone, 1951.
Burgess, E.W., and H.J. Locke. *The Family: From Institution to Companionship*. New York: American Book Company, 1945.
Burt, Cyril. *The Young Delinquent*. London: University of London Press, 1925.
Brannen, Julia, and Jean Collard. *Marriages in Trouble: The Process of Seeking Help*. London: Tavistock Publications, 1982.
Bridger, Harold. "The Discovery of the Therapeutic Community: The Northfield Experiments." In *The Social Engagement of Social Science*, edited by Eric Trist and Hugh Murray, 68–87. London: Free Association Books, 1990.
British Medical Association. *Venereal Disease and Young People: A Report by a Committee of the British Medical Association on the Problem of Venereal Disease Particularly among Young People*. London: British Medical Association, 1964.
Brown, William. *War and Peace: Essays in Psychological Analysis*. London: A&C Black, 1939.
Burns, Charles L.C. *Maladjusted Children*. London: Hollis & Carter, 1955.
Caffey, J. "Multiple Fracture of the Long Bones of Infants Suffering from Chronic Subdural Haematoma." *American Journal of Roentgenology* 56 (1946): 163–173.
Campaign for Homosexual Equality. *Women Together: Report of a Meeting of Women from the Gay Movement and from the Women's Movement*. Manchester, UK: Campaign for Homosexual Equality, 1975.
Campbell, Elaine. *The Childless Marriage: An Exploratory Study of Couples Who Do Not Want Children*. London: Tavistock Publications, 1985.
Cass, Henry, dir. *No Place for Jennifer*. UK: Associated British Picture Corporation, 1950.
Chartham, Robert. *You, Your Children and Sex: What to Tell Them, How, and When*. London: Leslie Frewin Publishers, 1973.
Comer, Lee. "The Motherhood Myth." *Australian Left Review* (March 1972): 28–34.

Comer, Lee. *Wedlocked Women*. Leeds, UK: Feminist Books Ltd., 1974.
Comerford, John. *Health the Unknown: The Story of the Peckham Experiment*. London: Hamish Hamilton, 1947.
Committee on Homosexual Offences and Prostitution. *Report of the Committee on Homosexual Offences and Prostitution*. London: HMSO, 1957.
Commonwealth Fund. *The Commonwealth Fund: Historical Sketch, 1918–1962*. New York: The Fund, 1963.
Cooper, David. *Psychiatry and Anti-Psychiatry*. London: Tavistock Publications, 1967.
Cooper, David. *The Death of the Family*. New York: Pantheon Books, 1970.
Cooper, David. *The Grammar of Living*. London: Allen Lane, 1974.
Cooper, David. *To Free a Generation: The Dialectics of Liberation*. New York: Collier Books, 1968.
Crane, Paul. *Gays and the Law*. London: Pluto Press Ltd., 1982.
Criminal Law Revision Committee. *Fifteenth Report: Sexual Offences*. London: HMSO, 1984.
Criminal Law Revision Committee. *Working Paper on Offences Relating to Prostitution and Allied Offences*. London: HMSO, 1982.
Curtis, Myra. *Report of the Care of Children Committee*. London: HMSO, 1946.
Dallas, Dorothy. *Exploring Sex Education in School and Society*. Slough, UK: National Foundation for Education Research in England and Wales, 1972.
Denborough, David, ed. *Queer Counselling and Narrative Practice*. Adelaide: Dulwich Centre Publications, 2002.
Denning, Alfred Thompson. *Final Report of the Committee on Procedure in Matrimonial Causes*. London: HMSO, 1947.
Department of Education and Science. *Report of the Committee on Maladjusted Children*. London, HMSO: 1955.
Department of Health and Social Security. *Teenage Mothers and Their Partners*. London: HMSO Publications, 1986.
Department of Health and Social Security. *The Family in Society: Preparation for Parenthood*. London: HMSO, 1974.
Departmental Committee on Human Artificial Insemination. *Report of the Departmental Committee on Human Artificial Insemination*. London: HMSO, 1960.
Devlin, Patrick. *The Enforcement of Morals*. The 1959 Maccabean Lecture in Jurisprudence of the British Academy. Oxford: Oxford University Press, 1959.
Dicks, Henry V. *Fifty Years of the Tavistock Clinic*. London: Routledge and Kegan Paul, 1970.
Dicks, Henry V. *Licensed Mass Murder: A Socio-psychological Study of Some SS Killers*. London: Heinemann, 1972.
Dicks, Henry V. *Marital Tensions: Clinical Studies towards a Psychological Theory of Interaction*. New York: Basic Books, Inc., 1967.
Dicks, Henry V. "Personality Traits and National Socialist Ideology." *Human Relations* 3, no. 2 (June 1950): 111–155.
Dicks, Henry V. *The Psychological Foundations of the Wehrmacht*. London: War Office, 1944.
Dinkmeyer, Don, and Gary D. McKay. *Raising a Responsible Child: Practical Steps to Successful Family Relationships*. New York: Simon and Schuster, 1973.
Dix, Carol. *The New Mother Syndrome: Coping with Stress and Depression*. Garden City, NY: Doubleday, 1985.
Dixon, C. Madeleine. *Keep Them Human: The Young Child at Home*. New York: John Day Co., 1942.
Doll, Edgar. *Vineland Social Maturity Scale: Manual of Directions*. Minneapolis, MN: Educational Test Bureau, 1947.
Edelston, Harry. *Teenagers Talking*. London: Pitman Medical Publishing Co. Ltd., 1963.
Endfield, Cy. *Child in the House*. London: Eros Films, 1956.

Erikson, Erik. *Childhood and Society*. New York: W.W. Norton and Co., 1950.
Fairbairn, W.R.D. *Psychoanalytic Studies of the Personality*. London: Routledge and Kegan Paul, 1952.
Family Planning Association. *Family Planning in the Sixties: Report of the Family Planning Association Working Party*. London: Family Planning Association, 1963.
Family Planning Association. *Learning to Live with Sex: A Handbook of Sex Education for Teenagers*. London: The Family Planning Association, 1972.
Feversham Committee. *The Voluntary Mental Health Services: The Report of the Feversham Committee*. London: The Committee, 1939.
Fogelman, Ken, ed. *Growing Up in Great Britain: Papers from the National Child Development Study*. London: Macmillan Press Ltd., 1983.
Ford, Donald. *The Deprived Child and the Community*. London: Constable, 1955.
Foss, B.M., ed. *Determinants of Infant Behaviour: Tavistock Study Group on Mother-Infant Interaction*. Vol. 1–4. Tavistock Publications: London, 1969–1965.
Freud, Anna. "Adolescence." *Psychoanalytical Study of the Child* 13 (1958): 255–278.
Freud, Anna. *Normality and Pathology in Childhood: Assessments of Development*. New York: International Universities Press, 1965.
Freud, Anna. "Discussion of Dr. John Bowlby's Paper." *The Psychoanalytic Study of the Child* 15 (1960): 53–62.
Freud, Anna. *Psychoanalysis for Teachers and Parents*. New York: Emerson Books, Inc., 1947.
Freud, Anna. *War and Children*. New York: Medical War Books, 1943.
Freud, Anna, and Dorothy Burlingham. *Infants without Families: The Case for and against Residential Nurseries*. London: Allen & Unwin, 1943.
Freud, Anna, and Dorothy Burlingham. *Young Children in War-Time*. London: Imago Publishing Co., 1949.
Freud, Sigmund. *Group Psychology and the Analysis of the Ego*. Translated by James Strachey. New York: W.W. Norton and Co., 1959 [1922].
Freud, Sigmund. *Three Essays on the Theory of Sexuality*. Translated by James Strachey. London: Hogarth Press, 1905.
Friedan, Betty. *The Feminine Mystique*. New York: W.W. Norton and Co., 1963.
Gavron, Hannah. *The Captive Wife*. London: Routledge & Kegan Paul, 1966.
Gelles, Richard J. *The Violent Home: A Study of Physical Aggression between Husbands and Wives*. New York: Sage Publications, 1974.
Gesell, Arthur. *Infant and Child in the Culture of Today: The Guidance of Development in Home and Nursery School*. New York: Harper and Bros., 1943.
Ginott, Haim. *Between Parents and Teenagers*. London: Cassell, 1973.
Glover, Edward. *War, Sadism and Pacifism: Three Essays*. London: George Allen and Unwin, 1933.
Gorer, Geoffrey. *Sex and Marriage in England Today: A Study of the Views and Experience of the Under-45s*. London: Thomas Nelson and Sons, Ltd., 1971.
Gorer, Geoffrey, and John Rickman. *The People of Great Russia: A Psychological Study*. London: Cresset Press, 1949.
Gough, Donald. *Schoolgirl Unmarried Mothers*. London: National Council for the Unmarried Mother and Her Child, 1967.
Great Britain. *Children Act 1948*. London: HMSO, 1948.
Great Britain. *Children Act 1958*. London: HMSO, 1958.
Greengross, Wendy. *Entitled to Love: The Sexual and Emotional Needs of the Handicapped*. London: National Marriage Guidance Council, 1976.
Grey, Antony. *Speaking Out: Writings on Sex, Law, Politics, and Society*. London: Cassell, 1997.
Grey, Antony. *The Albany Trust and Its Work*. London: Albany Trust, 1971.

Grey, Antony. *Quest for Justice: Towards Homosexual Emancipation*. London: Sinclair-Stevenson, 1992.
Griffith, Edward F. *A Sex Guide to Happy Marriage*. New York: Emerson Books, 1952.
Griffith, Edward F. *Marriage and the Unconscious*. London: Secker and Warburg, 1957.
Griffith, Edward F. *Modern Marriage and Birth Control*. London: V. Gollancz, 1937.
Griffith, Edward F. *Sex in Everyday Life*. London: Allen & Unwin, 1938.
Griffith, Edward F. *Sex and Citizenship*. London: V. Gollancz, 1941.
Griffith, Edward F. *The Pioneer Spirit*. Upton Grey, UK: Green Leaves Press, 1981.
Griffith, Edward F. *The Road to Maturity*. London: Methuen, 1944.
Griffith, Edward F. *Voluntary Parenthood*. London: William Heinemann Ltd., 1937.
Hacker, Rose. *Telling the Teenagers: A Guide for Parents, Teachers and Youth Leaders*. London: Andre Deutsch Ltd., 1966.
Hall, G. Stanley. *Adolescence: Its Psychology and Its Relation to Physiology, Anthropology, Sociology, Sex, Crime, Religion, and Education*. New York: D. Appleton and Co., 1904.
Halliday, James L. *Psychosocial Medicine: A Study of the Sick Society*. New York: W.W. Norton and Co., 1948.
Halmos, Paul. *Solitude and Privacy: A Study of Social Isolation, Its Causes and Therapy*. London: Routledge and Kegan Paul, 1952.
Hargreaves, G.R. *Psychiatry and the Public Health*. London: Oxford University Press, 1958.
Harris, Alan. *Questions about Sex*. London: Hutchinson Educational, 1968.
Harris, Sidney. *Report of the Departmental Committee on Grants for the Development of Marriage Guidance*. London: HMSO, 1948.
Hart, H.L.A. *Law, Liberty and Morality*. Stanford: Stanford University Press, 1963.
Hatton, Sidney F. *London's Bad Boys*. London: Chapman & Hall Ltd., 1931.
Havil, Anthony. *The Techniques of Sex: Towards a Better Understanding of the Sexual Relationship*. London: Wales Publishing Co., 1939.
Henriques, Basil. *The Indiscretions of a Warden*. London: Methuen and Co., 1950.
Herbert, A.P. *Holy Deadlock*. London: Methuen, 1934.
Heywood, Jean S. *The Deprived Child and the Nation*. London: Epworth, 1964.
Hilliard, Marion. *Problems of Adolescence: A Woman Doctor's Advice on Growing Up*. London: Macmillan and Co. Ltd., 1958.
Holt, Nancy. *Counselling in Marriage Problems*. London: The National Marriage Guidance Council, 1971.
House of Commons Select Committee on Violence in Marriage. *Report from the Select Committee on Violence in Marriage, together with the Proceedings of the Committee, Session 1974–75*, Vol. 1–2. London: HMSO, 1975.
Howells, John G. *Family Psychiatry*. Springfield, IL: Charles C. Thomas Publishers, 1963.
Ingleby, Alan H.B. *Learning to Love: A Wider View of Sex Education*. London: Robert Hale Limited, 1961.
International Congress on Mental Health. *Mental Health and World Citizenship: A Statement Prepared for the International Congress on Mental Health, London 1948*. London: World Federation for Mental Health, 1948.
International Planned Parenthood Federation. *A Survey on the Status of Sex Education in European Member Countries*. London: International Planned Parenthood Federation, 1975.
Isaacs, Susan, ed. *The Cambridge Evacuation Survey: A Wartime Study in Social Welfare and Education*. London: Methuen & Co., 1941.
Isaacs, Susan. *Troubles of Children and Parents*. London: Methuen, 1948.
James, Selma. *Women, the Unions and Work, or. . . What Is Not to Be Done*. London: Crest Press, 1975.
Joint Committee of the British Medical Association and the Magistrates' Association. *Cruelty to and Neglect of Children*. London: British Medical Association, 1956.

Select Bibliography

Joint Council for Gay Teenagers. *Breaking the Silence*. London: Joint Council for Gay Teenagers, 1980.

Joint Council for Gay Teenagers. *I Know What I Am: Gay Teenagers and the Law*. Liverpool: Joint Council for Gay Teenagers, 1980.

Joint Working Party on Pregnant Schoolgirls and Schoolgirl Mothers. *Pregnant at School*. London: National Council for One Parent Families, 1979.

Jones, Anne. *Counselling Adolescents: School and After*. London: Kogan Page Ltd., 1984.

Jones, Anne. *School Counselling in Practice*. London: Ward Lock Educational Co. Ltd., 1970.

Jones, Maxwell. *Social Psychiatry: A Study of Therapeutic Communities*. London: Tavistock Publications, Ltd., 1952.

Jones, Maxwell. "The Therapeutic Community, Social Learning and Social Change." In *Therapeutic Communities: Reflections and Progress*, edited by R.D. Hinshelwood and Nick Manning, 1–9. London: Routledge, 1979.

Kavanaugh, Kenneth. *Sex Education: Its Uses and Abuses*. London: The Responsible Society, 1975.

Kellmer Pringle, Mia. *Early Child Care in Britain*. London: Gordon and Breach, 1975.

Kellmer Pringle, Mia. *The Needs of Children*. London: Hutchinson and Co., 1974.

Kellmer Pringle, Mia. *11,000 Seven-Year-Olds: First Report of the National Child Development Study*. London: Longmans, 1966.

Kempe, C.H., Frederic N. Silverman, Brandt F. Steele, William Droegemuller, and Henry K. Silver. "The Battered Child Syndrome." *Journal of the American Medical Association* 181 (1962): 17–24.

Kennedy, Roger, Ann Heymans, and Lydia Tischler, eds. *The Family as In-Patient: Working with Families and Adolescents at the Cassel Hospital*. London: Free Association Books, 1987.

Key, Ellen. *The Century of the Child*. New York and London: Putnam's Sons, 1909.

Khan, Verity Saifullah, ed. *Minority Families in Britain: Support and Stress*. Basingstoke: Macmillan Press, 1979.

King, Joan. *The Probation Service*. London: Butterworth & Co. Ltd., 1958.

Klein, Josephine. *Samples from English Cultures*. Vol. 2: *Child-Rearing Practices*. London: Routledge and Kegan Paul, 1965.

Laing, R.D. *The Divided Self: A Study of Sanity and Madness*. Harmondsworth, UK: Penguin Books, 1965 [1960].

Laing, R.D. *The Self and Others: Further Studies in Sanity and Madness*. London: Tavistock Publications, 1962.

Laing, R.D. *The Politics of Experience*. New York: Pantheon Books, 1967.

Laing, R.D. *Wisdom, Madness, and Folly: The Making of a Psychiatrist*. New York: McGraw-Hill Book Co., 1985.

Laing, R.D., and Aaron Esterson. *Sanity, Madness, and the Family*. London: Tavistock Publications, 1964.

Lampl-de-Groot, Jeanne. "On Adolescence." *The Psychoanalytic Study of the Child* 15 (1960): 95–103.

Lane, Homer. *Talks to Teachers and Parents*. London: Allen & Unwin, 1928.

Lane, Mary Beauchamp. *Learning about Life: A Child-Centred Approach to Sex Education*. London: Evans Brothers Ltd., 1973.

Lasch, Christopher. *Haven in a Heartless World: The Family Besieged*. New York: Basic Books, 1977.

Lasch, Christopher. *The Culture of Narcissism: American Life in an Age of Diminishing Expectations*. New York: Norton, 1978.

Latey Committee on the Age of Majority. *Report of the Latey Committee on the Age of Majority*. London: HMSO, 1967.

Laufer, Moses. "A Psychoanalytical Approach to Work with Adolescents." Sixth International Congress of Psychotherapy, London 1964. *Psychotherapy and Psychosomatics* 13 (1965): 292–298.
Laufer, Moses, and M. Eglé Laufer. *Adolescence and Developmental Breakdown: A Psychoanalytic View*. New Haven, CT: Yale University Press, 1984.
Lawton, Denis. *Population Education and the Younger Generation*. London: International Planned Parenthood Federation, 1971.
Leach, Edmund. *A Runaway World?* The Reith Lectures 1967. London: British Broadcasting Corporation, 1968.
League of Nations. *The Placing of Children in Families*. Geneva: League of Nations, 1938.
Le Bon, Gustave. *The Crowd: A Study of the Popular Mind*. London: Berg, 1947.
Lewis, Aubrey. "Health as a Social Concept." *British Journal of Sociology* 4 (1955): 109–124.
Lewis, Hilda. *Deprived Children: The Mersham Experiment: A Social and Clinical Study*. Oxford: Oxford University Press, 1954.
Lidz, Theodore. *Schizophrenia and the Family*. New York: International Universities Press, Inc., 1965.
Mace, David. *Coming Home: A Series of Five Broadcast Talks*. New York; London: Staples Press Ltd., 1946.
Mace, David. *Marriage Counseling: The First Full Account of the Remedial Work of the Marriage Guidance Councils*. London: Churchill, 1948.
Mace, David. "Marriage Guidance in England." *Marriage and Family Living* 7, no. 1 (February 1945): 1–5.
Mace, David, and Vera Mace. *The Soviet Family*. New York: Doubleday and Co., 1963.
Main, T.F. *The Ailment and Other Psychoanalytic Essays*. Edited by Jennifer Johns. London: Free Association Books, 1989.
Main, T.F. et al. *The Cassel Hospital: Reports for the Five Years, 1953–1958*. Surrey, UK: Cassel Hospital, 1958.
Main, T.F. "Mutual Projection in a Marriage." *Comprehensive Psychiatry* 7, no. 5 (1966): 432–449.
Marshall, T.H. *Citizenship and Social Class and Other Essays*. Cambridge: Cambridge University Press, 1950.
Martin, Doreen. "The Beginnings of the Growth and Development of an Adolescent Unit in the Cassel Hospital." Sixth International Congress of Psychotherapy, London 1964. *Psychotherapy and Psychosomatics* 13 (1965): 309–313.
Marris, Peter. *Widows and Their Families*. London: Routledge & Kegan Paul, 1958.
Mawby, R.I. "Policing the Age of Consent." *Journal of Adolescence* 2 (1979): 41–49.
Mead, Margaret. *Coming of Age in Samoa: A Psychological Study of Primitive Youth for Western Civilization*. New York: William Morrow and Co., 1928.
Mead, Margaret. *Male and Female: A Study of the Sexes in a Changing World*. New York: William Morrow and Co., 1967.
Mead, Margaret. "Some Theoretical Considerations on the Problem of Mother-Child Separation." *American Journal of Orthopsychiatry* 24 (3) July 1954: 471–483.
Mead, Margaret, Geoffrey Gorer, and John Rickman. *Russian Culture*. Oxford: Berghahn Books, 2001.
Mead, Margaret, and Martha Wolfenstein, eds. *Childhood in Contemporary Cultures*. Chicago: University of Chicago Press, 1954.
McDougall, William. *The Group Mind*. Cambridge: The University Press, 1920.
McGregor, O.R. "Towards Divorce Law Reform." *British Journal of Sociology* 18 (1967): 91–99.
Middlemore, Merell. *The Nursing Couple*. London: Hamish Hamilton Medical Books, 1941.
Miller, Derek. *Growth to Freedom: The Psychosocial Treatment of Delinquent Youth*. London: Tavistock Publications, 1964.
Mitchell, A.R.K. *Violence in the Family*. Hove, UK: Wayland, 1978.

Mitchell, Juliet. *Psychoanalysis and Feminism*. London: Allen Lane, 1974.
Mitchell, Juliet. *Woman's Estate*. Harmondsworth, UK: Penguin, 1971.
Mitchell, Juliet. *Women: The Longest Revolution: Essays on Feminism, Literature, and Psychoanalysis*. London: Virago, 1984.
Morgan, Patricia. *Child Care: Sense and Fable*. London: Temple Smith, 1975.
Morgan, Patricia. *Farewell to the Family? Public Policy and Family Breakdown in Britain and the USA*. London: IEA Health and Welfare Unit, 1995.
Myrdal, Alva, and Viola Klein. *Women's Two Roles*. London: Routledge and K. Paul, 1956.
National Association for Mental Health. *Mental Health and Personal Responsibility*. London: National Association for Mental Health, 1956.
National Association for Mental Health. *Ninth Child Guidance Inter-Clinic Conference: Follow up on Child Guidance Cases, 24 November 1951*. London: National Association for Mental Health, 1952.
National Association for Mental Health. *The Family Approach to Child Guidance—Therapeutic Techniques: XIth Inter-Clinic Conference for Staffs of Child Guidance Clinics*. London: National Association for Mental Health, 1955.
National Council for Civil Liberties. *Homosexuality and the Teaching Profession: NCCL Report*. London: National Council for Civil Liberties, 1975.
National Council for Civil Liberties. *Sexual Offences: Evidence to the Criminal Law Revision Committee*. London: National Council for Civil Liberties, 1976.
National Marriage Guidance Council. *Counsellor Basic Training Prospectus*. London: NMGC, 1985.
National Marriage Guidance Council. *Your Teenagers: Help with Parents' Problems*. London: National Marriage Guidance Council, 1965.
National Marriage Guidance Council. *Sex Education in Perspective: A Symposium on Work in Progress*. London: National Marriage Guidance Council, 1972.
Neill, A.S. *Freedom—Not License!* New York: Hart Publishing Co., 1966.
Newson, John, and Elizabeth Newson. *Infant Care in an Urban Community*. London: Allen and Unwin, 1963.
Oakley, Ann. *Housewife*. London: Penguin, Ltd., 1974.
Odlum, Doris. *You and Your Children: BBC Talks by a Woman Medical Psychologist*. London: HMSO, 1946.
Odlum, Doris. *Journey Through Adolescence*. London: Delisle, 1957.
Odlum, Doris. *The Mind of Your Child*. London: Foyle, 1960.
Padley, Richard, and Margaret Cole. *Evacuation Survey: A Report to the Fabian Society*. London: Routledge and Sons, Ltd., 1940.
Parsons, Talcott, and Robert F. Bales. *Family Socialization and Interaction Process*. Glencoe, IL: Free Press, 1955.
Pasmore, Jean, and Margaret Blair. "Family Planning for the Unmarried." *Journal of the Royal College of General Practitioners* 18, no. 87 (1969): 214–218.
Pearse, Innes Hope. *The Quality of Life: The Peckham Approach to Human Ethology*. Edinburgh: Scottish Academic Press, 1979.
Pearse, Innes, and Lucy H. Crocker. *The Peckham Experiment: A Study in the Living Structure of Society*. London: George, Allen & Unwin, 1943.
Pearse, Innes, and G. Scott Williamson. *Biologists in Search of Material: An Interim Report on the Work of the Pioneer Health Centre*. London: Faber and Faber, 1938.
Pearse, Innes, and G. Scott Williamson. *The Case for Action: A Survey of Everyday Life under Modern Industrial Conditions, with Special Reference to the Question of Health*. London: Faber and Faber, Ltd., 1931.
Pfeffer, Naomi. *The Experience of Infertility*. London: Virago, 1983.
Phillipson, Herbert. *The Object Relations Technique*. Glencoe, IL: The Free Press, 1955.

Pincus, Lily, ed. *Marriage: Studies in Emotional Conflict and Growth*. 2nd. ed. London: Tavistock Institute of Human Relations, 1973.
Pizzey, Erin. *Infernal Child: A Memoir*. London: V. Gollancz, 1978.
Pizzey, Erin. *Scream Quietly or the Neighbours Will Hear*. Harmondsworth: Penguin Books, 1974.
Pizzey, Erin. *The Emotional Terrorist and the Violence-Prone*. Ottawa: Commoners, 1998.
Pizzey, Erin. *This Way to the Revolution: A Memoir*. London: Peter Owen Books, 2011.
Platt, Harry. *The Welfare of Children in Hospital: Report of the Committee*. London: HMSO, 1959.
Playne, Caroline. *The Neuroses of Nations*. London: George, Allen & Unwin Ltd., 1925.
Plummer, Kenneth. *Sexual Stigma: An Interactionist Account*. London: Routledge and Kegan Paul, 1975.
Policy Advisory Committee on Sexual Offences. *Report on the Age of Consent in Relation to Sexual Offences*. London: HMSO, April 1981.
Policy Advisory Committee on Sexual Offences. *Working Paper on the Age of Consent in Relation to Sexual Offences*. London: HMSO, June 1979.
Powers, G.P., and Wade Baskin, eds. *Sex Education in a Changing Culture*. London: Peter Owen Ltd., 1969.
Prince, Gordon Stewart. *Teenagers Today*. London: National Association for Mental Health, 1968.
Rapoport, Rhona, and Robert Rapoport. *Dual-Career Families*. Harmondsworth, UK: Penguin Books, 1971.
Rapoport, Robert. *Community as Doctor: New Perspectives on a Therapeutic Community*. London: Tavistock Publications, 1960.
Rees, John R. *Experiences of Neurosis and Backwardness in the War-Time Army: Can They Help with Civilian Problems?* National Association for Mental Health Conference Report, 1946.
Rees, John R. *Reflections: A Personal History and an Account of the Growth of the World Federation for Mental Health*. New York: World Federation for Mental Health, 1966.
Rees, John R., ed. *The Case of Rudolf Hess: A Problem in Diagnosis and Forensic Psychiatry*. London: William Heinemann, Ltd., 1947.
Rees, John R. *The Health of the Mind*. New York: W.W. Norton and Co., 1951.
Rees, John R. *The Shaping of Psychiatry by War*. New York: W.W. Norton and Co., 1945.
Renvoize, Jean. *Web of Violence: A Study of Family Violence*. London: Routledge and Kegan Paul, 1978.
Responsible Society Research and Education Trust. *Sex Education in Schools—What Every Parent Should Know*. Milton Keynes: The Trust, 1982.
Richter, Horst. *The Family as Patient: The Origin, Structure, and Therapy of Marital and Family Conflict*. Translated by Denver and Helen Lindley. New York: Farrar, Straus, and Giroux, 1974.
Robertson, James. *A Two-Year-Old Goes to Hospital, A Guide to the Film*. London: Tavistock Publications, 1953.
Robertson, James. *Going to Hospital with Mother, A Guide to the Documentary Film*. London: Tavistock Child Development Research Unit, 1958.
Robertson, James. *Hospitals and Children: A Parent's-Eye View: A Review of Letters from Parents to the Observer and the BBC*. London: Tavistock Publications, 1962.
Robertson, James. *Young Children in Hospitals*. New York: Basic Books, 1958.
Rogers, Carl. *Becoming a Person*. Oberlin: Board of Trustees of Oberlin College, 1954.
Rogers, Rex S, ed. *Sex Education: Rationale and Reaction*. Cambridge: Cambridge University Press, 1974.
Rowbotham, Sheila. *Promise of a Dream: Remembering the Sixties*. London: Penguin, 2001.
Rowbotham, Sheila. "To Be or Not to Be: The Dilemmas of Mothering." *Feminist Review*, 31 (1989): 82–93.

Select Bibliography

Royal Commission on Marriage and Divorce. *Report, 1951–55*. London: HMSO, 1956.

Royal Society of Health. *Sex Education of School Children*. London: Royal Society for the Promotion of Health, 1971.

Russell, Bertrand. *Marriage and Morals*. London: G. Allen and Unwin, 1929.

Rutter, Michael. *Changing Youth in a Changing Society: Patterns of Adolescent Development and Disorder*. London: Nuffield Provincial Hospitals Trust, 1979.

Sage, Lorna. *Bad Blood*. London: Fourth Estate Ltd., 2000.

Salk, Lee. *What Every Child Would Like His Parents to Know, To Help Him with the Emotional Problems of His Everyday Life*. London: Robert Hale and Co., 1972.

Schaffer, Rudolf, and Peggy Emerson. *The Development of Social Attachments in Infancy*. Lafayette, IN: Child Development Publications, 1964.

Schofield, Michael. *Sociological Aspects of Homosexuality*. London: The Camelot Press, Ltd., 1965.

Schofield, Michael. *The Sexual Behaviour of Young People*. London: Longmans, Green and Co. Ltd., 1965.

Schur, Max. "Discussion of Dr. John Bowlby's Paper." *The Psychoanalytic Study of the Child* 15 (1960): 63–84.

Schween, Peter, and Alexander Gralnick. "Factors Affecting Family Therapy in the Hospital Setting." *Comprehensive Psychiatry* 7 (5) 1966: 424–431.

Sexual Law Reform Society. *Report of the Working Party on the Law in Relation to Sexual Behaviour*. London: Sexual Law Reform Society, September 1974.

Skinner, Angela, and Raymond Castle. *78 Battered Children: A Retrospective Study*. London: National Society for the Prevention of Cruelty to Children, 1969.

Slater, Eliot, and Moya Woodside. *Patterns of Marriage: A Study of Marriage Relationships in the Urban Working Classes*. London: Cassell and Co. Ltd., 1951.

Smith, Cyril S. *Adolescence: An Introduction to the Problems of Order and the Opportunities for Continuity Presented by Adolescence in Britain*. London: Longmans, Green and Co. Ltd., 1968.

Soddy, Kenneth, ed. *Mental Health and Infant Development: Proceedings of the International Seminar held by the World Federation for Mental Health at Chichester, England*. Vol. 1. New York: Basic Books, Inc., 1955.

Soddy, Kenneth, ed. *Mental Health and Infant Development: Proceedings of the International Seminar Held by the World Federation for Mental Health at Chichester, England*. Vol. 2. New York: Basic Books, Inc., 1956.

Spence, James. *The Purpose of the Family: A Guide to the Care of Children*. London: National Children's Home, 1947.

Spinley, B.M. *The Deprived and the Privileged: Personality Development in English Society*. London: Routledge and Kegan Paul, 1953.

Spitz, Réne. "Discussion of Dr. John Bowlby's Paper." *The Psychoanalytic Study of the Child* 15 (1960): 85–94.

Spitz, Réne. "Hospitalism: An Inquiry in the Genesis of Psychiatric Conditions in Early Childhood." *Psychoanalytic Study of the Child* 1 (1945): 53–74.

Spitz, Réne. *The First Year of Life*. New York: International Universities Press, 1965.

Spock, Benjamin. *Baby and Child Care*. New York: Duell, Sloan and Pearce, 1946.

Stallibrass, Alison. *Being Me and Also Us: Lessons from the Peckham Experiment*. Edinburgh: Scottish Academic Press, 1989.

Steinmetz, Suzanne K., and Murray A. Straus, eds. *Violence in the Family*. New York: Dodd, Mead and Co., 1974.

Stopes, Marie Carmichael. *Marriage in My Time*. London: Rich & Cowan, 1935.

Stopes, Marie Carmichael. *Married Love: A New Contribution to the Solution of Sex Difficulties*. London: Putnam, 1926 [1918].

Strachey, Amy St. Loe. *Borrowed Children: A Popular Account of Some Evacuation Problems and Their Remedies*. New York: Commonwealth Fund, 1940.
Strachey, Amy St. Loe. *These Two Strange Years: Letters from England, October 1939–September 1941*. New York: Commonwealth Fund, 1942.
Suttie, Ian D. *The Origins of Love and Hate*. London: K. Paul, Trench, and Trubner, 1935.
Tanner, J.M. *Education and Physical Growth: Implications of the Study of Children's Growth for Educational Theory and Practice*. London: University of London Press, 1961.
Tanner, J.M. *Growth at Adolescence*. Oxford: Blackwell Scientific Publications, 1962.
Titmuss, Richard. *Essays on the Welfare State*. London: Allen and Unwin, 1958.
Titmuss, Richard. "Industrialization and the Family." *Social Service Review* 31, no. 1 (March 1957): 54–62.
Trotter, Wilfred. *Instincts of the Herd in Peace and War*. London: T.F. Unwin, 1916.
Tweedie, Jill. *Eating Children*. Harmondsworth: Penguin, 1994.
Tyler, Mary. *Advisory and Counselling Services for Young People*. London: HMSO, 1978.
Tyndall, Nicholas, ed. *Sex Education in Perspective*. London: National Marriage Guidance Council, 1972.
Van de Velde, Theo. *Ideal Marriage: Its Physiology and Technique*. London: William Heinemann Medical Books, Ltd., 1928.
Van der Eyken, Willem. *Home-Start: A Four-Year Evaluation*. Leicester: Home-Start Consultancy, 1982.
Vaughan, T.D, ed. *Concepts of Counselling: Papers Prepared by a Working Party of the Standing Conference for the Advancement of Counselling*. London: Bedford Square Press, 1975.
Walker, Lenore. *The Battered Woman*. New York: Harper & Row, 1979.
Wallis, J.H., and H.S. Booker. *Marriage Counselling: A Description and Analysis of the Remedial Work of the National Marriage Guidance Council*. London: Routledge and Kegan Paul, 1958.
Walmsley, Roy, and Karen White. *Sexual Offences, Consent, and Sentencing*. London: HMSO, 1979.
Weddell, Doreen. "Psychology and Nursing." *Nursing Times* 51 (1955): 63–65.
White, Margaret, and Jennet Kidd, *Sound Sex Education: A Handbook for Parents, Teachers, and Education Authorities*. London: Order of Christian Unity, 1976.
Whitehouse, Mary. *Cleaning Up TV: From Protest to Participation*. London: Blandford Press, 1967.
Wills, David. *Throw Away Thy Rod*. London: Victor Gollancz, 1960.
Winch, Robert. *The Modern Family*. New York: Holt, 1952.
Winnicott, Donald Woods. *Getting to Know Your Baby*. London: Heinemann, 1945.
Winnicott, Donald Woods. *The Child, the Family, and the Outside World*. Harmondsworth, UK: Penguin Books, 1964.
Winnicott, Donald Woods. "Thoughts on the Meaning of the Word Democracy." *Human Relations* 4 (1950): 171–185.
Winterson, Jeannette. *Written on the Body*. London: Jonathan Cape, 1992.
Wolf, Katherine. "Evacuation of Children in Wartime." *Psychoanalytic Study of the Child* (1945): 389–404.
Wolfenden, John. *Turning Points: The Memoirs of Lord Wolfenden*. London: Bodley Head Ltd., 1976.
Wolkon, G.H., et al. "Ethnicity and Social Class in the Delivery of Services: Analysis of a Child Guidance Clinic." *American Journal of Public Health* 64, no. 7 (July 1974): 709–712.
Women's Group on Public Welfare. *Our Towns: A Close Up, A Study Made in 1939–1942*. London: Oxford University Press, 1943.
Women's Group on Public Welfare. *The Neglected Child and His Family: A Study made in 1946–7 of the Problem of the Child Neglected in His Own Home*. London: Oxford University Press, 1948.

Women's Liberal Federation. *The Great Partnership*. London: Women's Liberal Federation, 1949.
Wright, Helena. *The Sex Factor in Marriage: A Book for Those Who Are or Are About to Be Married*. London: Douglas, 1932.
Young, Leontine. *Out of Wedlock: A Study of the Problems of the Unmarried Mother and her Child*. London and New York: McGraw-Hill Book Co., 1954.
Young, Michael, and Peter Willmott. *Family and Kinship in East London*. London: Routledge and Kegan Paul, 1957.
Younghusband, Eileen. *Social Work and Social Change*. London: Allen and Unwin, 1964.
Younghusband, Eileen. *Social Work and Social Values*. London: Allen and Unwin, 1967.
Younghusband, Eileen. "Statutes: The Children Act 1948." *The Modern Law Review* 12 (1) 1949: 65–69.

Secondary Sources

Allan, Graham, ed. *The Sociology of the Family*. Oxford: Blackwell Publishers Ltd., 1999.
Apple, Rima. "Constructing Mothers: Scientific Motherhood in the Nineteenth and Twentieth Centuries." *Social History of Medicine* 8, no. 2 (August 1995): 161–178.
Ariès, Philippe. *Centuries of Childhood: A Social History of Family Life*. New York: Alfred A. Knopf, 1962.
Ariès, Philippe, and Georges Duby. *A History of Private Life*. Cambridge, MA: Belknap Press of Harvard University Press, 1991.
Armstrong, David. *The Political Anatomy of the Body*. Cambridge: Cambridge University Press, 1983.
Bailkin, Jordanna. *The Afterlife of Empire*. Berkeley: University of California Press, 2012.
Bailkin, Jordanna. "The Postcolonial Family? West African Children, Private Fostering and the British State." *The Journal of Modern History* 81, no. 1 (2009): 87–121.
Bar-Haim, Shaul. *The Maternalists: Psychoanalysis, Motherhood, and the British Welfare State*. Philadelphia: University of Pennsylvania Press, 2021.
Baughan, Emily. "International Adoption and Anglo-American Internationalism, c. 1918–1925." *Past and Present* 239, no. 1 (2018): 181–217.
Baughan, Emily, and Juliano Fiori. "Save the Children, the Humanitarian Project, and the Politics of Solidarity: Reviving Dorothy Buxton's Vision." *Disasters* 39, s.2 (2015): s129–s145.
Beck, Ulrich. *Risk Society: Towards a New Modernity*. London: Sage Publications, 1992.
Beekman, Daniel. *The Mechanical Baby: A Popular History of the Theory and Practice of Child Raising*. Westport, CT: Lawrence, Hill and Co., 1977.
Berlant, Lauren. *Compassion: The Culture and Politics of an Emotion*. London: Routledge, 2014.
Berlant, Lauren, ed. *Intimacy*. Chicago: University of Chicago Press, 2000.
Bernini, Stefania. *Family Life and Individual Welfare in Postwar Europe: Britain and Italy Compared*. Basingstoke, UK: Palgrave Macmillan, 2007.
Boris, Eileen, and Rhacel Salazar Parrenas, eds. *Intimate Labors: Culture, Technologies and the Politics of Care*. Stanford: Stanford University Press, 2010.
Bourke, Joanna. "Fear and Anxiety: Writing about Emotion in Modern History." *History Workshop Journal* 55, no. 1 (2003): 111–133.
Bourke, Joanna. *Rape: Sex, Violence, History*. Berkeley: Counterpoint, 2007.
Briggs, Dennie. *A Life Well Lived: Maxwell Jones, a Memoir*. London: Jessica Kingsley Publishers, 2002.
British Film Institute. *The Joy of Sex Education*. London: British Film Institute, 2009.
Buhle, Mari Jo. *Feminism and Its Discontents: A Century of Struggle with Psychoanalysis*. Cambridge, MA: Harvard University Press, 1998.

Butler, Lise. "Michael Young, the Institute of Community Studies, and the Politics of Kinship." *Twentieth Century British History* 26, no.2 (May 2015): 203–224.

Burney, Ian. "War on Fear: Solly Zuckerman and Civilian Nerve in the Second World War." *History of the Human Sciences*, 25, no. 5 (2012): 49–72.

Brody, E.B. *The Search for Mental Health: A History and Memoir of the WFMH, 1948–1997*. Baltimore, MD: Williams and Wilkins, 1998.

Brooke, Stephen. *Sexual Politics: Sexuality, Family Planning, and the British Left from the 1880s to the Present Day*. Oxford: Oxford University Press, 2011.

Brown, Callum. *The Death of Christian Britain: Understanding Secularisation, 1800–2000*. 2nd. ed. London: Routledge, 2009.

Burley, Sarah Cunningham, and Lynn Jamieson, eds. *Families and the State: Changing Relationships*. London: Palgrave Macmillan, 2003.

Burton, Antoinette. *Burdens of History: British Feminists, Indian Women, and Imperial Culture, 1865–1915*. Chapel Hill: University of North Carolina Press, 1994.

Canaday, Margot. *The Straight State: Sexuality and Citizenship in Twentieth-Century America*. Princeton, NJ: Princeton University Press, 2009.

Celello, Kristin. *Making Marriage Work: A History of Marriage and Divorce in the Twentieth-Century United States*. Chapel Hill: University of North Carolina Press, 2009.

Cocks, Harry. "Conspiracy to Corrupt Public Morals and the 'Unlawful' Status of Homosexuality in Britain after 1967." *Social History* 41, no. 3 (2016): 267–284.

Cohen, Deborah. *Family Secrets: Shame and Privacy in Modern Britain*. Oxford: Oxford University Press, 2013.

Cohen-Cole, Jamie. *The Open Mind: Cold War Politics and the Sciences of Human Nature*. Chicago, IL: University of Chicago Press, 2014.

Collins, Marcus. *Modern Love: An Intimate History of Men and Women in Twentieth-Century Britain*. London: Atlantic Books, 2003.

Conekin, Becky, Frank Mort, and Chris Waters, eds. *Moments of Modernity: Reconstructing Britain, 1945–1964*. London: Rivers Oram Press, 1999.

Cook, Hera. *The Long Sexual Revolution: English Women, Sex and Contraception, 1800–1975*. Oxford: Oxford University Press, 2004.

Cook, Matt. *Queer Domesticities: Homosexuality and Home Life in Twentieth-Century London*. Basingstoke, UK: Palgrave Macmillan, 2014.

Cooper, Melinda. *Family Values: Between Neoliberalism and the New Social Conservatism*. New York: Zone Books, 2017.

Cowman, Krista. *Women in British Politics, c.1689–1979*. Basingstoke, UK: Palgrave Macmillan, 2010.

Cox, Pamela. *Gender, Justice and Welfare: Bad Girls in Britain, 1900–1950*. Basingstoke, UK: Palgrave Macmillan, 2003.

Cretney, Stephen. *Law, Law Reform and the Family*. Oxford: Clarendon Press, 1998.

Cretney, Stephen. *Same Sex Relationships: From "Odious Crime" to "Gay Marriage."* Oxford: Oxford University Press, 2006.

Crossley, Nick. *Contesting Psychiatry: Social Movements in Mental Health*. London: Routledge, 2006.

Cvetkovich, Ann. *Depression: A Public Feeling*. Durham, NC: Duke University Press, 2012.

Dally, Ann. *Inventing Motherhood: The Consequences of an Ideal*. New York: Schocken Books, 1982.

Danto, Elizabeth Ann. *Freud's Free Clinics: Psychoanalysis and Social Justice, 1918–1938*. New York: Columbia University Press, 2007.

Davis, Angela. "A Critical Perspective on British Social Surveys and Community Studies and Their Accounts of Married Life c.1945–70." *Cultural and Social History* 6 (2009): 47–64.

Davis, Angela. *Modern Motherhood: Women and Family in England, 1945–2000*. Manchester, UK: Manchester University Press, 2012.

Davis, Rebecca. *More Perfect Unions: The American Search for Marital Bliss*. Cambridge, MA: Harvard University Press, 2010.

De Certeau, Michel. *The Practice of Everyday Life*. Berkeley: University of California Press, 1984.

De Orio, Scott. "The Creation of the Modern Sex Offender." In *The War on Sex*, edited by David Halperin and Trevor Hoppe, 247–267. Durham, NC: Duke University Press, 2017.

Dickinson, Tommy. *"Curing Queers": Mental Nurses and Their Patients, 1935–74*. Manchester, UK: Manchester University Press, 2015.

Digby, Anne. *Madness, Morality and Medicine: A Study of the York Retreat, 1796–1914*. Cambridge: Cambridge University Press, 1985.

Dintenfass, Michael. *The Decline of Industrial Britain, 1870–1980*. London: Routledge, 1992.

Dixon, Joy. *Divine Feminine: Theosophy and Feminism in England*. Baltimore, MD: Johns Hopkins Press, 2001.

Donzelot, Jacques. *The Policing of Families*. New York: Pantheon Books, 1979.

Doroshow, Deborah Blythe. *Emotionally Disturbed: A History of Caring for America's Troubled Children*. Chicago, IL: University of Chicago Press, 2019.

Downs, Laura Lee. *Childhood in the Promised Land: Working-Class Movements and the Colonies de Vacances in France, 1880–1960*. Raleigh, NC: Duke University Press, 2002.

Duggan, Lisa. "The New Homonormativity: The Sexual Politics of Neoliberalism." In *Materializing Democracy: Toward a Revitalized Cultural Politics*, edited by Russ Castronovo and Dana D. Nelson, 175–194. Durham, NC: Duke University Press, 2002.

Duncombe, Jean, and Dennis Marsden. "Whose Orgasm Is This Anyway? 'Sex Work' in Long-term Heterosexual Couple Relationships." In *Sexual Cultures*, edited by Jeffrey Weeks and Janet Holland, 220–238. New York: St Martin's Press, 1996.

Edelman, Lee. *No Future: Queer Theory and the Death Drive*. Durham, NC: Duke University Press, 2004.

Edgerton, David. *Science, Technology and the British Industrial "Decline," 1870–1970*. Cambridge: Cambridge University Press, 1996.

Ehrenreich, Barbara, and Deirdre English. *For Her Own Good: 150 Years of the Experts' Advice to Women*. New York: Anchor Books, 1978.

Ensalaco, Mark. "The Right of the Child to Development." In *Children's Human Rights: Progress and Challenges for Children Worldwide*, edited by Mark Ensalaco and Linda C. Majka, 14–36. Lanham, MD: Rowman and Littlefield Publishers, 2005.

Esping-Anderson, Gøsta. *The Three Worlds of Welfare Capitalism*. Cambridge: Polity Press, 1990.

Evans, Barbara. *Freedom to Choose: The Life and Work of Dr. Helena Wright, Pioneer of Contraception*. London: Bodley Head, 1984.

Finzsch, Norbert, and Robert Jutte, eds. *Institutions of Confinement*. Cambridge: Cambridge University Press, 1996.

Foucault, Michel. *Discipline and Punish: The Birth of the Prison*. New York: Pantheon Books, 1977.

Foucault, Michel. "Friendship as a Way of Life." In *Michel Foucault: Ethics, Subjectivity, and Truth*, vol. 1, edited by Paul Rabinow, 135–156. New York: The New Press, 1994.

Foucault, Michel. *History of Sexuality*. Vol. 1: *An Introduction*. New York: Pantheon Books, 1978.

Foucault, Michel. *Madness and Civilization: A History of Insanity in the Age of Reason*. London: Tavistock, 1961.

Franklin, Bob, ed. *The Rights of Children*. Oxford: Basil Blackwell, 1986.

Fraser, Derek. *The Evolution of the British Welfare State: A History of Social Policy Since the Industrial Revolution*. Basingstoke, UK: Palgrave Macmillan, 2003.

Select Bibliography   295

Freeman, Simon, and Barrie Penrose. *The Rise and Fall of Jeremy Thorpe*. London: Bloomsbury, 1996.
Furedi, Frank. "The Silent Ascendancy of Therapeutic Culture in Britain." In *Therapeutic Culture: Triumphs and Defeat*, edited by Jonathan B. Imber, 19–50. New Brunswick, NJ: Transaction Publishers, 2004.
Furedi, Frank. *Therapy Culture: Cultivating Vulnerability in an Uncertain Age*. London: Routledge, 2004.
Geppert, Alexander C.T. "Divine Sex, Happy Marriage, Regenerated Nation: Marie Stopes' Marital Manual Married Love and the Making of a Best-Seller, 1918–1955." *Journal of the History of Sexuality* 8 (1998): 389–433.
Gere, Cathy. *Pain, Pleasure, and the Greater Good: From the Panopticon to the Skinner Box and Beyond*. Chicago, IL: University of Chicago Press, 2017.
Giddens, Anthony. *The Transformation of Intimacy: Sexuality, Love and Eroticism in Modern Societies*. Stanford: Stanford University Press, 1992.
Gillis, John R. *For Better, For Worse: British Marriages, 1600 to the Present*. New York: Oxford University Press, 1985.
Gladstone, David. *The Twentieth-Century Welfare State*. London: Palgrave Macmillan, 1999.
Glennerster, Howard, ed. *The Future of the Welfare State: Remaking Social Policy*. London: Heinemann, 1983.
Goffman, Erving. *Asylums: Essays on the Social Situation of Mental Patient and Other Inmates*. Chicago, IL: Aldine, 1961.
Goldstein, Jan. *The Post-Revolutionary Self: Politics and Psyche in France, 1750–1850*. Cambridge, MA: Harvard University Press, 2005.
Hacking, Ian. *Historical Ontology*. Cambridge, MA: Harvard University Press, 2004.
Hacking, Ian. "How 'Natural' are 'Kinds' of Sexual Orientation?" *Law and Philosophy* 21, no. 1 (2002): 95–107.
Hacking, Ian. "Kinds of People: Moving Targets." *Proceedings of the British Academy* 151 (2007): 285–318.
Haggett, Ali. "Housewives, Neuroses, and the Domestic Environment in Britain, 1945–70." In *Health and the Modern Home*, edited by Mark Jackson, 84–109. London: Routledge, 2007.
Halberstam, Jack. *In a Queer Time and Place: Transgender Bodies, Subcultural Lives*. New York: New York University Press, 2005.
Hall, Stuart, and Tony Jefferson, eds. *Resistance through Rituals: Youth Subcultures in Post-War Britain*. London: Hutchinson and Co., 1976.
Halperin, David. *How to Be Gay*. Cambridge, MA: Belknap Press, 2012.
Harris, Jose. "Political Thought and the Welfare State 1870–1940: An Intellectual Framework for British Social Policy." *Past & Present* 135, no. 1 (May 1992): 116–141.
Harris, Jose. *Private Lives, Public Spirit: Britain, 1870–1914*. London: Penguin, 1994.
Harrington, Anne. *Mind Fixers: Psychiatry's Troubled Search for the Biology of Mental Illness*. New York: W.W. Norton, 2019.
Harrington, Anne. "Mother Love and Mental Illness: An Emotional History." *Osiris* 31 (2016): 94–115.
Harrison, Tom. *Bion, Rickman, Foulkes, and the Northfield Experiments: Advancing on a Different Front*. London: Jessica Kingsley Publishers, 1999.
Hayes, Sarah. "Rabbits and Rebels: The Medicalisation of Maladjusted Children in Mid-Twentieth-Century Britain." In *Health and the Modern Home*, edited by Mark Jackson, 128–152. London: Routledge, 2007.
Hayward, Rhodri. "Busman's Stomach and the Embodiment of Modernity." *Contemporary British History* 31, no. 1 (2017): 1–23.

Hayward, Rhodri. "Desperate Housewives and Model Amoebae: The Invention of Suburban Neurosis in Inter-War Britain." In *Health and the Modern Home*, edited by Mark Jackson, 42–62. London: Routledge, 2007.
Hayward, Rhodri. "The Invention of the Psychosocial: An Introduction." *History of the Human Sciences*, 25, no. 5 (2012): 3–12.
Hayward, Rhodri. "The Pursuit of Serenity." In *History and Psyche: Culture, Psychoanalysis and the Past*, edited by Sally Alexander and Barbara Taylor, 283–304. London: Palgrave Macmillan, 2012.
Hayward, Rhodri. *The Transformation of the Psyche in British Primary Care, 1880–1970*. London: Bloomsbury, 2014.
Hendrick, Harry. *Child Welfare: Historical Dimensions, Contemporary Debate*. Bristol, UK: Policy Press, 2003.
Hendrick, Harry. "Children's Emotional Well-Being and Mental Health in Early Post-Second World War Britain: The Case of Unrestricted Hospital Visiting." In *Cultures of Child Health in Britain and the Netherlands in the Twentieth Century*, edited by Marijke Gijswijt-Hofstra and Hilary Marland, 213–242. Amsterdam: Rodopi, 2003.
Herman, Ellen. *The Romance of American Psychology: Political Culture in the Age of Experts*. Berkeley: University of California Press, 1995.
Herzog, Dagmar. *Cold War Freud: Psychoanalysis in an Age of Catastrophes*. Cambridge: Cambridge University Press, 2017.
Herzog, Dagmar. *Sexuality in Europe: A Twentieth-Century History*. Cambridge: Cambridge University Press, 2013.
Hoare, Oliver, ed. *Camp 020: MI5 and the Nazi Spies*. Richmond, UK: Public Record Office, 2000.
Hochshild, Arlie. *The Managed Heart: Commercialization of Human Feeling*. Berkeley: University of California Press, 2012.
Hochshild, Arlie, and Barbara Ehrenreich. *Global Woman: Nannies, Maids, and Sex Workers in the New Economy*. New York: Henry Holt, 2002.
Holmes, Jeremy. *John Bowlby and Attachment Theory*. London: Routledge, 1993.
Horn, Pamela. *Young Offenders: Juvenile Delinquency, 1700–2000*. Stroud, UK: Amberley, 2010.
Hull, Andrew. "Glasgow's 'Sick Society'? James Halliday, Psychosocial Medicine and Medical Holism in Britain, c.1920–48." *History of the Human Sciences* 25, no. 5 (2012): 73–90.
Igo, Sarah. *The Averaged American: Surveys, Citizens, and the Making of a Mass Public*. Cambridge, MA: Harvard University Press, 2008.
Igo, Sarah. *The Known Citizen: A History of Privacy in Modern America*. Cambridge, MA: Harvard University Press, 2018.
Illouz, Eva. *Cold Intimacies: The Making of Emotional Capitalism*. Cambridge: Polity Press, 2007.
Illouz, Eva, ed. *Emotions as Commodities: Capitalism, Consumption, and Authenticity*. London: Routledge, 2018.
Illouz, Eva. *Saving the Modern Soul: Therapy, Emotions, and the Culture of Self-Help*. Berkeley: University of California Press, 2008.
Itzin, Catherine. *Stages in the Revolution: Political Theatre in Britain since 1968*. London: Methuen, 1980.
Jackson, Mark. "'Home Sweet Home': Historical Perspectives on Health and the Home." In *Health and the Modern Home*, edited by Mark Jackson, 1–17. London: Routledge, 2007.
Jones, Edgar. "'The Gut War': Functional Somatic Disorders in the UK During the Second World War." *History of the Human Sciences* 25, no. 5 (2012): 30–48.
Jones, Colin. "Raising the Anti: Jan Foudraine, Ronald Laing and Anti-Psychiatry." In *Cultures of Psychiatry and Mental Health in Postwar Britain and the Netherlands*, edited by Marijke Gijswijt-Hofstra and Roy Porter, 283–294. Amsterdam: Rodopi, 1998.

Jones, Kathleen. *Taming the Troublesome Child: American Families, Child Guidance, and the Limits of Psychiatric Authority*. Cambridge, MA: Harvard University Press, 2002.
Jordanova, Ludmilla. "The Social Construction of Medical Knowledge." In *Locating Medical History: Their Stories and Their Meanings*, edited by F. Huisman and J.H. Warner, 338–363. Baltimore, MD: Johns Hopkins University Press, 2004.
Joyce, Patrick. *Democratic Subjects: The Self and the Social in Nineteenth-Century England*. Cambridge: Cambridge University Press, 1994.
Joyce, Patrick. "What is the Social in Social History?" *Past and Present* 206 (2010): 213–248.
Kavanagh, Dennis. *Thatcherism and British Politics: The End of Consensus?* Oxford: Oxford University Press, 1987.
King, Laura. *Family Men: Fatherhood and Masculinity in Britain, c.1914–1960*. Oxford: Oxford University Press, 2015.
Kipnis, Laura. *Against Love: A Polemic*. New York: Pantheon Books, 2003.
Kline, Wendy. *Building a Better Race: Gender, Sexuality, and Eugenics from the Turn of the Century to the Baby Boom*. Berkeley: University of California Press, 2001.
Koven, Seth, and Sonya Michel, eds. *Mothers of a New World: Maternalist Politics and the Origins of Welfare States*. New York: Routledge, 1993.
Kunzel, Regina. "Queer History, Mad History, and the Politics of Health." *American Quarterly* 69, no. 2 (June 2017): 315–319.
Ladd-Taylor, Molly. *Mother-Work: Women, Child Welfare and the State, 1890–1930*. Urbana: University of Illinois Press, 1994.
Ladd-Taylor, Molly, and Lauri Umansky, eds. *"Bad" Mothers: The Politics of Blame in Twentieth-Century America*. New York: New York University Press, 1998.
Langford, Wendy. *Revolutions of the Heart: Gender, Power, and the Delusions of Love*. London: Routledge, 2002.
Langhamer, Claire. *The English in Love*. Oxford: Oxford University Press, 2013.
Latour, Bruno. *Reassembling the Social: An Introduction to Actor-Network-Theory*. Oxford: Oxford University Press, 2005.
LeMahieu, Daniel. *A Culture for Democracy: Mass Communication and the Cultivated Mind in Britain Between the Wars*. Oxford: Clarendon Press, 1988.
Lewis, Helen. *Difficult Women: A History of Feminism in 11 Fights*. London: Penguin, 2020.
Lewis, Jane. *The End of Marriage? Individualism and Intimate Relations*. Cheltenham, UK: Edward Elgar, 2001.
Lewis, Jane, Kathleen Kiernan, and Hilary Land. *Lone Motherhood in Twentieth-Century Britain: From Footnote to Front Page*. Oxford: Clarendon Press, 1998.
Lewis, Jane, and David Morgan. *"Whom God Hath Joined Together": The Work of Marriage Guidance*. London: Tavistock, 1992.
Leys, Ruth. *Trauma: A Genealogy*. Chicago: University of Chicago Press, 2000.
Linstrum, Erik. *Ruling Minds: Psychology in the British Empire*. Cambridge, MA: Harvard University Press, 2016.
Linstrum, Erik. "The Politics of Psychology in the British Empire, 1898–1960." *Past and Present* 215 (2012): 195–233.
Loughran, Tracey. "Landscape for a Good Woman's Weekly." In *Women in Magazines: Research, Representation, Production and Consumption*, edited by Rachel Ritchie et al, 40–52. New York: Routledge, 2016.
Lowe, Rodney. *The Welfare State in Britain since 1945*. New York: St. Martin's Press, 1993.
Lowe, Rodney, and Helen Fawcett, eds. *Welfare Policy in Britain: The Road from 1945*. Basingstoke: Macmillan Press Ltd., 1999.
Luckhurst, Roger. *The Trauma Question*. New York: Routledge, 2008.
Lunbeck, Elizabeth. *The Psychiatric Persuasion: Knowledge, Gender, and Power in Modern America*. Princeton, NJ: Princeton University Press, 1994.

Lynch, Gordon. "Pathways to the 1946 Curtis Report and the Post-War Reconstruction of Children's Out of Home Care." *Contemporary British History* 34, no. 1 (2020): 22–43.
Lynch, Kathleen. "Love Labour as a Distinct and Non-Commodifiable Form of Care Labour." *The Sociological Review* 55, no. 3 (2007): 550–570.
Makepeace, Clare. *Captives of War: British Prisoners of War in Europe in the Second World War.* Cambridge: Cambridge University Press, 2017.
Mandler, Peter. *Return from the Natives: How Margaret Mead Won the Second World War and Lost the Cold War.* New Haven, CT: Yale University Press, 2013.
Marwick, Arthur. *British Society since 1945.* Harmondsworth: Penguin, 1982.
May, Elaine Tyler. *Homeward Bound: American Families in the Cold War Era.* New York: Basic Books, 1988.
McRae, Susan, ed. *Changing Britain: Families and Households in the 1990s.* Oxford: Oxford University Press, 1999.
Mecca, Tommy Avicolli. *Smash the Church, Smash the State!: The Early Years of Gay Liberation.* San Francisco: City Lights Books, 2009.
Metzl, Jonathan. "'Mother's Little Helper': The Crisis of Psychoanalysis and the Miltown Resolution," *Gender and History* 15, no. 3 (August 2003): 240–267.
Metzl, Jonathan. *Prozac on the Couch: Prescribing Gender in the Era of Wonder Drugs.* Durham: Duke University Press, 2005.
Metzl, Jonathan. *The Protest Psychosis: How Schizophrenia Became a Black Disease.* Boston: Beacon Press, 2014.
Meyerowitz, Joanne. "'How Common Culture Shapes the Separate Lives': Sexuality, Race, and Mid-Twentieth-Century Social Constructionist Thought." *The Journal of American History* 96, no. 4 (2010): 1057–1084.
Michel, Sonya, and Rianne Mahon. *Child Care Policy at the Crossroads: Gender and Welfare State Restructuring.* London: Routledge, 2002.
Milam, Erika Lorraine. *Creatures of Cain: The Hunt for Human Nature in Cold War America.* Princeton, NJ: Princeton University Press, 2019.
Minton, Henry. *Departing from Deviance: A History of Homosexual Rights and Emancipatory Science in America.* Chicago, IL: University of Chicago Press, 2002.
Moran, Jeffrey P. *Teaching Sex: The Shaping of Adolescence in the 20th Century.* Cambridge, MA: Harvard University Press, 2000.
Mort, Frank. *Dangerous Sexualities: Medico-Moral Politics in England since 1830.* London: Routledge & Kegan Paul, 1987.
Mort, Frank. "Mapping Sexual London: The Wolfenden Committee on Homosexual Offences and Prostitution." *New Formations* 37 (1999): 92–113.
Nelson, Deborah. *Pursuing Privacy in Cold War America.* New York: Columbia University Press, 2002.
Nuttall, Jeremy. *Psychological Socialism: The Labour Party and Qualities of Mind and Character, 1931 to the Present.* Manchester, UK: Manchester University Press, 2013.
Oosterhuis, Harry. *Stepchildren of Nature: Krafft-Ebing, Psychiatry, and the Making of Sexual Identity.* Chicago, IL: University of Chicago Press, 2000.
Orloff, Ann Shola. "Gender in the Welfare State." *Annual Review of Sociology* 22 (1996): 51–78.
Orloff, Ann Shola. "Gendering the Comparative Analysis of Welfare States: An Unfinished Agenda." *Sociological Theory* 27, no. 3 (September 2009): 317–343.
Ortolano, Guy. *Thatcher's Progress: From Social Democracy to Market Liberalism through an English New Town.* Cambridge: Cambridge University Press, 2019.
Ortolano, Guy. *The Two Cultures Controversy: Science, Literature and Cultural Politics in Postwar Britain.* Cambridge: Cambridge University Press, 2009.
Osgerby, Bill. *Youth in Britain since 1945.* Oxford: Blackwell Publishers, Ltd., 1998.

Owen, Alex. *The Place of Enchantment: British Occultism and the Culture of the Modern.* Chicago, IL: University of Chicago Press, 2004.
Pedersen, Susan. *After the Victorians: Private Conscience and Public Duty in Modern Britain.* London: Routledge, 1994.
Pedersen, Susan. *Family, Dependence and the Origins of the Welfare State.* Cambridge: Cambridge University Press, 1993.
Perkin, Harold. *The Rise of Professional Society: England Since 1880.* London: Routledge, 1989.
Phillips, Roderick. *Putting Asunder: A History of Divorce in Western Society.* Cambridge: Cambridge University Press, 1988.
Pick, Daniel. *The Pursuit of the Nazi Mind: Hitler, Hess, and the Analysts.* Oxford: Oxford University Press, 2014.
Pilcher, Jane, and Stephen Wagg. *Thatcher's Children? Politics, Childhood and Society in the 1980s and 1990s.* London: Falmer Press, 1996.
Pines, Malcolm. "The Development of the Psychodynamic Movement." In *150 Years of British Psychiatry*, edited by German Berrios and Hugh Freeman, 198–231. London: Gaskell, 1991.
Plant, Rebecca Jo. *Mom: The Transformation of Motherhood in Modern America.* Chicago, IL: University of Chicago Press, 2010.
Pugh, Martin. *State and Society: A Social and Political History of Britain, 1870–1997.* London: Arnold, 1994.
Pugh, Martin. *Women and the Women's Movement in Britain, 1914–1959.* London: Macmillan, 1992.
Rapp, Dean. "The Reception of Freud by the British Press: General Interest and Literary Magazines, 1920–1925." *Journal of the History of the Behavioral Sciences* 24, no. 2 (April 1998): 191–201.
Rayner, Eric. *The Independent Mind in British Psychoanalysis.* Northvale, NJ: Jason Aronson Inc., 1991.
Raz, Mical. *What's Wrong with the Poor? Psychiatry, Race, and the War on Poverty.* Chapel Hill: University of North Carolina Press, 2013.
Renwick, Chris. *British Sociology's Lost Biological Roots: A History of Futures Past.* Basingstoke: Palgrave Macmillan, 2012.
Rieff, Philip. *Freud: The Mind of the Moralist.* New York: Viking Press, 1959.
Rieff, Philip. *The Triumph of the Therapeutic: Uses of Faith after Freud.* New York: Harper and Row, 1966.
Riley, Denise. *Am I That Name? Feminism and the Category of "Women" in History.* Minneapolis: University of Minnesota Press, 1988.
Riley, Denise. *War in the Nursery: Theories of the Child and Mother.* London: Virago Press, 1983.
Robcis, Camille. *The Law of Kinship: Anthropology, Psychoanalysis, and the Family in France.* Ithaca, NY: Cornell University Press, 2013.
Rose, Jacqueline. *Mothers: An Essay on Love and Cruelty.* New York: Farrar, Straus and Giroux, 2014.
Rose, Nikolas. *Governing the Soul: The Shaping of the Private Self.* London: Free Association Books, 1999.
Rose, Nikolas. *Inventing Our Selves: Psychology, Power and Personhood.* Cambridge: Cambridge University Press, 1996.
Rose, Nikolas. *The Psychological Complex: Psychology, Politics and Society in England, 1869–1939.* London: Routledge & Kegan Paul, 1985.
Rose, Sonya. *Which People's War? National Identity and Citizenship in Britain, 1939–1945.* Oxford: Oxford University Press, 2003.
Rubin, Gayle. "Thinking Sex: Notes for a Radical Theory of the Politics of Sexuality." In *Pleasure and Danger: Exploring Female Sexuality*, edited by Carole S. Vance, 267–293. London: Pandora, 1992.

Rusterholz, Caroline. "'You Can't Dismiss That as Being Less Happy, You See it is Different': Sexual Counselling in 1950s England." *Twentieth Century British History* 30, no. 3 (September 2019): 375–398.

Schorske, Carl. *Fin-de-siècle Vienna: Politics and Culture*. New York: Knopf, 1979.

Scull, Andrew. *Madness in Civilization: A Cultural History of Insanity from the Bible to Freud, From the Madhouse to Modern Medicine*. Princeton, NJ: Princeton University Press, 2016.

Scull, Andrew. *Museums of Madness: The Social Organization of Insanity in Nineteenth-Century England*. New York: St. Martin's Press, 1979.

Sedgwick, Peter. *Psycho-Politics: Laing, Foucault, Goffman, Szasz and the Future of Mass Psychiatry*. New York: Harper and Row, 1982.

Seldon, Anthony, and Kevin Hickson, eds. *New Labour, Old Labour: The Wilson and Callaghan Governments, 1974–79*. London: Routledge, 2004.

Shamdasani, Sonu. "The Psychoanalytic Body." In *Medicine in the Twentieth Century*, edited by R. Cooter and J. Pickstone, 307–322. Amsterdam: Overseas Publishers Association, 2000.

Shapira, Michal. "Psychoanalysts on the Radio: Domestic Citizenship and Motherhood in Postwar Britain." In *Women and Gender in Postwar Europe*, edited by Bonnie Smith and Joanna Regulska, 71–86. London: Routledge, 2011.

Shapira, Michal. "The Psychological Study of Anxiety in the Era of the Second World War." *Twentieth Century British History* 24, no. 1 (March 2013): 31–57.

Shapira, Michal. *The War Inside: Psychoanalysis, Total War, and the Making of the Democratic Self in Postwar Britain*. Cambridge: Cambridge University Press, 2013.

Sheehy, Peter. "The Triumph of Group Therapeutics: Therapy, the Social Self, and Liberalism in America, 1910–1960." Unpublished PhD dissertation. University of Virginia, 2002.

Shephard, Ben. *A War of Nerves: Soldiers and Psychiatrists in the Twentieth Century*. Cambridge, MA: Harvard University Press, 2001.

Simic, Zora. "From Battered Wives to Domestic Violence: The Transnational Circulation of Chiswick Women's Aid and Erin Pizzey's *Scream Quietly or the Neighbours Will Hear* (1974)." *Australian Historical Studies* 51, no. 2 (2020): 107–126.

Skidelsky, Robert. *English Progressive Schools*. Harmondsworth, UK: Penguin, 1969.

Smith, Roger. *Being Human: Historical Knowledge and the Creation of Human Nature*. New York: Columbia University Press, 2007.

Smith, Roger. *Inhibition: History and Meaning in the Sciences of Mind and Brain*. Berkeley: University of California Press, 1992.

Staub, Michael. *Madness is Civilization: When the Diagnosis Was Social, 1948–1980*. Chicago, IL: University of Chicago Press, 2011.

Steedman, Carolyn. *Childhood, Culture and Class in Britain: Margaret McMillan, 1860–1931*. New Brunswick, NJ: Rutgers University Press, 1990.

Steedman, Carolyn. *Strange Dislocations: Childhood and the Idea of Human Interiority, 1780–1930*. Cambridge, MA: Harvard University Press, 1995.

Stewart, John. *Child Guidance in Britain, 1918–1955: The Dangerous Age of Childhood*. London: Pickering & Chatto, 2013.

Stewart, John. "'I Thought You Would Want to Come and See His Home': Child Guidance and Psychiatric Social Work in Inter-War Britain." In *Health and the Modern Home*, edited by Mark Jackson, 111–125. London: Routledge, 2007.

Stewart-Steinberg, Suzanne. *Impious Fidelity: Anna Freud, Psychoanalysis, Politics*. Ithaca, NY: Cornell University Press, 2011.

Stone, Lawrence. *The Family, Sex and Marriage in England, 1500–1800*. New York: Harper & Row, 1977.

Szreter, Simon, and Kate Fisher. *Sex Before the Sexual Revolution: Intimate Life in England, 1918–1963*. Cambridge: Cambridge University Press, 2010.

Tambe, Ashwini. *Defining Girlhood in India: A Transnational History of Sexual Maturity Laws.* Urbana: University of Illinois Press, 2019.

Tantum, Digby. "The Anti-Psychiatry Movement." In *150 Years of British Psychiatry*, edited by German Berrios and Hugh Freeman, 333–347. London: Gaskell, 1991.

Tebbutt, Melanie. *Making Youth: A History of Youth in Modern Britain.* London: Palgrave, 2016.

Thane, Pat. *Foundations of the Welfare State.* London: Longman, 1982.

Thane, Pat. *Sinners? Scroungers? Saints?: Unmarried Motherhood in Twentieth-Century England.* Oxford: Oxford University Press, 2012.

Thane, Pat. "'The Big Society' and the 'Big State': Creative Tension or Crowding Out?" *Twentieth Century British History* 23, no. 3 (September 2012): 408–429.

Thom, Deborah. "Wishes, Anxieties, Play and Gestures: Child Guidance in Inter-War England." In *In the Name of the Child: Health and Welfare, 1880–1940*, edited by Roger Cooter, 200–220. London: Routledge, 1992.

Thomson, Mathew. *Lost Freedom: The Landscape of the Child and the British Post-War Settlement.* Oxford: Oxford University Press, 2013.

Thomson, Mathew. *Psychological Subjects: Identity, Culture, and Health in Twentieth-Century Britain.* Oxford: Oxford University Press, 2006.

Thomson, Mathew. *The Problem of Mental Deficiency: Eugenics, Democracy and Social Policy in Britain, c.1870–1959.* Oxford: Clarendon, 1998.

Thomson, Mathew. "The Psychological Body." In *Medicine in the Twentieth Century*, edited by Roger Cooter and John Pickstone, 291–306. Amsterdam: Overseas Publishers Association, 2000.

Thompson, Charis. *Making Parents: The Ontological Choreography of Reproductive Technologies.* Cambridge, MA: MIT Press, 2005.

Toms, Jonathan. *Mental Hygiene and Psychiatry in Modern Britain.* Basingstoke, UK: Palgrave Macmillan, 2013.

Toms, Jonathan. "Political Dimensions of 'the Psychosocial': The 1948 International Congress on Mental Health and the Mental Hygiene Movement." *History of the Human Sciences*, 25, no. 5 (2012): 91–106.

Tone, Andrea. *The Age of Anxiety: A History of America's Turbulent Affair with Tranquilizers.* New York: Basic Books, 2009.

Unwin, Cathy, and Elaine Sharland. "From Bodies to Minds in Childcare Literature: Advice to Parents in Inter-war Britain." In *In the Name of the Child: Health and Welfare, 1880–1940*, edited by Roger Cooter, 174–199. London: Routledge, 1992.

Van der Horst, Frank C.P., and Rene van der Veer. "Separation and Divergence: The Untold Story of James Robertson's and John Bowlby's Theoretical Dispute on Mother-Child Separation." *Journal of the History of the Behavioral Sciences.* 45, no. 3 (2009): 236–252.

Van der Horst, Frank C.P. *John Bowlby—From Psychoanalysis to Ethology: Unraveling the Roots of Attachment Theory.* Chichester, UK: Wiley-Blackwell, 2011.

Vernon, James. "The Mirage of Modernity." *Social History* 22, no. 2 (1997): 208–215.

Vicedo, Marga. "Mothers, Machines and Morals: Harry Harlow's Work on Primate Love from Lab to Legend." *Journal of the History of the Behavioral Sciences* 45, no. 3 (2009): 193–218.

Vicedo, Marga. *The Nature and Nurture of Love: From Imprinting to Attachment in Cold War America.* Chicago, IL: University of Chicago Press, 2013.

Vicedo, Marga. "The Social Nature of the Mother's Tie to Her Child: John Bowlby's Theory of Attachment in Post-War America." *British Journal of the History of Science* 44, no. 3 (2011): 401–426.

Wallach Scott, Joan. "The Evidence of Experience." In *Questions of Evidence: Proof, Practice, and Persuasion across the Disciplines*, edited by James Chandler, Arnold I. Davidson, and Harry Harootunian, 363–387. Chicago, IL: University of Chicago Press, 1994.

Warner, Michael. *Publics and Counterpublics.* New York: Zone Books, 2002.

Waters, Chris. "The Homosexual as a Social Being in Britain, 1945–1968," *Journal of British Studies* 51, no. 3 (December 2012): 687–710.

Webster, Wendy. *Imagining Home: Gender, "Race" and National Identity, 1945–64*. London: UCL Press, 1998.

Weinstein, Deborah. "The 'Make Love, Not War' Ape: Bonobos and Late Twentieth-Century Explanations for War and Peace." *Endeavour* 40, no. 4 (2016): 256–267.

Weinstein, Deborah. *The Pathological Family: Postwar America and the Rise of Family Therapy*. Ithaca, NY: Cornell University Press, 2013.

Weinstein, Deborah. "Sexuality, Therapeutic Culture, and Family Ties in the United States after 1973." *History of Psychology* 21, no. 3 (2018): 273–289.

Weeks, Jeffrey. *Coming Out: Homosexual Politics in Britain from the Nineteenth Century to the Present*. London: Quartet Books, 1977.

Weeks, Jeffrey. *The World We Have Won: The Remaking of Erotic and Intimate Life*. London: Routledge, 2007.

Weeks, Jeffrey, Brian Heaphy, and Catherine Donovan. *Same Sex Intimacies: Families of Choice and Other Life Experiments*. London: Routledge, 2001.

Wellings, Kaye, and Roslyn Kane. "Trends in Teenage Pregnancy in England and Wales: How Can We Explain Them?" *Journal of the Royal Society of Medicine*, 92 (June 1999): 277–282.

Welshman, John. "Recuperation, Rehabilitation and the Residential Option: The Brentwood Centre for Mothers and Children." *Twentieth Century British History* 19, no.4 (2008): 502–529.

Williamson, Charlotte. *Towards the Emancipation of Patients: Patients' Experiences and the Patient Movement*. Bristol, UK: The Policy Press, 2010.

Winter, Alison. *Mesmerized: Powers of Mind in Victorian Britain*. Chicago, IL: University of Chicago Press, 1998.

Yoshino, Kenji. "The Epistemic Contract of Bisexual Erasure." *Stanford Law Review* 52, no. 2 (January 2000): 353–461.

Zahra, Tara. *The Lost Children: Reconstructing Europe's Families after World War II*. Cambridge, MA: Harvard University Press, 2011.

Zahra, Tara. "'The Psychological Marshall Plan': Displacement, Gender, and Human Rights after World War II." *Central European History* 44, no. 1 (2011): 37–62.

Zaretsky, Eli. *Political Freud: A History*. New York: Columbia University Press, 2015.

Zaretsky, Eli. *Secrets of the Soul: A Social and Cultural History of Psychoanalysis*. New York: Knopf, 2004.

Zelizer, Viviana. *Pricing the Priceless Child: The Changing Social Value of Children*. New York: Basic Books, 1985.

Zelizer, Viviana. *The Purchase of Intimacy*. Princeton, NJ: Princeton University Press, 2005.

Index

For the benefit of digital users, indexed terms that span two pages (e.g., 52–53) may, on occasion, appear on only one of those pages.
Figures are indicated by *f* following the page number

abortion, 112, 135, 170–71, 179, 180, 193, 235
Abse, Leo, 132–34, 135
adolescent counseling, 175–76
adolescent sexuality
    abortion and, 170–71, 179, 180, 193, 235
    age of consent and, 21, 170–73, 182–93, 195–96, 269n.96
    birth control and, 5–6, 21, 178–79, 180–82, 193, 194, 195–96
    class considerations of, 185, 188, 195
    dangers associated with, 173, 177–78, 180–82, 185, 192–93, 196
    democratic citizens and, 196
    emotional deprivation and, 188
    emotional development and, 21, 170–71, 173, 179, 185, 188, 192–93, 195–96
    emotional maturity and, 21, 170–71, 172–76, 182–92, 194–95
    family values and, 180, 182, 192–96
    freedom and, 21, 171, 172–73, 196
    homosexuality and, 170–71, 181–82, 186–87, 188–92, 193
    international views on, 268n.76
    interwar period and, 174
    intimate relationships and, 5, 170–71, 193, 196
    media portrayal of sex and, 179–80, 182
    monogamy and, 5–6, 173, 186, 191, 196
    nuclear family and, 195–96
    parenting teenagers and, 175–76, 177
    premarital sex and, 177–78, 193
    privacy and, 172, 173, 184, 192–93, 194–96
    promiscuity and, 177, 178, 191
    prostitution and, 185–86, 196
    psychiatry and, 21, 172–76
    puberty and, 170, 184, 187, 188
    public morals and, 183
    sex education and, 178–80, 181–82
    sexual assault and, 185–86, 196
    sexual revolution and, 21, 172–73, 192–93
    STIs and, 178–79, 183
    teen pregnancy and, 170–71, 172, 177, 178–79, 180–81
adoption, 1–2, 19, 54, 65–66, 79, 110–11, 193, 238

Adoption of Children Act (1949), 65–66
adulthood, 5, 10–13, 21, 97, 121–22, 138, 173, 194–95, 196, 230. *See also* emotional maturity
age of consent, 21, 170–73, 181–93, 195–96, 269n.96
Ainsworth, Mary, 72, 78
Albany Trust
    approach to counseling of, 153–55, 158, 162–63, 169
    creation of, 144–45, 152–53
    emotional development and, 154
    ending of counseling services at, 158–59
    equality and, 153
    goals of, 152–53
    growth of, 157
    heteronormativity and, 154–55
    intimate relationships and, 154–56, 162–63
    monogamous relationships and, 162–63, 169
    public funding lost at, 167
    queer counseling at, 145–47, 153–54, 158, 169
    sexual promiscuity and, 154–55, 156–58
    social reform and, 153, 154, 158
    social stigma and, 152–53, 158–59
Allen, Marjory, 52, 60, 61–63
Anionwu, Elizabeth, 8–9
anti-hospital therapy, 200, 201–2, 204
antipsychiatry movement
    development of, 201–2
    emotional development and, 200, 201–6
    family violence and, 21–22, 199–206
    feminism and, 206–9, 211
    influence of, 7, 10, 206
    intimate relationships and, 2, 201–2
    motherhood and, 200–1, 203–6
    nuclear family and, 199–201, 203
    psychopolitics and, 7, 10, 201, 205–6
    schizophrenia and, 199–206, 207, 228–29
    therapeutic communities and, 201–2
Arendt, Hannah, 10
asylums, 29–32, 44
authoritarianism
    democratic citizens and, 28, 49
    efforts to eliminate, 19, 26–27, 49, 120, 200–1
    emotional development and, 33, 49–50, 53, 176

authoritarianism (*cont.*)
  family structure as basis of, 8, 26, 120, 132, 176
  fatherhood and, 26, 46, 47
  homosexuality and, 167
  psychiatry and, 8, 26–27, 49, 88–89, 120
  queer counseling and, 168
  therapeutic communities and, 44
  welfare state and, 119
aversion therapy, 20–21, 144–45, 153–54

Baden-Powell, Robert, 174, 188–89
Barnes, Mary, 204–6
Bateson, Gregory, 201
Beaumont, Tim, 184–85
Beauvoir, Simone de, 207
befriending services, 18, 20–21, 146–47, 159, 160–61, 162, 168, 169
Behan, Christopher, 168
Bell, Enid Moberly, 62
Benedek, Therese, 98
Benedict, Ruth, 26
Bennett, Alan, 8–9
Berke, Joseph, 204–6
Berlant, Lauren, 15, 161, 229–30, 235–36
Beveridge, William
  childhood and, 54, 56
  democratic citizens and, 50–51
  motherhood and, 99–100, 105–6, 107
  nuclear family and, 50–51
  welfare state and, 6–7, 54, 99, 100
Beyfus, Drusilla, 129
Bierer, Joshua, 32
Bion, Wilfred, 26–27, 40–41, 43
birth control
  adolescent sexuality and, 5–6, 21, 178–79, 180–82, 193, 194, 195–96
  campaigns against, 125–26, 180–81, 194
  emotional development and, 136
  family values and, 122
  marriage counseling and, 116–17, 124, 125, 137
  nuclear family and, 229
  overpopulation and, 182
  welfare state and, 180–81
Birth Control Campaign (BCC), 180, 182–83
bisexuality, 20–21, 157, 169, 189–90, 237
Bodman, Frank, 62
Bott, Elizabeth, 105–6
Bowlby, John
  animal research and, 72
  authoritarianism and, 8
  Bowlbyism and, 78–79, 209, 213
  child homelessness and, 68–69, 78
  criticism of, 1–2, 70, 75–76, 209
  democratic citizens and, 1, 8, 25, 26–27, 28, 79
  emotional deprivation and, 11, 12, 52, 66, 67–70, 71
  family violence and, 207–8, 215–17, 224
  feminism and, 207–8
  influence of, 1–2, 68, 70–71, 73–76, 78–79
  interwar period and, 29
  intimate relationships and, 1–2, 8, 11, 69, 75–76, 78–79
  juvenile delinquency and, 78
  mother-child relationship and, 1–2, 11–12, 57, 61, 67–69, 70, 72–73, 75–76, 78–79, 209
  nuclear family and, 72–73, 75–76
  policy recommendations of, 69–71, 72–73
  psychology of war and, 29, 61
  relationality and, 11–12, 75
  separation experiences and, 57, 61, 67–68, 70–76, 90
  welfare state and, 8, 66, 72–73, 75
  working mothers and, 103–5
Boyle, Helen, 30
Brentwood Recuperation Centre for Mothers and Children, 85–87, 98, 99, 109, 110–11
Bridger, Harold, 41
British Medical Association (BMA), 85–86, 91, 99
British Psychoanalytical Society, 39–40, 57, 75, 121, 208
British War Office, 26, 27
Britton, Clare, 66
Burbidge, Micky, 194–95
Burlingham, Dorothy, 61
Burns, Charles, 57–58
Burt, Cyril, 11
Butler, Josephine, 185–86, 196
Butt, Ronald, 184–85

Cambridge Evacuation Survey, 61
Campaign for Homosexual Equality (CHE), 144–45, 159, 160, 171, 185, 189
Cassel Hospital, 93–98
  adolescent counseling and, 175
  emotional maturity and, 19–20, 94–95
  influence of, 98–99, 108–9
  intimate relationships and, 108
  marriage counseling and, 127–28
  motherhood and, 19–20, 87–96, 108–10
  naturalness of motherhood and, 109–10
  nuclear family and, 97–98
  post-partum mental illness and, 95–96, 106, 109
  psychosocial nursing at, 93–94
  rehabilitating mothers at, 93–98
  separation experiences and, 90
  social reform and, 98–99, 110
  therapeutic community at, 19–20, 88–90, 97–98, 99, 109
Catholic Marriage Advisory Center, 125–26
Certeau, Michel de, 17
Chesser, Eustace, 112
Child Care and the Growth of Love (Bowlby), 1–2, 69
child guidance, 3, 8, 13, 14, 18–19, 49–50, 54, 56–62, 68–70, 76, 117–18, 174,

Index

childhood
  abuse during, 64–65, 199–200, 212–17
  class dimensions of, 55, 56, 60
  democratic citizens and, 58, 79
  development theories of, 3, 11–12, 13, 55, 63, 66–67, 76
  displaced children and, 52–53, 60–63, 68
  divorce and, 20, 76, 131, 230–31
  emotional deprivation and, 3, 13–14, 19, 53–55, 59–63, 66–67, 69–70, 75–77, 82–83
  emotional development and, 3, 5, 12, 19–20, 53–54, 58, 61–62, 66–67, 78–79, 81–82, 119–20, 200
  emotional maturity and, 12–13, 62
  family violence and, 64, 199–200, 212–17, 222–24, 225–26, 229
  fatherhood and, 75–76, 85, 197–98, 209, 229
  feminism and, 211
  foster care prioritized and, 54, 62, 64–65
  future orientation of, 13, 53–54, 55–56, 77, 229
  heterosexuality and, 77, 152
  homelessness and, 4, 54–55, 62–63, 65–66, 68–69, 78
  institutionalization and, 53, 54–55, 62–63
  interwar period and, 56–59
  intimate relationships and, 2–3, 6, 11–12, 13, 54–56, 63, 76–78, 199
  juvenile delinquency and, 9, 11, 13–14, 19, 56, 58–59, 71–72, 78
  maladjustment and, 11, 56–58, 59, 63, 71, 77, 116
  marriage counseling and, 116, 119–20, 126–27
  mother-child relationship and, 1–2, 11–12, 19–20, 54–55, 58, 67–76, 78–79, 81–83, 92–93, 105, 197–200
  nuclear family and, 3–4, 10–11, 53–55, 57, 60–61, 63–64, 66, 68–70, 78–79, 97, 200
  politicization of, 58–59, 98–108
  psychoanalysis and, 57
  relationality and, 11–12, 77–79
  residential schools for, 57–58, 60, 61–62, 64
  separation experiences and, 57, 61, 67–68, 70–76, 90
  social conditions and, 53–54, 56–57, 58
  social reform and, 67–77
  welfare state and, 3, 5–6, 13, 19, 54–56, 58–59, 62–67, 77–79, 98–108
  World War II and, 52–53, 60–63
childlessness, 108, 110–11, 138–39, 219
Children Act (1908), 58–59
Children Act (1948), 3, 63–66, 78, 79
Children and Young Persons Act (1933), 63–64
Chiswick Women's Aid (CWA), 199, 211–12, 217, 219, 221–23, 224–25
citizenry. *See* democratic citizens
Citizens' Advice Bureau, 121
Civil Resettlement Units (CRUs), 42–44

classless society aim of welfare state, 20, 55–56, 78, 113–14, 124–25, 234
Clean Up TV Campaign, 179–80, 182
Cole, Martin, 179–80
Comer, Lee, 198, 209, 210–11
Committee on Grants for the Development of Marriage Guidance (1948), 119–20
Committee on Procedure in Matrimonial Causes (1947), 119
Committee on the Care of Children (1946), 62–63
Commonwealth Fund, 56
Congress for the Dialectics of Liberation (1967), 207, 234
contraception. *See* birth control
Cooper, David, 2, 201–2, 205–7, 234
counseling. *See* adolescent counseling; marriage counseling; queer counseling
Counter-Psychiatry Group, 144–45
Cretney, Stephen, 65
Criminal Law Revision Committee, 172, 192, 195–96
Curtis, Myra, 62–63
Curtis Report (1946), 62–63, 64, 65–66, 69–70, 84

democratic citizens
  adolescent sexuality and, 196
  childhood and, 58, 79
  divorce and, 132, 133
  emotional development and, 10, 15–16, 17, 18–19, 49–50, 79, 98–99, 133, 137–38
  emotional maturity and, 139
  freedom and, 10, 133, 138, 196
  future orientation of, 28
  heterosexuality and, 15–16, 77
  intimate relationships and, 2, 4, 9, 15, 18, 19, 55–56, 114, 133, 138, 139, 151–52, 238
  maladjustment and, 58
  marriage counseling and, 2, 49–50, 118, 138–39
  mental health's relation to, 9, 26–27, 32–39, 40, 42, 50
  motherhood and, 1–2, 98, 108
  nuclear family and, 4, 28, 47, 49–51, 55–56, 79, 138, 234–35
  privacy and, 21, 151–52
  psychiatry and, 18–19, 27, 49, 50–51
  psychopolitics and, 1–2, 27, 135
  queer counseling and, 145–46
  relationality and, 50–51
  sexual revolution and, 5, 21, 138
  social conditions and, 18–19, 27, 50–51
  therapeutic communities and, 26–27, 42, 44, 98–99, 120
  welfare state and, 19, 20, 113, 118, 151–52
  World War II and, 26–27
Denning, Alfred Thompson, 119, 152–53
deprivation. *See* emotional deprivation

development. *See* adolescent sexuality; childhood; emotional development
Devlin, Patrick, 149–50, 151–52
Dicks, Henry
 authoritarianism and, 26–27, 46–50
 democratic citizens and, 47–48, 49–50
 emotional development and, 25–26, 45–49, 53–54
 family life emphasis of, 45–47
 influence of, 2, 48, 49–50
 interrogation methods and, 47–48
 marriage counseling and, 2, 120–21, 122–23
 motherhood and, 2
 Nazi POW assessment by, 25–26, 45–49
 psychological warfare and, 26
 women and, 47
Divided Self, The (Laing), 201, 202–3, 206, 208–9
divorce
 childhood and, 20, 76, 131, 230–31
 custody decisions following, 197–98, 230–31
 democratic citizens and, 132, 133
 divorce epidemic, 112, 119, 136–37
 emotional deprivation and, 76
 emotional development and, 20, 76, 114–15, 130–37
 family violence and, 220
 fatherhood and, 197–98, 230–31, 235
 feminism and, 231
 financial impact of, 134–35
 heterosexuality and, 151
 increased rates of, 4, 112, 117, 119, 132, 136–37
 intimate relationships and, 5, 6, 20, 114–15, 132, 133, 135, 136–37, 230
 legal reform of, 20, 112–40
 marriage breakdown model of, 119–20, 130, 133–34, 135
 marriage counseling and, 20, 113–14, 115, 117, 119, 122–23, 130, 131, 136–37, 156
 media portrayal of, 112–13, 130, 131
 mutual consent model of, 131, 132–33
 offense model of, 130–31, 132, 133–34
 psychiatry and, 113–14, 130
 public support for, 132, 135–36
 resistance to legal reform of, 133–34, 135
 social problems tied to, 112–13
 unhappy marriages and, 116, 125, 131–32
 welfare state and, 3, 8, 63, 119, 228–29
 World War II and, 131
Divorce Reform Bill (1968), 132–35, 136–37
domestic violence. *See* family violence
Domestic Violence and Matrimonial Proceedings Act (1976), 225
Dukes, Ethel, 116
Duncombe, Jean, 107
Durbin, Evan, 1, 28, 79

Dyson, Tony, 152–53

Edelman, Lee, 77, 78–79, 161, 229
Eichholtz, Enid, 121
Elithorn, Alick, 197
emotional deprivation
 adolescent sexuality and, 188
 childhood and, 3, 13–14, 19, 53–55, 59–63, 66–67, 69–70, 75–77, 82–83
 divorce and, 76
 family violence and, 225–26
 fatherhood and, 85, 230–31
 feminism and, 83
 institutionalization and, 67–68, 70
 maladjustment and, 59
 media portrayal of, 74, 76–77
 motherhood and, 11–12, 75–76, 78, 82–83, 84–93, 98–99, 198, 225–26
 nuclear family and, 53–54, 67
 social conditions and, 55
 social ills and, 59, 63, 76
 welfare state and, 3, 54–55, 63–64, 66–67, 78
emotional development
 adolescent sexuality and, 21, 170–71, 173, 179, 185, 188, 192–93, 195–96
 antipsychiatry movement and, 200, 201–6
 authoritarianism and, 33, 49–50, 53, 176
 birth control and, 136
 childhood and, 3, 5, 12, 19–20, 53–54, 58, 61–62, 66–67, 78–79, 81–82, 119–20, 200
 democratic citizens and, 10, 15–16, 17, 18–19, 49–50, 79, 98–99, 133, 137–38
 divorce and, 20, 76, 114–15, 130–37
 family violence and, 199–201, 211–12, 219, 223, 225–26
 fatherhood and, 75–76, 197, 209, 231
 feminism and, 200, 206–11
 freedom and, 17, 133
 homosexuality and, 15–16, 171
 idealized model of, 2, 5, 12
 marriage counseling and, 4, 20, 113–15, 119–25, 126, 130–31, 132, 135–40
 monogamy and, 12, 136–37, 139
 motherhood and, 14–15, 19–20, 70, 75–76, 81–82, 83–84, 86–87, 90–91, 232
 nuclear family and, 11, 14–15, 66–67, 97, 200, 225, 229
 psychiatry and, 2, 9, 12, 66
 queer counseling and, 161–64, 165
 relationality and, 13–14, 18, 136–37
 separation experiences and, 72
 social conditions and, 53–54, 120
 social reform and, 67–77
 welfare state and, 5, 12, 19, 63–67, 78, 139
emotional intimacy. *See* intimate relationships

emotional life. *See* intimate relationships
emotional maturity
   adolescent sexuality and, 21, 170–71, 172–76, 182–92, 194–95
   childhood and, 12–13, 62
   democratic citizens and, 139
   family violence and, 203, 215–16, 217, 218–19, 226
   freedom and, 21
   future orientation of, 12–13
   intimate relationships and, 5, 12, 171, 230
   marriage counseling and, 5, 125, 127–28, 137, 139, 145
   monogamy and, 145
   motherhood and, 15, 19–20, 83, 84, 90–92, 94–95, 107, 109, 110–11, 229
   nuclear family and, 94, 97
   queer counseling and, 145
   therapeutic communities and, 19–20
   welfare state and, 13, 21, 139–40, 173
eugenics, 18–19, 28, 258n.24

Fairbairn, Ronald, 121
Families Need Fathers (FNF), 197–98, 230, 231
the family. *See* nuclear family
family breakdown, 58, 112–13, 119–20, 235. *See also* divorce
Family Discussion Bureau (FDB), 118, 120–22, 123, 125–27, 128–29
Family Planning Act (1967), 172, 180
Family Planning Association (FPA), 124, 158–59
family therapy, 6–7, 8, 20, 106, 107, 234–35
family values, 122, 171, 180, 182, 192–96, 235, 237–38
family violence
   antipsychiatry movement and, 21–22, 199–206
   battered woman syndrome and, 220–21
   campaigns to end, 211–28
   childhood and, 64, 199–200, 212–17, 222–24, 225–26, 229
   cycle of violence and, 211–28
   divorce and, 220
   emotional deprivation and, 225–26
   emotional development and, 199–201, 211–12, 219, 223, 225–26
   emotional maturity and, 203, 215–16, 217, 218–19, 226
   fatherhood and, 199, 219–20, 222–23
   feminism and, 21–22, 199–200, 206–11, 221, 223–24, 226
   intimate relationships and, 21–22, 199
   marriage counseling and, 218–19, 220, 230
   media portrayal of violence and, 212, 221
   men as perpetrators and women as victims in, 212, 219–21, 224–25, 228
   motherhood and, 21–22, 199–200, 209–10, 212–17, 225–26, 228
   nuclear family and, 21–22, 199–201, 223, 225, 228–29
   prevalence of, 212, 221–22
   privacy and, 220, 230
   relationality and, 225–26, 228, 229–30, 231–32
   shelters for women fleeing from, 21–22, 199, 211–12, 219, 223–25, 226, 230
   social conditions and, 221
   social ills as result of, 212
   therapeutic communities and, 224–25
   underreporting of, 220
   welfare state and, 221–25, 230
   women's role in, 199, 212–13, 217, 226–28
fatherhood
   authoritarianism and, 26, 46, 47
   childhood and, 75–76, 85, 197–98, 209, 229
   divorce and, 197–98, 230–31, 235
   emotional deprivation and, 85, 230–31
   emotional development and, 75–76, 197, 209, 231
   family violence and, 199, 219–20, 222–23
   feminism and, 198
   motherhood and, 85, 93, 96–97, 197–98, 231
   welfare state and, 234–35
Feminine Mystique, The (Friedan), 253n.18
feminism
   antipsychiatry movement and, 206–9, 211
   childhood and, 211
   consciousness raising and, 159–60, 209–10
   divorce and, 231
   emotional deprivation and, 83
   emotional development and, 200, 206–11
   emotional labor of women and, 12, 14–15, 21–22, 200–1
   family violence and, 21–22, 199–200, 206–11, 221, 223–24, 226
   fatherhood and, 198
   freedom and, 211
   intimate relationships and, 236–37
   motherhood and, 12, 75–76, 82, 91, 100, 198, 208, 209–11
   nuclear family and, 82, 199–201, 207–8
   personal is political and, 2, 159–60, 207–8, 211
   psychoanalysis and, 207–8, 209–10
Feversham Report (1939), 32, 58–59
Fisher, Geoffrey, 149, 151
foster care, 1–2, 19, 54, 62, 64–65, 66–67, 76–77
Foucault, Michel, 5–6, 10, 17, 137–38, 192–93, 239
Foulkes, S.H., 25, 26–27, 41
Fraser, Derek, 7–8
freedom
   adolescent sexuality and, 21, 171, 172–73, 196
   democratic citizens and, 10, 133, 138, 196

freedom (cont.)
   emotional development and, 17, 133
   emotional maturity and, 21
   feminism and, 211
   homosexuality and, 147–48, 149–50
   intimate relationships and, 20, 22, 138
   liberal conception of, 6–7, 10
   marriage counseling and, 114–15, 127–28, 130
   motherhood and, 209
   nuclear family and, 233–34
   queer counseling and, 167–68
   social reform and, 229–30
   therapeutic communities and, 33, 37, 40
   welfare state and, 6–7, 10, 238
Freud, Anna, 11–12, 61, 90, 121, 175, 176
Freud, Sigmund, 11, 29, 174, 185–86, 207
Friend (organization)
   approach of, 159, 160, 165–66
   communication encouraged by, 162–64
   concerns about services of, 163–64, 165–66
   counseling expertise and, 159
   emotional development and, 162–64
   establishment of, 144–45, 159
   fetishes and, 163–65
   intimate relationships and, 162–63, 169
   queer initiation and, 165
   race and class dimensions of, 14
   relaunching of, 160
   services of, 146–47, 159, 160, 162
   social reform and, 168–69
Fromm-Reichmann, Frieda, 271n.12
future orientation
   childhood and, 13, 53–54, 55–56, 77, 229
   democratic citizens and, 28
   emotional maturity and, 12–13
   heterosexuality and, 12–13, 77
   intimate relationships and, 15
   marriage counseling and, 114
   motherhood and, 98–99, 229
   welfare state and, 13, 55–56, 78
Fyfe, David Maxwell, 147–48

Gavron, Hannah, 207
Gayford, John, 221–22, 225
Gay Liberation Front (GLF), 144–45, 159–60
gay liberation movement, 144–45, 146–47, 158, 159–60, 169
Gay Switchboard, 144–45, 146–47, 168–69, 189–90
Gay Youth Movement (GYM), 193–94
Gesell, Arnold, 98
Giddens, Anthony, 138
Gillick, Victoria, 194, 195–96
Glover, Edward, 29
Going to Hospital with Mother (film), 73, 74
Goldstein, Jan, 10, 126
Gorer, Geoffrey, 135–36

Grand, Elaine, 80–81
Great Partnership, The (Women's Liberal Federation), 80
Grey, Antony, 2, 143–44, 153, 154–56, 157, 158, 167–68, 181
Griffith, Edward, 112–13, 115–16, 117–18, 170, 213, 231–32
group therapy, 25, 26–27, 41, 42, 120
Growing Up (film), 179–80

Hacking, Ian, 17
Halberstam, Jack, 12
Hall, G. Stanley, 174
Halperin, David, 165
Hargreaves, Ronald, 68, 70
Harlow, Harry, 2–3, 75–76
Harris, Alan, 268n.75
Harris, Sidney, 119–20
Harris Committee, 120–21
Hart, Herbert, 149–50, 153, 158
Hayward, Rhodri, 7
Hendrick, Harry, 58–59
Hess, Rudolf, 45–46
heterosexuality
   childhood and, 77, 152
   democratic citizens and, 15–16, 77
   divorce and, 151
   intimate relationships and, 15–16, 144, 151, 158
   marriage counseling and, 114–15, 129–30, 137, 145
   normativity of, 5–6, 12, 15–16, 77, 94, 144, 151, 154–55, 169, 229–30
   welfare state and, 148
Hitler, Adolf, 45
Hochschild, Arlie, 78, 81–82
Holy Deadlock (Herbert), 130–31
homelessness, 4, 54–55, 62–63, 65–66, 68–69, 78
Homeless Person's Act (1977), 225
Home-Start, 217
homosexuality. *See also* befriending services; queer counseling
   adolescent sexuality and, 170–71, 181–82, 186–87, 188–92, 193
   age of consent and, 170–72, 182–83, 186–87, 188–92
   AIDS crisis and, 194
   aversion therapy and, 20–21, 144–45, 153–54
   decriminalization of, 4, 20–21, 135, 137, 143–45, 146–52, 172, 186
   emotional development and, 15–16, 171
   equality and, 145, 150
   freedom and, 147–48, 149–50
   harms of criminalization of, 149–50, 158, 171, 190–91
   heteronormativity and, 12, 151–52, 190

Index

intimate relationships and, 5–6, 143–44, 145, 152, 169, 193
nuclear family and, 5–6, 77, 112–13, 144, 151
privacy and, 144, 148–52, 172
promiscuity and, 145, 156, 191
psychiatry and, 12, 77, 145, 154, 159–60
public morals and, 148–50, 151–52, 167
relationality and, 5–6
sexual revolution and, 20–21
social stigma against, 18, 20–21, 46, 144–45, 147–53, 154–55, 156, 159, 171, 190–91, 194
welfare state and, 148–49, 151–52
Homosexual Law Reform Society (HLRS), 144–45, 150, 152–53
Horney, Karen, 209–10
Howells, J.G., 75–76
Hubback, Eva, 83, 85, 109
Huxley, Julian, 36, 152–53

Icebreakers, 144–45, 159–60, 166
Igo, Sarah, 151–52
I Know What I Am (JCGT), 189–92
Illouz, Eva, 78, 114–15
Infernal Child (Pizzey), 197, 227
Ingleby, Alan, 177–78
Institute of Marital Studies (IMS), 126, 136, 137, 138–39
institutionalization, 44, 53, 54–55, 62–63, 70, 74, 85–87, 234, 239
interwar period, 28–32, 51, 56–59, 115–18, 174–77
intimate relationships
  adolescent sexuality and, 5, 170–71, 193, 196
  antipsychiatry movement and, 2, 201–2
  childhood and, 2–3, 6, 11–12, 13, 54–56, 63, 76–78, 199
  democratic citizens and, 2, 4, 9, 15, 18, 19, 55–56, 114, 133, 138, 139, 151–52, 238
  development of focus on, 2–6, 7, 11–12, 16–17, 45, 51, 113
  divorce and, 5, 6, 20, 114–15, 132, 133, 135, 136–37, 230
  emotional maturity and, 5, 12, 171, 230
  family violence and, 21–22, 199
  feminism and, 236–37
  freedom and, 20, 22, 138
  future orientation of, 15
  gender and class and, 13–16
  heterosexuality and, 15–16, 144, 151, 158
  homosexuality and, 5–6, 143–44, 145, 152, 169, 193
  marriage counseling and, 4, 16, 20, 113–18, 120–21, 124–25, 126, 136–37, 138–39, 235–36
  monogamy and, 136–37, 138, 237
  motherhood and, 2, 11–12, 14–15, 17–18, 19–20, 54, 79, 83, 199–201, 229–30, 237–38
  nuclear family and, 3–5, 14–15, 51, 55–56, 100–3, 139, 199, 229, 231–32, 237–38
  overview of, 1–6, 7, 18–22, 233–39
  politicization of, 2, 5–6, 7–8, 15, 18, 113, 114, 139, 161, 230, 238
  privacy and, 21–22, 138–39, 152, 169, 229–30
  psychopolitics and, 13, 16–17, 238
  public and private life in, 16–18, 161
  queer counseling and, 2, 5–7, 20–21, 145–46, 155, 158–69
  relationality and, 2, 4–5, 13–14, 18, 161, 163, 238
  sexual revolution and, 4–6, 238
  subjectivities through, 13–16
  therapeutic communities and, 13–14, 18, 97–98
  welfare state and, 3–8, 19, 54–56, 78, 79, 119–25, 139, 230, 238
In Two Minds (Mercer), 202–3
Isaacs, Susan, 11, 53, 61, 66

Jeger, Lena, 222
Jenkins, Roy, 171, 184
Joint Council for Gay Teenagers (JCGT), 189–91
Jones, Marjorie, 184
Jones, Maxwell, 26–27, 42
Joseph, Keith, 180–81, 185, 195
juvenile delinquency, 9, 11, 13–14, 19, 56, 58–59, 71–72, 78

Kempe, C. Henry, 212–13
Key, Ellen, 11
Kiernan, Kathleen, 137–38
King, Ambrose, 184
King, Joan, 122–23
Kingsley Hall, 204–5
Kinnock, Neil, 235
Klein, Melanie, 57, 91, 109, 121
Klein, Viola, 91, 105–7, 108, 109–10
Kline, Wendy, 258n.24

Labouchere Amendment (1885), 147–48
Laing, Ronald D., 201–4, 205–6, 207, 208–9, 211
Land, Hilary, 137–38
Lane, Homer, 58
Latey Committee on the Age of Majority, 186–87, 194–95
Laufer, Moses (Moe), 175
Leach, Edmund, 201
Le Bon, Gustave, 29
Lewis, Jane, 137–38
LGBTQ+ people, 5–6, 13–14, 20–21, 145–46, 157, 171, 236–37. *See also* befriending services; homosexuality; queer counseling
Lidz, Theodore, 271n.12
Loach, Ken, 202
Logan, Bill, 168
Lomas, Peter, 106

Lorenz, Konrad, 2–3, 72
Lynch, Kathleen, 107

Maccabean Lecture (1959), 149
Mace, David, 117–18, 123, 155, 167
Main, Tom
  child-centered culture and, 92–93
  democratic citizens and, 42
  emotional maturity and, 91, 109
  fatherhood and, 93, 96–97
  marriage counseling and, 97, 127
  morale cultivation by, 26–27, 40–41
  motherhood and, 80, 83, 90–92, 105–6, 108, 109
  separation experiences and, 90
  therapeutic communities and, 88–90
  working mothers and, 105–6
Major, John, 235
maladjustment, 11, 56–58, 59, 63, 71, 77, 116
marriage counseling
  accessibility of, 122–23
  birth control and, 116–17, 124, 125, 137
  childhood and, 116, 119–20, 126–27
  class dimensions of, 14, 122–23
  democratic citizens and, 2, 49–50, 118, 138–39
  depth psychology and, 113, 122–23
  development of, 6, 20, 112–13, 115–18, 120–21
  divorce and, 20, 113–14, 115, 117, 119, 122–23, 130, 131, 136–37, 156
  dysfunctional marriages and, 112–13, 136–37, 229
  emotional development and, 4, 20, 113–15, 119–25, 126, 130–31, 132, 135–40
  emotional maturity and, 5, 125, 127–28, 137, 139, 145
  family breakdown and, 58, 112–13, 119–20, 235
  family violence and, 218–19, 220, 230
  freedom and, 114–15, 127–28, 130
  future orientation of, 114
  heterosexuality and, 114–15, 129–30, 137, 145
  interwar period and, 115–18
  intimate relationships and, 4, 16, 20, 113–18, 120–21, 124–25, 126, 136–37, 138–39, 235–36
  marriage breakdown, 112–13, 130, 134, 259n.60
  marital roles and, 125–26, 128–30
  monogamy and, 14, 114–15, 129–30, 135–37
  mutual cause of problems and, 127–28
  nuclear family and, 6, 14, 125–26, 127, 138, 235
  personality as issue in, 125–27
  privacy and, 138–39
  professionalization and, 123–24
  psychiatry and, 115, 116, 118, 120–21, 124, 138–39
  psychoanalysis and, 121
  public perception of, 135–37
  queer counseling and, 20–21, 167
  relationality and, 121–22, 125–30
  relationship as object of therapy in, 120–22

  sexual dissatisfaction and, 115–17, 125–26, 127–28
  sexual revolution and, 127, 135–36
  social reform and, 116–17, 137–38
  welfare state and, 3, 4, 6, 20, 112–15, 119–25, 138–40
Married Women's Association (MWA), 99–100, 134
Marsden, Dennis, 107
Marshall, T.H., 113, 139
Martin, Mary E., 95–96
Maternal Care and Mental Health (Bowlby), 1–2, 52, 68–69
Matrimonial Causes Act (1937), 130–31
Matrimonial Causes and Reconciliation Bill (1963), 133
maturity. *See* emotional maturity
Maudsley, Henry, 30
McMillan, Margaret, 55
Mead, Margaret, 26, 75–76
media influence, 74, 76–77, 81, 100, 112–13, 130, 131, 179–80, 182, 212, 221
mental hospitals, 29–32. *See also* Cassel Hospital; Northfield military hospital
Mental Treatment Act (1930), 29–30, 31–32
Mercer, David, 202–3
Meyerowitz, Joanne, 27
middle-class families. *See* intimate relationships; nuclear family
Middlemore, Merrell, 81
Mill Hill Hospital, 42–43
"Miserable Married Women" *(Observer)*, 80–81, 131–32
Mitchell, Juliet, 206–10
monogamy
  adolescent sexuality and, 5–6, 173, 186, 191, 196
  emotional development and, 12, 136–37, 139
  emotional maturity and, 145
  intimate relationships and, 136–37, 138, 237
  marriage counseling and, 14, 114–15, 129–30, 135–37
  queer counseling and, 154–55, 156–57, 158, 161, 162–63, 168–69
  relationality and, 158
  welfare state and, 148
Montagu, Ashley, 52
Montessori, Maria, 11
Moore-Brabazon, John, 143–44
Morgan, Patricia, 213–16
motherhood
  advertisements emphasizing, 101*f*, 102*f*, 103*f*, 104*f*, 214*f*, 215*f*, 216*f*
  antipsychiatry movement and, 200–1, 203–6
  "bad" mothers, 19–20, 83, 199
  Bowlbian framework for, 1–2, 11–12, 57, 61, 67–69, 70, 72–73, 75–76, 78–79, 209

mother-child relationship and, 1–2, 11–12, 19–20, 54–55, 58, 67–76, 78–79, 81–83, 92–93, 105, 197–200
  class dimensions of, 103–4, 105
  criticism of prioritization of, 1–2, 70, 75–76, 91, 209
  democratic citizens and, 1–2, 98, 108
  dissatisfaction in, 80–83, 96, 105
  emotional deprivation and, 11–12, 75–76, 78, 82–83, 84–93, 98–99, 198, 225–26
  emotional development and, 14–15, 19–20, 70, 75–76, 81–82, 83–84, 85, 86–87, 90–91, 107, 108, 232
  emotional maturity and, 15, 19–20, 83, 84, 90–92, 94–95, 107, 109, 110–11, 229
  family violence and, 21–22, 199–200, 209–10, 212–17, 225–26, 228
  fatherhood and, 85, 93, 96–97, 197–98, 231
  feminism and, 12, 75–76, 82, 91, 100, 198, 208, 209–11
  freedom and, 209
  future orientation of, 98–99, 229
  housework and, 99–100, 106–7, 110, 207–8, 210
  intimate relationships and, 2, 11–12, 14–15, 17–18, 19–20, 54, 79, 83, 199–201, 229–30, 237–38
  labor involved in, 12, 14–15, 21–22, 90–91, 107–8, 200–1
  media portrayal of, 81, 100
  mother-baby units and, 49–50, 87–88, 95–97
  mother-child units and, 73, 93–94, 98
  naturalness of, 19–20, 81–82, 84, 91, 92, 98, 109–10, 197–99, 200
  neglect as psychological problem in, 87–93
  nuclear family and, 14–15, 72–73, 82, 97, 100–3, 231–32
  politicization of, 2–3, 15, 98–108, 200
  poverty and, 84–87
  psychopolitics and, 15
  relationality and, 15, 82, 225–26, 228, 229–30, 231–32
  schizophrenia and, 199–206, 207, 228–29
  separation experiences and, 57, 61, 67–68, 70–76, 90
  shame in, 1–2, 12, 17–18, 80–81, 91
  social reform and, 84, 98–99, 110–11
  therapeutic communities and, 82–84
  welfare state and, 66, 72–73, 78, 85, 87, 98–108, 208
  working mothers and, 54, 66, 78, 103–5, 106–7
  World War II and, 81
Myrdal, Alva, 91, 105–7, 108, 109–10

National Association of Mental Health (NAMH), 9, 62, 76, 175–76
National Council for Civil Liberties (NCCL), 170, 171, 184, 185
National Federation of Women's Institutes (WI), 99–100
National Health Service (NHS), 8–9, 21, 66, 88, 92, 108–9, 222
National Marriage Guidance Council (NMGC), 116–17, 119, 120–21, 123–24, 125–26, 129, 155, 168–69, 177
National Society for the Prevention of Cruelty to Children (NSPCC), 67, 85
National Women's Aid Federation (later Women's Aid), 12, 221–22, 223
Nazi Germany. *See also* authoritarianism
  denazification following, 18–19, 26, 48
  eugenics and, 28
  family structure informing, 18–19, 25–26, 27, 45–49, 120, 121
  POW assessment and, 25–26, 27, 45–49
neglect. *See* emotional deprivation
Nelson, Deborah, 161
Newson, Elizabeth, 105–6
Newson, John, 105–6
No Difference to Me (Hambledon), 76, 252n.102
No Place for Jennifer (film), 76, 252n.102
Northfield military hospital, 39–45
  democratic citizens and, 40–41, 42
  disarray at, 40–41
  first experiment at, 40–41
  freedom of movement and, 40
  Hospital Club experiment at, 41
  therapeutic community at, 18–19, 27, 40, 41–42
nuclear family
  adolescent sexuality and, 195–96
  antipsychiatry movement and, 199–201, 203
  birth control and, 229
  childhood and, 3–4, 10–11, 53–55, 57, 60–61, 63–64, 66, 68–70, 78–79, 97, 200
  criticism of, 4, 21–22, 82, 199–201, 203, 206
  democratic citizens and, 4, 28, 47, 49–50, 55–56, 79, 234–35
  emotional deprivation and, 53–54, 67
  emotional development and, 11, 14–15, 66–67, 97, 200, 225, 229
  emotional maturity and, 94, 97
  family violence and, 21–22, 199–201, 223, 225, 228–29
  feminism and, 82, 199–201, 207–8
  freedom and, 233–34
  homosexuality and, 5–6, 77, 112–13, 144, 151
  intimate relationships and, 3–5, 14–15, 51, 55–56, 100–3, 139, 199, 229, 231–32, 237–38
  marriage counseling and, 6, 14, 125–26, 127, 138, 235
  motherhood and, 14–15, 72–73, 82, 97, 100–3, 231–32
  politicization of, 3–4, 10–11, 22, 28, 229, 233–35
  privacy and, 97–98, 233–34
  psychopolitics and, 201, 206

nuclear family (*cont.*)
    queer counseling and, 161
    sexual revolution and, 4
    welfare state and, 4, 6, 54, 66, 72–73, 75–76, 78–79, 112–13, 139

Oakley, Ann, 91, 210
occupational therapy, 32, 38, 41, 42
Odlum, Doris, 81, 175–76, 177–78, 185–86
O'Neill, Denis, 64–65

Pakenham, Frank, 148–49
Parkin, Keith, 197, 198, 230
Parsons, Talcott, 100–3
Pasmore, Jean, 127
Pearse, Innes, 32–33, 35–36, 37, 38, 41
Peckham Experiment, 32–38
    democratic nature of, 32–38, 50
    depictions of, 34f, 37f, 38f, 39f
    development of, 32–33, 35–36
    disarray in, 34–35
    ending of, 39
    experimental design of, 32–38
    freedom in, 37
    group interactions in, 38
    reception of, 33, 36
    social basis of mental health and, 32–33, 37
Pedersen, Susan, 10–11
Pincus, Lily, 127, 128
Pioneer Health Centre. *See* Peckham Experiment
Pitman, Isaac, 65, 67
Pizzey, Erin
    childhood and, 197, 224
    emotional development and, 211–12, 219
    family violence and, 211–12, 217–19, 221–22, 225, 226
    men's role in family violence and, 219–20, 224, 226
    social reform and, 221–22, 223–25
    therapeutic communities and, 224–25
    women's role in family violence and, 199, 223–24, 226–28, 273n.65
Platt Report (1959), 73, 74
Playne, Caroline, 46
Plummer, Ken, 191
Policy Advisory Committee on Sexual Offences (PAC), 171, 184, 188, 189, 191–92, 194–95
Politics of Experience, The (Laing), 209
Poor Law, 63–64, 65
Popenoe, Paul, 258n.24
post-partum mental illness, 4, 5, 19–20, 83, 87–88, 90–91, 95–96, 106, 109
POW assessment, 25–26, 27, 43–49
Pregnant at School (WPPSSM), 191–92
premarital sex, 136, 151, 177–78, 193
Priestley, J.B., 87, 152–53

privacy
    adolescent sexuality and, 172, 173, 184, 192–93, 194–96
    class dimensions of, 138–39
    democratic citizens and, 21, 151–52
    family violence and, 220, 230
    homosexuality and, 144, 148–52, 172
    intimate relationships and, 21–22, 138–39, 152, 169, 229–30
    marriage counseling and, 138–39
    nuclear family and, 97–98, 233–34
promiscuity, 20–21, 145, 155, 156, 158, 177, 178, 191
Prone to Violence (Pizzey), 199, 226
prostitution, 77–78, 147–48, 158, 185–87, 196
psychiatry. *See also* antipsychiatry movement
    adolescent sexuality and, 21, 172–76
    authoritarianism and, 8, 26–27, 49, 88–89, 120
    democratic citizens and, 18–19, 27, 49, 50–51
    development of, 19, 28–32, 49–50
    divorce and, 113–14, 130
    emotional development and, 2, 9, 12, 66
    group psychiatry, 19, 28–29
    homosexuality and, 12, 77, 145, 154, 159–60
    interwar period and, 28–32
    marriage counseling and, 115, 116, 118, 120–21, 124, 138–39
    psychopolitics and, 26–27, 44
    relationality and, 49
    social psychiatry and, 18–19, 25–32, 39–40, 49
    World War II and, 39–40, 49–50
psychoanalysis, 14, 57, 121, 207–8, 209–10
Psychoanalysis and Feminism (Mitchell), 207, 208
psychopolitics
    antipsychiatry movement and, 7, 10, 201, 205–6
    democratic citizens and, 1–2, 27, 135
    intimate relationships and, 13, 16–17, 238
    motherhood and, 15
    nuclear family and, 201, 206
    psychiatry and, 26–27, 44
    therapeutic communities and, 44
    World War II and, 27
psychosexual counseling. *See* queer counseling
public morals, 148–50, 151–52, 167, 183

queer counseling
    age of consent and, 190
    approaches in, 146–47, 153–54, 162–65, 167–68
    authoritarianism and, 168
    democratic citizens and, 145–46
    development of, 144–47, 152–59, 160–61
    emotional development and, 161–64, 165
    emotional maturity and, 145
    freedom and, 167–68
    internalized homophobia and, 159, 168–69, 237

intimate relationships and, 2, 5–7, 20–21, 145–46, 155, 158–69
  marriage counseling and, 20–21, 167
  monogamy and, 154–55, 156–57, 158, 161, 162–63, 168–69
  network of relationships in, 163
  nuclear family and, 161
  relationality and, 161, 163, 168–69
  sexual revolution and, 20–21, 147
  social reform and, 145–47, 160–61, 168–69
  social stigma and, 146–47, 162, 167–68
queer liberation, 2, 20–21, 146, 147, 159–60

Rapoport, Robert, 44
Rees, John Rawlings, 51
Rees-Mog, William, 170
relationality
  childhood and, 11–12, 77–79
  democratic citizens and, 50–51
  emotional development and, 13–14, 18, 136–37
  family violence and, 225–26, 228, 229–30, 231–32
  homosexuality and, 5–6
  intimate relationships and, 2, 4–5, 13–14, 18, 161, 163, 238
  marriage counseling and, 121–22, 125–30
  monogamy and, 158
  motherhood and, 15, 82, 225–26, 228, 229–30, 231–32
  psychiatry and, 49
  publicness and, 161
  queer counseling and, 161, 163, 168–69
  therapeutic communities and, 13–14
  welfare state and, 77–79
Responsible Society, The, 180, 182, 183–84
Rickman, John, 29, 39–40, 121
Riley, Denise, 66
Robertson, James, 67–68, 70, 71–73, 74, 78
Robinson, Kenneth, 143
Rose, Nikolas, 10
Rosenbluth, Dina, 72
Rowbotham, Sheila, 178, 200, 206, 208–9, 211
Rubin, Gayle, 15–16
Rutter, Michael, 176

Sage, Lorna, 195
Sanity, Madness and the Family (Laing), 202–3, 207
Sargant, William, 202–3
schizophrenia, 199–206, 207, 228–29
Schofield, Michael, 156, 187
School Meals Act (1906), 58–59
Scott, Joan Wallach, 17
Scream Quietly or the Neighbours Will Hear (Pizzey), 224, 226
Select Committee on Violence in Marriage, 197, 212, 219, 221–22, 223, 225–26

separation experiences, 57, 61, 67–68, 70–76, 90
sex education, 21, 116, 177, 178–80, 181–82, 191, 196, 222
sexuality. *See* adolescent sexuality; heterosexuality; homosexuality; queer counseling
Sexual Law Reform Society (SLRS), 171, 183–85
sexually transmitted infections (STIs), 112, 178–79, 183, 193
Sexual Offences Act (1967), 144, 150–51, 158, 186–87, 192–93
sexual revolution
  adolescent sexuality and, 21, 172–73, 192–93
  democratic citizens and, 5, 21, 138
  homosexuality and, 20–21
  intimate relationships and, 2, 4–6, 238
  marriage counseling and, 127, 135–36
  nuclear family and, 4
  queer counseling and, 20–21, 147
Shackleton, Edward, 167
Shaftesbury, Lord, 185
Shaw, Frederic Charles, 149–50
Sheridan, Mary, 86
Shils, Edward, 25–26, 46, 53–54
social psychiatry, 18–19, 25–32, 39–40, 49
social therapy, 42, 44, 224–25
Spare Rib (magazine), 12, 199, 207, 210, 211, 236–37
Spence, James, 51, 90, 100–3
Spitz, René, 67–68
Spock, Benjamin, 81–82, 98, 231
Standing Conference for the Advancement of Counselling, 167, 168
Stead, W.T., 185, 196
Steedman, Carolyn, 77
Stewart, John, 57
Stonewall riots, 158, 159
Stopes, Marie, 35, 115–16, 125
subjectivities. *See* intimate relationships
Summerskill, Edith, 99–100, 106–7, 109–10, 134–35
Super Marital Sex (Pearsall), 235–36
Sutherland, J.D., 124–25
Suttie, Ian, 11, 121

Tanner, J.M., 269n.107
Tavistock Clinic
  adolescent unit at, 175
  ethos of, 70
  family violence and, 220
  marriage counseling at, 14, 48–49, 118, 120–22, 125–26, 132, 220
Taylor, Stephen, 31
teenage sexuality. *See* adolescent sexuality
teen pregnancy, 170–71, 172, 177, 178–79, 180–81, 183, 191
Thane, Pat, 255n.82

Thatcher, Margaret, 167, 179–80, 194, 233–34, 235–36
therapeutic communities. *See also* Cassel Hospital; Northfield military hospital
  antipsychiatry movement and, 201–2
  authoritarianism and, 44
  autonomy and, 44
  democratic citizens and, 26–27, 42, 44, 98–99, 120
  development of, 13–14, 18–19, 32, 39–40, 43–44, 88, 89–90, 120
  emotional maturity and, 19–20
  family violence and, 224–25
  freedom and, 33, 37, 40
  intimate relationships and, 13–14, 18, 97–98
  morale cultivation in, 40
  motherhood and, 82–84
  psychopolitics and, 44
  relationality and, 13–14
  World War II and, 26–27, 39–40, 43–44
therapy. *See* adolescent counseling; anti-hospital therapy; aversion therapy; family therapy; group therapy; marriage counseling; occupational therapy; queer counseling; social therapy
Thompson, E.P., 17
Thorpe, Jeremy, 182–83
Tindall, Gillian, 132
Titmuss, Richard, 7–8, 50–51
totalitarianism. *See* authoritarianism
transphobia, 18, 20–21, 147, 158–59, 167–68, 238
Trotter, Wilfred, 29, 36
Tweedie, Jill, 198, 223–25, 231
Two Accounts of a Journey through Madness (Barnes and Berke), 204
Two-Year-Old Goes to Hospital, A (film), 71–72, 73, 74

Van der Eyken, Willem, 217
Villa 21, 201–2
violence, domestic. *See* family violence

Walker, Kenneth, 152–53
Walker, Lenore, 220–21
Wallis, John, 123–24
Wandor, Michelene, 210–11
Warner, Michael, 161, 229–30
Waters, Chris, 156
Weddell, Doreen, 93, 98–99
Weeks, Jeffrey, 151, 160–61
welfare state
  authoritarianism and, 119
  birth control and, 180–81
  childhood and, 3, 5–6, 13, 19, 54–56, 58–59, 62–67, 77–79, 98–108
  classless society as aim of, 20, 55–56, 78, 113–14, 124–25, 234
  democratic citizens and, 19, 20, 113, 118, 151–52
  development of, 3–4, 6–8, 55, 58–59, 63
  divorce and, 3, 8, 63, 119, 228–29
  emotional deprivation and, 3, 54–55, 63–64, 66–67
  emotional development and, 5, 12, 19, 63–67, 78, 139
  emotional maturity and, 13, 21, 139–40, 173
  family violence and, 221–25, 230
  fatherhood and, 234–35
  freedom and, 6–7, 10, 238
  future orientation of, 13, 55–56, 78
  goals of, 4, 6–8, 20
  heterosexuality and, 148
  homelessness and, 54–55
  homosexuality and, 148–49, 151–52
  intimate relationships and, 3–8, 19, 54–56, 78, 79, 119–25, 139, 230, 238
  marriage counseling and, 3, 4, 6, 20, 112–15, 119–25, 138–40
  meaning of health expanded in, 8–10
  monogamy and, 148
  motherhood and, 66, 72–73, 78, 85, 87, 98–108, 208
  nuclear family and, 4, 6, 54, 66, 72–73, 75–76, 78–79, 112–13, 139
  overview of, 6–8
  relationality and, 77–79
  scholarship on, 7–9, 55, 139
Whitehouse, Mary, 167, 179–80, 182, 183–84
Williamson, George, 32–36, 37, 38
Willmott, Peter, 105, 106, 256n.96
Wilson, A.T.M. (Tommy), 43–44
Winnicott, Donald
  asylums and, 44
  authoritarianism and, 8, 44
  childhood and, 11–12, 61
  democratic citizens and, 8
  emotional development and, 61
  interpersonal intimacy and, 8
  mother-child relationship and, 11–12, 81–82, 83, 98
  welfare state and, 8, 66
  World War II and, 61
Wise, Audrey, 222
Wolf, Katherine, 61
Wolfenden, John, 147–48, 149
Wolfenden Committee on Homosexual Offences and Prostitution, 143–44, 147–49, 152–53, 154, 186–87
Woman's Estate (Mitchell), 206–7
Women's Group on Public Welfare, 83, 84–86, 87
Women's Liberation Movement, 206

Woodruff, Caroline, 180
Wooley, P.V., 212–13
World War I, 27, 29, 43, 56, 119, 174, 185–86
World War II
   childhood and, 52–53, 60–63
   democratic citizens and, 26–27
   divorce and, 131
   intimacy ideal and, 51
   motherhood and, 81
   Nazi POW assessment in, 25–26, 27, 45–49
   psychopolitics and, 27
   therapeutic communities and, 26–27, 39–40, 43–44

Wright, Helena, 115–16, 125

Yoshino, Kenji, 237
Young, Michael, 105, 256n.96
Young Liberals, 182–83
Young People's Consultation Centre, 175
youth sexuality. *See* adolescent sexuality

Zahra, Tara, 68
Zelizer, Viviana, 78
Zero Population Growth, 182
Zinkin, Nancy, 178–79